CROSSING THE QUALITY CHASM

A New Health System for the 21st Century

Committee on Quality of Health Care in America

INSTITUTE OF MEDICINE

NATIONAL ACADEMY PRESS
Washington, D.C.

NATIONAL ACADEMY PRESS • 2101 Constitution Avenue, N.W. • Washington, DC 20418

NOTICE: The project that is the subject of this report was approved by the Governing Board of the National Research Council, whose members are drawn from the councils of the National Academy of Sciences, the National Academy of Engineering, and the Institute of Medicine. The members of the committee responsible for the report were chosen for their special competences and with regard for appropriate balance.

Support for this project was provided by: the Institute of Medicine; the National Research Council; The Robert Wood Johnson Foundation; the California Health Care Foundation; the Commonwealth Fund; and the Department of Health and Human Services' Health Care Financing Administration and Agency for Healthcare Research and Quality. The views presented in this report are those of the Institute of Medicine Committee on the Quality of Health Care in America and are not necessarily those of the funding agencies.

Library of Congress Cataloging-in-Publication Data

Crossing the quality chasm : a new health system for the 21st century / Committee on Quality Health Care in America, Institute of Medicine.
      p. ; cm.
   Includes bibliographical references and index.
   ISBN 0-309-07280-8
      1. Medical care—United States. 2. Health care reform—United States. 3. Medical care—United States—Quality control. I. Institute of Medicine (U.S.). Committee on Quality of Health Care in America.
      [DNLM: 1. Health Care Reform—methods—United States. 2. Quality of Health Care—United States. WA 540 AA1 C937 2001]
   RA395.A3 C855 2001
   362.1¢0973—dc21

                                                                        2001030775

Additional copies of this report are available for sale from the National Academy Press, 2101 Constitution Avenue, N.W., Box 285, Washington, D.C. 20055. Call (800) 624-6242 or (202) 334-3313 (in the Washington metropolitan area), or visit the NAP's home page at **www.nap.edu.** The full text of this report is available at **www.nap.edu.**

For more information about the Institute of Medicine, visit the IOM home page at: **www.iom.edu.**

Printed in the United States of America.

The serpent has been a symbol of long life, healing, and knowledge among almost all cultures and religions since the beginning of recorded history. The serpent adopted as a logotype by the Institute of Medicine is a relief carving from ancient Greece, now held by the Staatliche Museen in Berlin.

First Printing, July 2001   Fifth Printing, June 2004
Second Printing, September 2001   Sixth Printing, May 2005
Third Printing, February 2002   Seventh Printing, August 2007
Fourth Printing, February 2003

"Knowing is not enough; we must apply.
Willing is not enough; we must do."
—Goethe

INSTITUTE OF MEDICINE

Shaping the Future for Health

THE NATIONAL ACADEMIES

National Academy of Sciences
National Academy of Engineering
Institute of Medicine
National Research Council

The **National Academy of Sciences** is a private, nonprofit, self-perpetuating society of distinguished scholars engaged in scientific and engineering research, dedicated to the furtherance of science and technology and to their use for the general welfare. Upon the authority of the charter granted to it by the Congress in 1863, the Academy has a mandate that requires it to advise the federal government on scientific and technical matters. Dr. Bruce M. Alberts is president of the National Academy of Sciences.

The **National Academy of Engineering** was established in 1964, under the charter of the National Academy of Sciences, as a parallel organization of outstanding engineers. It is autonomous in its administration and in the selection of its members, sharing with the National Academy of Sciences the responsibility for advising the federal government. The National Academy of Engineering also sponsors engineering programs aimed at meeting national needs, encourages education and research, and recognizes the superior achievements of engineers. Dr. William A. Wulf is president of the National Academy of Engineering.

The **Institute of Medicine** was established in 1970 by the National Academy of Sciences to secure the services of eminent members of appropriate professions in the examination of policy matters pertaining to the health of the public. The Institute acts under the responsibility given to the National Academy of Sciences by its congressional charter to be an adviser to the federal government and, upon its own initiative, to identify issues of medical care, research, and education. Dr. Kenneth I. Shine is president of the Institute of Medicine.

The **National Research Council** was organized by the National Academy of Sciences in 1916 to associate the broad community of science and technology with the Academy's purposes of furthering knowledge and advising the federal government. Functioning in accordance with general policies determined by the Academy, the Council has become the principal operating agency of both the National Academy of Sciences and the National Academy of Engineering in providing services to the government, the public, and the scientific and engineering communities. The Council is administered jointly by both Academies and the Institute of Medicine. Dr. Bruce M. Alberts and Dr. William A. Wulf are chairman and vice chairman, respectively, of the National Research Council.

Study Staff

JANET M. CORRIGAN
    Director, Quality of Health Care in America Project
    Director, Board on Health Care Services
MOLLA S. DONALDSON, Project Codirector
LINDA T. KOHN, Project Codirector
SHARI K. MAGUIRE, Research Assistant
KELLY C. PIKE, Senior Project Assistant

Auxiliary Staff

ANTHONY BURTON, Administrative Assistant
MIKE EDINGTON, Managing Editor
JENNIFER CANGCO, Financial Advisor

Consultant/Editor

RONA BRIERE, Briere Associates, Inc.

Reviewers

The report was reviewed by individuals chosen for their diverse perspectives and technical expertise in accordance with procedures approved by the National Research Council's Report Review Committee. The purpose of this independent review is to provide candid and critical comments to assist the authors and the Institute of Medicine in making the published report as sound as possible and to ensure that the report meets institutional standards for objectivity, evidence, and responsiveness to the study charge. The content of the review comments and the draft manuscript remain confidential to protect the integrity of the deliberative process. The committee wishes to thank the following individuals for their participation in the report review process:

TERRY CLEMMER, Intermountain Health Care, Salt Lake City, UT
SUSAN EDGMAN-LEVITAN, The Picker Institute, Boston, MA
ANN GREINER, Center for Studying Health System Change, Washington, D.C.
DAVID LANSKY, The Foundation for Accountability, Portland, OR
DAVID MECHANIC, Rutgers, The State University of New Jersey,
    New Brunswick, NJ
L. GORDON MOORE, Brighton Family Medicine, Rochester, NY
DAVID G. NATHAN, Dana-Farber Cancer Institute (Emeritus), Boston, MA
VINOD K. SAHNEY, Henry Ford Health System, Detroit, MI
WILLIAM STEAD, Vanderbilt University, Nashville, TN
EDWARD WAGNER, Group Health Center for Health Studies, Seattle, WA

Although the reviewers listed above have provided many constructive comments and suggestions, they were not asked to endorse the conclusions or recommendations nor did they see the final draft of the report before its release. The review of this report was overseen by **WILLIAM H. DANFORTH**, Washington University, St. Louis, Missouri, and **EDWARD B. PERRIN**, University of Washington and VA Puget Sound Health Care System, Seattle, Washington. Appointed by the National Research Council and the Institute of Medicine, they were responsible for making certain that an independent examination of this report was carried out in accordance with institutional procedures and that all review comments were carefully considered. Responsibility for the final content of this report rests entirely with the authoring committee and the institution.

Preface

This is the second and final report of the Committee on the Quality of Health Care in America, which was appointed in 1998 to identify strategies for achieving a substantial improvement in the quality of health care delivered to Americans. The committee's first report, *To Err Is Human: Building a Safer Health System*, was released in 1999 and focused on a specific quality concern—patient safety. This second report focuses more broadly on how the health care delivery system can be designed to innovate and improve care.

This report does not recommend specific organizational approaches to achieve the aims set forth. Rather than being an organizational construct, redesign refers to a new perspective on the purpose and aims of the health care system, how patients and their clinicians should relate, and how care processes can be designed to optimize responsiveness to patient needs. The principles and guidance for redesign that are offered in this report represent fundamental changes in the way the system meets the needs of the people it serves.

Redesign is not aimed only at the health care organizations and professionals that comprise the delivery system. Change is also required in the structures and processes of the environment in which those organizations and professionals function. Such change includes setting national priorities for improvement, creating better methods for disseminating and applying knowledge to practice, fostering the use of information technology in clinical care, creating payment policies that encourage innovation and reward improvement in performance, and enhancing educational programs to strengthen the health care workforce.

The Quality of Health Care in America project is supported largely by the income from an endowment established within the Institute of Medicine by the

Howard Hughes Medical Institute and income from an endowment established for the National Research Council by the W. K. Kellogg Foundation. Generous support was provided by the Commonwealth Fund for a workshop on applying information technology to improve the quality of clinical care, by the Health Care Financing Administration for a workshop aimed at exploring the relationship between payment policy and quality improvement, by the Robert Wood Johnson Foundation for a survey of exemplary systems of care, by the California Health Care Foundation for a workshop to explore methods for communicating with the public about quality in health care, and by the Agency for Healthcare Research and Quality for a workshop on the relationship between patient outcomes and provider volume.

Although the committee takes full responsibility for the content of this report, many people have made important contributions. The Subcommittee on Designing the Health System of the 21st Century, under the direction of Donald Berwick, combined a depth of knowledge and creativity to propose a vision on how health care could be delivered in the 21st century. The Subcommittee on Creating an External Environment for Quality, under the direction of J. Cris Bisgard and Molly Joel Coye, provided expert guidance and a wealth of experience on how the external environment could support improved delivery of care. Lastly, the IOM staff, under the direction of Janet Corrigan, have provided excellent research, analysis and writing.

Now is the right time for the changes proposed in this report. Technological advances make it possible to accomplish things today that were impossible only a few years ago. Patients, health care professionals, and policy makers are becoming all too painfully aware of the shortcomings of our current care delivery systems and the importance of finding better approaches to meeting the health care needs of all Americans. The committee does not offer a simple prescription, but a vision of what is possible and the path that can be taken. It will not be an easy road, but it will be most worthwhile.

William C. Richardson, Ph.D.
Chair
March 2001

Foreword

This is the second and final report of the Committee on the Quality of Health Care in America. Response to the committee's first report, *To Err is Human: Building a Safer Health System*, has been swift, positive, and ongoing from many health care organizations, practitioners, researchers, and policy makers.

The present report addresses quality-related issues more broadly, providing a strategic direction for redesigning the health care delivery system of the 21st century. Fundamental reform of health care is needed to ensure that all Americans receive care that is safe, effective, patient centered, timely, efficient, and equitable.

As this report is being released, we are reflecting on the recent loss of a great 20th-century leader in the field of health care quality. Avedis Donabedian, member of the Institute of Medicine, leaves behind a rich body of work on the conceptualization and measurement of quality. His extraordinary intellectual contributions will continue to guide efforts to improve quality well into the coming century.

The Quality of Health Care in America project continues the Institute of Medicine's long-standing focus on quality-of-care issues. The Institute's National Roundtable on Health Care Quality has described the variability of the quality of health care in the United States and highlighted the urgent need for improvement. The report *Ensuring Quality Cancer Care* issued by the Institute's National Cancer Policy Board, offers the conclusion that there is a wide gulf between ideal cancer care and the reality experienced by many Americans. And a forthcoming report from the Institute's Committee on the National Quality

Report on Health Care Delivery will offer a framework for periodic reporting to the nation on the state of quality of care.

This report reinforces the conviction of these and other concerned groups that we cannot wait any longer to address the serious quality-of-care challenges facing our nation. A comprehensive and strong response is needed now.

Kenneth I. Shine, M.D.
President, Institute of Medicine
March 2001

Acknowledgments

The Committee on the Quality of Health Care in America first and foremost acknowledges the tremendous contribution by the members of two subcommittees, both of which spent many hours working on exceedingly complex issues. Although individual subcommittee members put forth differing perspectives on a variety of issues, there was no disagreement on the ultimate goal of providing the leadership, strategic direction, and analytic tools needed to achieve a substantial improvement in health care quality during the next decade. We take this opportunity to thank each subcommittee member for his or her contribution.

Subcommittee on Creating an Environment for Quality in Health Care: J. Cris Bisgard (*Cochair*), Delta Air Lines, Inc.; Molly Joel Coye, (*Cochair*), Institute for the Future; Phyllis C. Borzi, The George Washington University; Charles R. Buck, General Electric Company; Jon Christianson, University of Minnesota; Mary Jane England, Washington Business Group on Health; George J. Isham, HealthPartners; Brent James, Intermountain Health Care; Roz D. Lasker, New York Academy of Medicine; Lucian L. Leape, Harvard School of Public Health; Patricia A. Riley, National Academy of State Health Policy; Gerald M. Shea, American Federation of Labor and Congress of Industrial Organizations; Gail L. Warden, Henry Ford Health System; and A. Eugene Washington, University of California, San Francisco School of Medicine.

Subcommittee on Building the 21st Century Health Care System: Don M. Berwick (*Chair*), Institute for Healthcare Improvement; Christine K. Cassel, Mount Sinai School of Medicine; Rodney Dueck, HealthSystem Minnesota;

Jerome H. Grossman, John F. Kennedy School of Government, Harvard University; John E. Kelsch, Consultant in Total Quality; Risa Lavizzo-Mourey, University of Pennsylvania; Arthur Levin, Center for Medical Consumers; Eugene C. Nelson, Hitchcock Medical Center; Thomas Nolan, Associates in Process Improvement; Gail J. Povar, Cameron Medical Group; James L. Reinertsen, CareGroup; Joseph E. Scherger, University of California, Irvine; Stephen M. Shortell, University of California, Berkeley; Mary Wakefield, George Mason University; and Kevin Weiss, Rush Primary Care Institute. Paul Plsek served as an expert consultant to the subcommittee.

In addition, a number of people willingly and generously contributed their time and expertise as the committee and both subcommittees conducted their deliberations.

The planning committee for the Workshop on Using Information Technology to Improve the Quality of Care did an excellent job of organizing the workshop. This committee consisted of E. Andrew Balas, University of Missouri School of Medicine; Don E. Detmer, University of Cambridge; Jerome H. Grossman, John F. Kennedy School of Government, Harvard University; and Brent James, Intermountain Health Care. **The participants in this workshop** provided a great deal of useful information that is reflected in this report. These participants were E. Andrew Balas, University of Missouri School of Medicine; David W. Bates, Brigham Internal Medicine Associates; Mark Braunstein, Patient Care Technologies; Charles R. Buck, General Electric Company; Maj. Gen. Paul K. Carlton, Jr., Air Force Medical Operations Agency; David C. Classen, University of Utah; Paul D. Clayton, Intermountain Health Care; Kathryn L. Coltin, Harvard Pilgrim Health Care; Louis H. Diamond, The MEDSTAT Group; J. Michael Fitzmaurice, Agency for Health Care Policy and Research; Janlori Goldman, Georgetown University; Jerome H. Grossman, John F. Kennedy School of Government, Harvard University; David Gustafson, University of Wisconsin-Madison; Betsy L. Humphreys, U.S. National Library of Medicine; Brent James, Intermountain Health Care; John T. Kelly, AETNA/U.S. Healthcare; David B. Kendall, Progressive Policy Institute; Robert Kolodner, Department of Veterans Affairs; George D. Lundberg, Northwestern University; Robert Mayes, Health Care Financing Administration; Ned McCulloch, IBM, formerly Office of Senator Joseph Lieberman; Elizabeth A. McGlynn, The RAND Corporation; Blackford Middleton, MedicaLogic; Gregg S. Meyer, Agency for Health Care Policy and Research; Arnold Milstein, Pacific Business Group on Health; Donald Moran, The Moran Company; Michael Nerlich, University of Regensburg; William C. Richardson, W. K. Kellogg Foundation; Richard D. Rubin, Foundation for Health Care Quality; Charles Saunders, Healtheon/WebMD; Joseph E. Scherger, University of California, Irvine; Kenneth Smithson, VHA, Inc.; William W. Stead, Vanderbilt University; Stuart Sugarman, Mount Sinai/NYU Health; Paul C. Tang,

Palo Alto Medical Clinic; and Jan H. van Bemmel, Erasmus University Rotterdam.

The technical advisory panel on the Communication of Quality of Care Information organized a successful Workshop on Communicating with the Public About Quality of Care. This panel consisted of Mary Wakefield (*Chair*), George Mason University; Robert J. Blendon, Harvard School of Public Health and Kennedy School of Government; Charles R. Buck, General Electric Company; Molly Joel Coye, Institute for the Future; Arthur Levin, Center for Medical Consumers; Lee N. Newcomer, Vivius, Inc., formerly with United HealthCare Corporation; and Richard Sorian, Georgetown University. **Participants in the Workshop on Communicating with the Public about Quality of Care** provided many useful insights reflected in this report. They included Lisa Aliferis, Dateline NBC; Carol Blakeslee, News Hour with Jim Lehrer; Robert J. Blendon, Harvard School of Public Health and Kennedy School of Government; Charles R. Buck, General Electric Company; Christine Cassel, Mount Sinai School of Medicine; Molly Joel Coye, Institute for the Future; W. Douglas Davidson, Foundation for Accountability; Susan Dentzer, News Hour with Jim Lehrer; Mason Essif, HealthWeek Public Television; David Glass, Kaiser-Permanente; Ann Greiner, Center for Studying Health System Change; Madge Kaplan, WGBH Radio; Richard Knox, *Boston Globe*; Arthur Levin, Center for Medical Consumers; Trudy Lieberman, *Consumer Reports*; Lani Luciano, *Money Magazine*; Laura Meckler, Associated Press; Duncan Moore, *Modern Healthcare*; Lee N. Newcomer, Vivius, Inc., formerly with United HealthCare Corporation; William Richardson, W.K. Kellogg Foundation; Marty Rosen, *New York Daily News*; Sabin Russell, *San Francisco Chronicle*; Stuart Schear, The Robert Wood Johnson Foundation; Richard Sorian, Georgetown University; Abigail Trafford, *Washington Post*; Mary Wakefield, George Mason University; Lawrence Wallack, Portland State University; Michael Weinstein, *New York Times*; and Ronald Winslow, *Wall Street Journal*.

The technical advisory panel on the State of Quality in America, through their findings, based on a commissioned paper from Mark Schuster at RAND, provided important input to the committee's deliberations. The panel included Mark R. Chassin, The Mount Sinai School of Medicine; Arnold Epstein, Harvard School of Public Health; Brent James, Intermountain Health Care; James P. Logerfo, University of Washington, Seattle; Harold Luft, University of California, San Francisco; R. Heather Palmer, Harvard School of Public Health; and Kenneth B. Wells, University of California, Los Angeles.

Participants in the one-day Workshop on the Effects of Financing Policies on Quality of Care also provided important input to the committee's deliberations. They included Robert Berenson, Health Care Financing Administration; Don Berwick, Institute for Healthcare Improvement; J. Cris Bisgard, Delta Air Lines, Inc.; Phyllis Borzi, The George Washington University; David Bradley, Sentinel Health Partners Inc.; Lonnie Bristow, Former President, American Medical Association; Charles R. Buck, General Electric Company; Kathleen Buto, Health Care Financing Administration; Lawrence Casalino, The University of Chicago; Molly Joel Coye, Institute for the Future; Rick Curtis, Institute for Health Policy Solutions; Charles Cutler, American Association of Health Plans; Geraldine Dallek, Georgetown University; Irene Fraser, Agency for Healthcare Research and Quality; Jerome H. Grossman, John F. Kennedy School of Government, Harvard University; Sam Ho, PacifiCare Health Systems; Thomas Hoyer, Health Care Financing Administration; Brent James, Intermountain Health Care; Glenn D. Littenberg, Practicing Gastroenterologist; James Mortimer, Midwest Business Group on Health; Don Nielsen, American Hospital Association; Ann Robinow, Buyers Health Care Action Group; Gerald Shea, AFL–CIO; David Shulkin, DoctorQuality.com; Bruce Taylor, GTE Service Corporation; and Gail R. Wilensky, Project Hope & MedPAC.

Participants in a workshop held to explore the relationship between volume and outcomes made valuable contributions to this study as well. They included   Richard Bae, University of California San Francisco; Colin Begg, Memorial Sloan-Kettering Cancer Center; Donald M. Berwick, Institute for Healthcare Improvement; Bruce Bradley, General Motors; Mark R. Chassin, The Mount Sinai School of Medicine; Steve Clauser, Health Care Financing Administration; Jan De la Mare, Agency for Healthcare Research and Quality; Suzanne DelBanco, The Leapfrog Group; R. Adams Dudley, University of California, San Francisco; John Eisenberg, Agency for Healthcare Research and Quality; Irene Fraser, Agency for Healthcare Research and Quality; Robert Galvin, General Electric Company; Ethan Halm, The Mount Sinai School of Medicine; Edward Hannan, State University of New York, Albany; Norman Hertzer, Cleveland Clinic; Bruce Hillner, Virginia Commonwealth University; Sam Ho, PacifiCare Health Systems; George J. Isham, HealthPartners; Clara Lee, The Mount Sinai School of Medicine; Arthur Levin, Center for Medical Consumers; Arnold Milstein, William M. Mercer, Inc.; Peggy McNamara, Agency for Healthcare Research and Quality; Don Nielsen, American Hospital Association; Diana Petitti, Kaiser Permanente of Southern California; Joseph Simone, Huntsman Cancer Foundation and Institute; Jane Sisk, Mount Sinai School of Medicine; and Ellen Stovall, National Coalition for Cancer Survivorship.

A steering group that provided invaluable advice and review of the design of the microsystems study included Paul B. Batalden, Dartmouth Medical School; Donald M. Berwick, Institute for Healthcare Improvement; Eugene C. Nelson, Dartmouth Medical Center; Thomas Nolan, Associates in Process Improvement; and Stephen M. Shortell, University of California, Berkeley. The assistance of Susan B. Hassimiller, Project Officer at The Robert Wood Johnson Foundation was critical to the undertaking of this study. **The following individuals provided assistance in formulating interview questions and identifying study sites:** E. Andrew Balas, University of Missouri-Columbia School of Medicine; Connie Davis, Center for Health Studies of the Group Health Cooperative of Puget Sound; Joanne Lynn, Center to Improve Care of the Dying; and Charles M. Kilo, Institute for Health Care Improvement. The committee also wishes to thank the individuals at the study sites who gave their time to provide information on their practice settings.

Several other individuals made important contributions to the committee's work. They include John Demakis and Lynn McQueen, Health Services Research and Development Service, Department of Veterans Affairs; Joy Grossman, Center for Studying Health System Change; Stephanie Maxwell, the Urban Institute; and Ann Gauthier, Academy for Health Services Research and Health Policy.

Support for this project was provided by the Institute of Medicine, the National Research Council, The Robert Wood Johnson Foundation (Study of Micro-Systems), the California Health Care Foundation (Workshop on Communicating with the Public about Quality of Care), the Commonwealth Fund (Workshop on Using Information and Technology to Improve the Quality of Care), and the Department of Health and Human Services' Health Care Financing Administration (Workshop on the Effects of Financing Policy on Quality of Care), and Agency for Healthcare Research and Quality (Volume/Outcomes Workshop).

Contents

CROSSING THE QUALITY CHASM

Executive Summary

The American health care delivery system is in need of fundamental change. Many patients, doctors, nurses, and health care leaders are concerned that the care delivered is not, essentially, the care we should receive (Donelan et al., 1999; Reed and St. Peter, 1997; Shindul-Rothschild et al., 1996; Taylor, 2001). The frustration levels of both patients and clinicians have probably never been higher. Yet the problems remain. Health care today harms too frequently and routinely fails to deliver its potential benefits.

Americans should be able to count on receiving care that meets their needs and is based on the best scientific knowledge. Yet there is strong evidence that this frequently is not the case.[1] Crucial reports from disciplined review bodies document the scale and gravity of the problems (Chassin et al., 1998; Institute of Medicine, 1999; Advisory Commission on Consumer Protection and Quality in the Health Care Industry, 1998). Quality problems are everywhere, affecting many patients. Between the health care we have and the care we could have lies not just a gap, but a chasm.

The Committee on the Quality of Health Care in America was formed in June 1998 and charged with developing a strategy that would result in a substantial improvement in the quality of health care over the next 10 years. In carrying out this charge, the committee commissioned a detailed review of the literature on the quality of care; convened a communications workshop to identify strategies for raising the awareness of the general public and key stakeholders of quality concerns; identified environmental forces that encourage or impede ef-

---

[1]See Appendix A of this report for a review of the literature on the quality of care.

forts to improve quality; developed strategies for fostering greater accountability for quality; and identified important areas of research that should be pursued to facilitate improvements in quality. The committee has focused on the personal health care delivery system, specifically, the provision of preventive, acute, chronic, and end-of-life health care for individuals. Although the committee recognizes the critical role of the public health system in protecting and improving the health of our communities, this issue lies beyond the purview of the present study.

The committee has already spoken to one urgent quality problem—patient safety. In our first report, *To Err Is Human: Building a Safer Health System*, we concluded that tens of thousands of Americans die each year from errors in their care, and hundreds of thousands suffer or barely escape from nonfatal injuries that a truly high-quality care system would largely prevent (Institute of Medicine, 2000b).

As disturbing as the committee's report on safety is, it reflects only a small part of the unfolding story of quality in American health care. Other defects are even more widespread and, taken together, detract still further from the health, functioning, dignity, comfort, satisfaction, and resources of Americans. This report addresses these additional quality problems. As the patient safety report was a call for action to make care safer, this report is a call for action to improve the American health care delivery system as a whole, in all its quality dimensions, for all Americans.

WHY ACTION IS NEEDED NOW

At no time in the history of medicine has the growth in knowledge and technologies been so profound. Since the first contemporary randomized controlled trial was conducted more than 50 years ago, the number of trials conducted has grown to nearly 10,000 annually (Chassin, 1998). Between 1993 and 1999, the budget of the National Institutes of Health increased from $10.9 to $15.6 billion, while investments by pharmaceutical firms in research and development increased from $12 to $24 billion (National Institutes of Health, 2000; Pharmaceutical Research and Manufacturers of America, 2000). Genomics and other new technologies on the horizon offer the promise of further increasing longevity, improving health and functioning, and alleviating pain and suffering. Advances in rehabilitation, cell restoration, and prosthetic devices hold potential for improving the heath and functioning of many with disabilities. Americans are justifiably proud of the great strides that have been made in the health and medical sciences.

As medical science and technology have advanced at a rapid pace, however, the health care delivery system has floundered in its ability to provide consistently high-quality care to all Americans. Research on the quality of care reveals a health care system that frequently falls short in its ability to translate knowledge into practice, and to apply new technology safely and appropriately. During the last decade alone, more than 70 publications in leading peer-reviewed journals have documented serious quality shortcomings (see Appendix A). The performance of the health care system varies considerably. It may be exemplary, but often is not, and millions of Americans fail to receive effective care. If the health care system cannot consistently deliver today's science and technology, we may conclude that it is even less prepared to respond to the extraordinary scientific advances that will surely emerge during the first half of the 21st century. And finally, more than 40 million Americans remain without health insurance, deprived of critically important access to basic care (U.S. Census Bureau, 2000).

The health care system as currently structured does not, as a whole, make the best use of its resources. There is little doubt that the aging population and increased patient demand for new services, technologies, and drugs are contributing to the steady increase in health care expenditures, but so, too, is waste. Many types of medical errors result in the subsequent need for additional health care services to treat patients who have been harmed (Institute of Medicine, 2000b). A highly fragmented delivery system that largely lacks even rudimentary clinical information capabilities results in poorly designed care processes characterized by unnecessary duplication of services and long waiting times and delays. And there is substantial evidence documenting overuse of many services—services for which the potential risk of harm outweighs the potential benefits (Chassin et al., 1998; Schuster et al., 1998).

What is perhaps most disturbing is the absence of real progress toward restructuring health care systems to address both quality and cost concerns, or toward applying advances in information technology to improve administrative and clinical processes. Despite the efforts of many talented leaders and dedicated professionals, the last quarter of the 20th century might best be described as the "era of Brownian motion in health care." Mergers, acquisitions, and affiliations have been commonplace within the health plan, hospital, and physician practice sectors (Colby, 1997). Yet all this organizational turmoil has resulted in little change in the way health care is delivered. Some of the new arrangements have failed following disappointing results. Leaders of health care institutions are under extraordinary pressure, trying on the one hand to strategically reposition their organizations for the future, and on the other to respond to today's challenges, such as reductions in third-party payments (Guterman, 1998), shortfalls in nurse staffing (Egger, 2000), and growing numbers of uninsured patients seeking uncompensated care (Institute of Medicine, 2000a).

For several decades, the needs of the American public have been shifting from predominantly acute, episodic care to care for chronic conditions. Chronic conditions are now the leading cause of illness, disability, and death; they affect almost half of the U.S. population and account for the majority of health care expenditures (Hoffman et al., 1996; The Robert Wood Johnson Foundation, 1996). As the need for community-based acute and long-term care services has grown, the portion of health care resources devoted to hospital care has declined, while that expended on pharmaceuticals has risen dramatically (Copeland, 1999). Yet there remains a dearth of clinical programs with the infrastructure required to provide the full complement of services needed by people with heart disease, diabetes, asthma, and other common chronic conditions (Wagner et al., 1996). The fact that more than 40 percent of people with chronic conditions have more than one such condition argues strongly for more sophisticated mechanisms to communicate and coordinate care (The Robert Wood Johnson Foundation, 1996). Yet physician groups, hospitals, and other health care organizations operate as silos, often providing care without the benefit of complete information about the patient's condition, medical history, services provided in other settings, or medications prescribed by other clinicians. For those without insurance, care is often unobtainable except in emergencies. It is not surprising, then, that studies of patient experience document that the health system for some is a "nightmare to navigate" (Picker Institute and American Hospital Association, 1996).

QUALITY AS A SYSTEM PROPERTY

The committee is confident that Americans can have a health care system of the quality they need, want, and deserve. But we are also confident that this higher level of quality cannot be achieved by further stressing current systems of care. The current care systems cannot do the job. Trying harder will not work. Changing systems of care will.

The committee's report on patient safety offers a similar conclusion in its narrower realm. Safety flaws are unacceptably common, but the effective remedy is not to browbeat the health care workforce by asking them to try harder to give safe care. Members of the health care workforce are already trying hard to do their jobs well. In fact, the courage, hard work, and commitment of doctors, nurses, and others in health care are today the only real means we have of stemming the flood of errors that are latent in our health care systems.

Health care has safety and quality problems because it relies on outmoded systems of work. Poor designs set the workforce up to fail, regardless of how hard they try. If we want safer, higher-quality care, we will need to have redesigned systems of care, including the use of information technology to support clinical and administrative processes.

Throughout this report, the committee offers a strategy and action plan for building a stronger health system over the coming decade, one that is capable of delivering on the promise of state-of-the-art health care to all Americans. In some areas, achieving this ideal will require crossing a large chasm between today's system and the possibilities of tomorrow.

AN AGENDA FOR CROSSING THE CHASM

The need for leadership in health care has never been greater. Transforming the health care system will not be an easy process. But the potential benefits are large as well. Narrowing the quality chasm will make it possible to bring the benefits of medical science and technology to all Americans in every community, and this in turn will mean less pain and suffering, less disability, greater longevity, and a more productive workforce. To this end, the committee proposes the following agenda for redesigning the 21st-century health care system:

- **That all health care constituencies, including policymakers, purchasers, regulators, health professionals, health care trustees and management, and consumers, commit to a national statement of purpose for the health care system as a whole and to a shared agenda of six aims for improvement that can raise the quality of care to unprecedented levels.**
- **That clinicians and patients, and the health care organizations that support care delivery, adopt a new set of principles to guide the redesign of care processes.**
- **That the Department of Health and Human Services identify a set of priority conditions upon which to focus initial efforts, provide resources to stimulate innovation, and initiate the change process.**
- **That health care organizations design and implement more effective organizational support processes to make change in the delivery of care possible.**
- **That purchasers, regulators, health professions, educational institutions, and the Department of Health and Human Services create an environment that fosters and rewards improvement by (1) creating an infrastructure to support evidence-based practice, (2) facilitating the use of information technology, (3) aligning payment incentives, and (4) preparing the workforce to better serve patients in a world of expanding knowledge and rapid change.**

The committee recognizes that implementing this agenda will be a complex process and that it will be important to periodically evaluate progress and reassess strategies for overcoming barriers.

Establishing Aims for the 21st-Century Health Care System

The committee proposes six aims for improvement to address key dimensions in which today's health care system functions at far lower levels than it can and should. Health care should be:

- *Safe*—avoiding injuries to patients from the care that is intended to help them.

- *Effective*—providing services based on scientific knowledge to all who could benefit and refraining from providing services to those not likely to benefit (avoiding underuse and overuse, respectively).
- *Patient-centered*—providing care that is respectful of and responsive to individual patient preferences, needs, and values and ensuring that patient values guide all clinical decisions.
- *Timely*—reducing waits and sometimes harmful delays for both those who receive and those who give care.
- *Efficient*—avoiding waste, including waste of equipment, supplies, ideas, and energy.
- *Equitable*—providing care that does not vary in quality because of personal characteristics such as gender, ethnicity, geographic location, and socioeconomic status.

A health care system that achieved major gains in these six dimensions would be far better at meeting patient needs. Patients would experience care that was safer, more reliable, more responsive, more integrated, and more available. Patients could count on receiving the full array of preventive, acute, and chronic services from which they are likely to benefit. Such a system would also be better for clinicians and others who would experience the satisfaction of providing care that was more reliable, more responsive to patients, and more coordinated than is the case today.

The entire enterprise of care would ideally be united across these aims by a single, overarching purpose for the American health care system as a whole. For this crucial statement of purpose, the committee endorses and adopts the phrasing of the Advisory Commission on Consumer Protection and Quality in the Health Care Industry (1998).

Recommendation 1: All health care organizations, professional groups, and private and public purchasers should adopt as their explicit purpose to continually reduce the burden of illness, injury, and disability, and to improve the health and functioning of the people of the United States.

Recommendation 2: All health care organizations, professional groups, and private and public purchasers should pursue six major aims; specifically, health care should be safe, effective, patient-centered, timely, efficient, and equitable.

Additionally, without ongoing tracking to assess progress in meeting the six aims, policy makers, leaders within the health professions and health organizations, purchasers, and consumers will be unable to determine progress or understand where improvement efforts have succeeded and where further work is most needed. The National Quality Report has the potential to play an important role in continuing to raise the awareness of the American public about the quality-of-care challenges facing the health care system. Public awareness of shortcomings in quality is critical to securing public support for the steps that must be taken to address these concerns.

Recommendation 3: Congress should continue to authorize and appropriate funds for, and the Department of Health and Human Services should move forward expeditiously with the establishment of, monitoring and tracking processes for use in evaluating the progress of the health system in pursuit of the above-cited aims of safety, effectiveness, patient-centeredness, timeliness, efficiency, and equity. The Secretary of the Department of Health and Human Services should report annually to Congress and the President on the quality of care provided to the American people.

The committee applauds Congress and the Administration for their current efforts to establish a National Quality Report for tracking the quality of care. Ongoing input from the many public- and private-sector associations, professional groups, and others involved in quality measurement and improvement will contribute to the success of these efforts. The establishment of specific goals for each of the six aims could further enhance the usefulness of this monitoring and tracking system as a stimulus for performance improvement. Continued funding for this activity should be ensured, as well as regular reports that communicate progress to all concerned. It should be noted that although this report focuses only on health care for individuals, the above overarching statement of purpose and six aims for improvement are sufficiently robust that they can be applied equally to decisions and evaluations at the population–health level.

Formulating New Rules to Redesign and Improve Care

As discussed earlier, improved performance will depend on new system designs. The committee believes it would be neither useful nor possible for us to specify in detail the design of 21st-century health care delivery systems. Imagination and valuable pluralism abound at the local level in the nation's health care enterprise. At the same time, we believe local efforts to implement innovation and achieve improvement can benefit from a set of simple rules to guide the redesign of the health care system.

In formulating these rules, the committee has been guided by the belief that care must be delivered by systems that are carefully and consciously designed to provide care that is safe, effective, patient-centered, timely, efficient, and equitable. Such systems must be designed to serve the needs of patients, and to ensure that they are fully informed, retain control and participate in care delivery whenever possible, and receive care that is respectful of their values and preferences. Such systems must facilitate the application of scientific knowledge to practice, and provide clinicians with the tools and supports necessary to deliver evidence-based care consistently and safely.

Recommendation 4: Private and public purchasers, health care organizations, clinicians, and patients should work together to redesign health care processes in accordance with the following rules:

1. Care based on continuous healing relationships. Patients should receive care whenever they need it and in many forms, not just face-to-face visits. This rule implies that the health care system should be responsive at all times (24 hours a day, every day) and that access to care should be provided over the Internet, by telephone, and by other means in addition to face-to-face visits.

2. Customization based on patient needs and values. The system of care should be designed to meet the most common types of needs, but have the capability to respond to individual patient choices and preferences.

3. The patient as the source of control. Patients should be given the necessary information and the opportunity to exercise the degree of control they choose over health care decisions that affect them. The health system should be able to accommodate differences in patient preferences and encourage shared decision making.

4. Shared knowledge and the free flow of information. Patients should have unfettered access to their own medical information and to clinical knowledge. Clinicians and patients should communicate effectively and share information.

5. Evidence-based decision making. Patients should receive care based on the best available scientific knowledge. Care should not vary illogically from clinician to clinician or from place to place.

6. Safety as a system property. Patients should be safe from injury caused by the care system. Reducing risk and ensuring safety require greater attention to systems that help prevent and mitigate errors.

7. The need for transparency. The health care system should make information available to patients and their families that allows them to make informed decisions when selecting a health plan, hospital, or clinical practice, or choosing among alternative treatments. This should include information describing the system's performance on safety, evidence-based practice, and patient satisfaction.

8. Anticipation of needs. The health system should anticipate patient needs, rather than simply reacting to events.

9. *Continuous decrease in waste.* **The health system should not waste resources or patient time.**

10. *Cooperation among clinicians.* **Clinicians and institutions should actively collaborate and communicate to ensure an appropriate exchange of information and coordination of care.**

The above rules will lead the redesign effort in the right direction, guiding the innovation required to achieve the aims for improvement outlined earlier. Widespread application of these ten rules, each grounded in both logic and varying degrees of evidence, will represent a new paradigm for health care delivery. As the redesign effort moves forward, it will be important to assess not only progress toward meeting the aims, but also the specific effects attributable to the new rules and to adapt the rules as appropriate.

Design ideas are not enough, however. To initiate the process of change, both an action agenda and resources are needed.

Taking the First Steps

The committee recognizes the enormity of the change that will be required to achieve a substantial improvement in the nation's health care system. Although steps can be taken immediately to apply the ten rules set forth above to the redesign of health care, widespread application will require commitment to the provision of evidence-based care that is responsive to individual patients' needs and preferences. Well-designed and well-run systems of care will be required as well. These changes will occur most rapidly in an environment in which public policy and market forces are aligned and in which the change process is supported by an appropriate information technology infrastructure.

To initiate the process of change, the committee believes the health care system must focus greater attention on the development of care processes for the common conditions that afflict many people. A limited number of such conditions, about 15 to 25, account for the majority of health care services (Centers for Disease Control and Prevention, 1999; Medical Expenditure Panel Survey, 2000; Ray et al., 2000). Nearly all of these conditions are chronic. By focusing attention on a limited number of common conditions, the committee believes it will be possible to make sizable improvements in the quality of care received by many individuals within the coming decade.

Health care for chronic conditions is very different from care for acute episodic illnesses. Care for the chronically ill needs to be a collaborative, multidisciplinary process. Effective methods of communication, both among caregivers and between caregivers and patients, are critical to providing high-quality care. Personal health information must accompany patients as they transition from home to clinical office setting to hospital to nursing home and back.

Carefully designed, evidence-based care processes, supported by automated clinical information and decision support systems, offer the greatest promise of achieving the best outcomes from care for chronic conditions. Some efforts are now under way to synthesize the clinical evidence pertaining to common chronic conditions and to make this information available to consumers and clinicians on the Web and by other means (Lindberg and Humphreys, 1999). In addition, evidence-based practice guidelines have been developed for many chronic conditions (Eisenberg, 2000). Yet studies of the quality of care document tremendous variability in practice for many such conditions. Given these variations and the prevalence of chronic conditions, these conditions represent an excellent starting point for efforts to better define optimum care or best practices, and to design care processes to meet patient needs. Moreover, such efforts to improve quality must be supported by payment methods that remove barriers to integrated care and provide strong incentives and rewards for improvement.

To facilitate this process, the Agency for Healthcare Research and Quality should identify a limited number of priority conditions that affect many people and account for a sizable portion of the national health burden and associated expenditures. In identifying these priority conditions, the agency should consider using the list of conditions identified through the Medical Expenditure Panel Survey (2000). According to the most recent survey data, the top 15 priority conditions are cancer, diabetes, emphysema, high cholesterol, HIV/AIDS, hypertension, ischemic heart disease, stroke, arthritis, asthma, gall bladder disease, stomach ulcers, back problems, Alzheimer's disease and other dementias, and depression and anxiety disorders. Health care organizations, clinicians, purchasers, and other stakeholders should then work together to (1) organize evidence-based care processes consistent with best practices, (2) organize major prevention programs to target key health risk behaviors associated with the onset or progression of these conditions, (3) develop the information infrastructure needed to support the provision of care and the ongoing measurement of care processes and patient outcomes, and (4) align the incentives inherent in payment and accountability processes with the goal of quality improvement.

Recommendation 5: The Agency for Healthcare Research and Quality should identify not fewer than 15 priority conditions, taking into account frequency of occurrence, health burden, and resource use. In collaboration with the National Quality Forum, the agency should convene stakeholders, including purchasers, consumers, health care organizations, professional groups, and others, to develop strategies, goals, and action plans for achieving substantial improvements in quality in the next 5 years for each of the priority conditions.

Redirecting the health care industry toward the implementation of well-designed care processes for priority conditions will require significant resources.

Capital will be required to invest in enhancing organizational capacity, building an information infrastructure, and training multidisciplinary care teams, among other things. The committee believes it is appropriate for the public sector to take the lead in establishing an innovation fund to seed promising projects, but not to shoulder the full burden of the transition. Private-sector organizations, including foundations, purchasers, health care organizations, and others, should also make investments. High priority should be given to projects that are likely to result in making available in the public domain new programs, tools, and technologies that are broadly applicable throughout the health care sector.

> **Recommendation 6:** Congress should establish a Health Care Qual-
> ity Innovation Fund to support projects targeted at (1) achieving the
> six aims of safety, effectiveness, patient-centeredness, timeliness, ef-
> ficiency, and equity; and/or (2) producing substantial improvements
> in quality for the priority conditions. The fund's resources should
> be invested in projects that will produce a public-domain portfolio
> of programs, tools, and technologies of widespread applicability.

Americans now invest annually $1.1 trillion, or 13.5 percent, of the nation's gross domestic product (GDP) in the health care sector (Health Care Financing Administration, 1999). This figure is expected to grow to more than $2 trillion, or 16 percent of GDP, by 2007 (Smith et al., 1998). The committee believes a sizable commitment, on the order of $1 billion over 3 to 5 years, is needed to strongly communicate the need for rapid and significant change in the health care system and to help initiate the transition. Just as a vigorous public commitment has led to the mapping of human DNA, a similar commitment is needed to help the nation's health care system achieve the aims for improvement outlined above.

Building Organizational Supports for Change

Supporting front-line teams that deliver care are many types of health care organizations. Today, these are hospitals, physician practices, clinics, integrated delivery systems, and health plans, but new forms will unquestionably emerge. Whatever those forms, care that is responsive to patient needs and makes consistent use of the best evidence requires far more conscious and careful organization than we find today.

Organizations will need to negotiate successfully six major challenges. The first is to redesign care processes to serve more effectively the needs of the chronically ill for coordinated, seamless care across settings and clinicians and over time. The use of tools to organize and deliver care has lagged far behind biomedical and clinical knowledge. A number of well-understood design principles, drawn from other industries as well as some of today's health care organizations, could help greatly in improving the care that is provided to patients.

A second challenge is making effective use of information technologies to automate clinical information and make it readily accessible to patients and all members of the care team. An improved information infrastructure is needed to establish effective and timely communication among clinicians and between patients and clinicians.

A third challenge is to manage the growing knowledge base and ensure that all those in the health care workforce have the skills they need. Making use of new knowledge requires that health professionals develop new skills or assume new roles. It requires that they use new tools to access and apply the expanding knowledge base. It also requires that training and ongoing licensure and certification reflect the need for lifelong learning and evaluation of competencies.

A fourth challenge for organizations is coordination of care across patient conditions, services, and settings over time. Excellent information technologies and well-thought-out and -implemented modes of ongoing communication can reduce the need to craft laborious, case-by-case strategies for coordinating patient care.

A fifth challenge is to continually advance the effectiveness of teams. Team practice is common, but the training of health professionals is typically isolated by discipline. Making the necessary changes in roles to improve the work of teams is often slowed or stymied by institutional, labor, and financial structures, and by law and custom.

Finally, all organizations—whether or not health care related—can improve their performance only by incorporating care process and outcome measures into their daily work. Use of such measures makes it possible to understand the degree to which performance is consistent with best practices, and the extent to which patients are being helped.

Recommendation 7: The Agency for Healthcare Research and Quality and private foundations should convene a series of workshops involving representatives from health care and other industries and the research community to identify, adapt, and implement state-of-the-art approaches to addressing the following challenges:

- **Redesign of care processes based on best practices**
- **Use of information technologies to improve access to clinical information and support clinical decision making**
- **Knowledge and skills management**
- **Development of effective teams**
- **Coordination of care across patient conditions, services, and settings over time**
- **Incorporation of performance and outcome measurements for improvement and accountability**

Establishing a New Environment for Care

To enable the profound changes in health care recommended in this report, the *environment* of care must also change. The committee believes the current environment often inhibits the changes needed to achieve quality improvement. Two types of environmental change are needed:

• *Focus and align the environment toward the six aims for improvement.* To effect this set of changes, purchasers and health plans, for example, should eliminate or modify payment practices that fragment the care system, and should establish incentives designed to encourage and reward innovations aimed at improving quality. Purchasers and regulators should also create precise streams of accountability and measurement reflecting achievements in the six aims. Moreover, efforts should be made to help health care consumers understand the aims, why they are important, and how to interpret the levels of performance of various health care systems.

• *Provide, where possible, assets and encouragement for positive change.* For example, national funding agencies could promote research on new designs for the care of priority conditions, state and national activities could be undertaken to facilitate the exchange of best practices and shared learning among health care delivery systems, and a national system for monitoring progress toward the six aims for improvement could help improvement efforts remain on track.

Such environmental changes need to occur in four major areas: the infrastructure that supports the dissemination and application of new clinical knowledge and technologies, the information technology infrastructure, payment policies, and preparation of the health care workforce.

Changes will also be needed in the quality oversight and accountability processes of public and private purchasers. This issue is not addressed here. The IOM will be issuing a separate report on federal quality measurement and improvement programs in Fall 2002. In addition, the National Quality Forum has an extensive effort under way to develop a national framework for quality measurement and accountability and will be issuing a report in Summer 2001.

Applying Evidence to Health Care Delivery

In the current health care system, scientific knowledge about best care is not applied systematically or expeditiously to clinical practice. An average of about 17 years is required for new knowledge generated by randomized controlled trials to be incorporated into practice, and even then application is highly uneven (Balas and Boren, 2000). The extreme variability in practice in clinical areas in which there is strong scientific evidence and a high degree of expert consensus about best practices indicates that current dissemination efforts fail to reach many clinicians and patients, and that there are insufficient tools and incentives to promote rapid adoption of best practices. The time has come to invest in the creation of a more effective infrastructure for the application of knowledge to health care delivery.

Recommendation 8: **The Secretary of the Department of Health and Human Services should be given the responsibility and necessary resources to establish and maintain a comprehensive program aimed at making scientific evidence more useful and accessible to clinicians and patients. In developing this program, the Secretary should work with federal agencies and in collaboration with professional and health care associations, the academic and research communities, and the National Quality Forum and other organizations involved in quality measurement and accountability.**

It is critical that leadership from the private sector, both professional and other health care leaders and consumer representatives, be involved in all aspects of this effort to ensure its applicability and acceptability to clinicians and patients. The infrastructure developed through this public- and private-sector partnership should focus initially on priority conditions and include:

- Ongoing analysis and synthesis of the medical evidence
- Delineation of specific practice guidelines
- Identification of best practices in the design of care processes
- Enhanced dissemination efforts to communicate evidence and guidelines to the general public and professional communities
- Development of decision support tools to assist clinicians and patients in applying the evidence
- Establishment of goals for improvement in care processes and outcomes
- Development of quality measures for priority conditions

More systematic approaches are needed to analyze and synthesize medical evidence for both clinicians and patients. Far more sophisticated clinical decision support systems will be required to assist clinicians and patients in selecting the best treatment options and delivering safe and effective care. Many promising private- and public-sector activities now under way can serve as excellent models and building blocks for a more expanded effort. In particular, the Cochrane Collaboration and the Agency for Healthcare Research and Quality's Evidence-Based Practice Centers represent important efforts to synthesize medical evidence. The growth of the Internet has also opened up many new opportunities to make evidence more accessible to clinicians and consumers. The efforts of the National Library of Medicine to facilitate access to the medical literature by both consumers and health care professionals and to design Web sites that organize large amounts of information on particular health needs are particularly promising.

The development of a more effective infrastructure to synthesize and organize evidence around priority conditions would also offer new opportunities to enhance quality measurement and reporting. A stronger and more organized evidence base should facilitate the adoption of best practices, as well as the development of valid and reliable quality measures for priority conditions that could be used for both internal quality improvement and external accountability.

Using Information Technology

Health care delivery has been relatively untouched by the revolution in information technology that has been transforming nearly every other aspect of society. The majority of patient and clinician encounters take place for purposes of exchanging clinical information: patients share information with clinicians about their general health, symptoms, and concerns, and clinicians use their knowledge and skills to respond with pertinent medical information, and in many cases reassurance. Yet it is estimated that only a small fraction of physicians offer e-mail interaction, a simple and convenient tool for efficient communication, to their patients (Hoffman, 1997).

The meticulous collection of personal health information throughout a patient's life can be one of the most important inputs to the provision of proper care. Yet for most individuals, that health information is dispersed in a collection of paper records that are poorly organized and often illegible, and frequently cannot be retrieved in a timely fashion, making it nearly impossible to manage many forms of chronic illness that require frequent monitoring and ongoing patient support.

Although growth in clinical knowledge and technology has been profound, many health care settings lack basic computer systems to provide clinical information or support clinical decision making. The development and application of more sophisticated information systems is essential to enhance quality and improve efficiency.

The Internet has enormous potential to transform health care through information technology applications in such areas as consumer health, clinical care, administrative and financial transactions, public health, professional education, and biomedical and health services research (National Research Council, 2000). Many of these applications are currently within reach, including remote medical consultation with patients in their homes or offices; consumer and clinician access to the medical literature; creation of "communities" of patients and clinicians with shared interests; consumer access to information on health plans, participating providers, eligibility for procedures, and covered drugs in a formulary; and videoconferencing among public health officials during emergency situations. Other applications are more experimental, such as simulation of surgical procedures; consultation among providers involving manipulation of digital images; and control of experimental equipment, such as electron microscopes.

The Internet also supports rising interest among consumers in information and convenience in all areas of commerce, including health care. The number of Americans who use the Internet to retrieve health-related information is estimated to be about 70 million (Cain et al., 2000). Consumers access health-related Web sites to research an illness or disease; seek information on nutrition and fitness; research drugs and their interactions; and search for doctors, hospitals, and online medical support groups.

The committee believes information technology must play a central role in the redesign of the health care system if a substantial improvement in quality is to be achieved over the coming decade. Automation of clinical, financial, and administrative transactions is essential to improving quality, preventing errors, enhancing consumer confidence in the health system, and improving efficiency.

Central to many information technology applications is the automation of patient-specific clinical information. A fully electronic medical record, including all types of patient information, is not needed to achieve many, if not most, of the benefits of automated clinical data. Sizable benefits can be derived in the near future from automating certain types of data, such as medication orders. Efforts to automate clinical information date back several decades, but progress has been slow (Institute of Medicine, 1991), in part because of the barriers and risks involved. An important constraint is that consumers and policy makers share concerns about the privacy and confidentiality of these data (Cain et al., 2000; Goldman, 1998). The United States also lacks national standards for the capture, storage, communication, processing, and presentation of health information (Work Group on Computerization of Patient Records, 2000).

The challenges of applying information technology to health care should not be underestimated. Health care is undoubtedly one of the most, if not the most, complex sector of the economy. The number of different types of transactions (i.e., patient needs, interactions, and services) is very large. Sizable capital investments and multiyear commitments to building systems will be required. Widespread adoption of many information technology applications will require behavioral adaptations on the part of large numbers of patients, clinicians, and organizations. Yet, the Internet is rapidly transforming many aspects of society, and many health-related processes stand to be reshaped as well.

In the absence of a national commitment and financial support to build a national health information infrastructure, the committee believes that progress on quality improvement will be painfully slow. The automation of clinical, financial, and administrative information and the electronic sharing of such information among clinicians, patients, and appropriate others within a secure environment are critical if the 21st-century health care system envisioned by the committee is to be realized.

Recommendation 9: **Congress, the executive branch, leaders of health care organizations, public and private purchasers, and health informatics associations and vendors should make a renewed national commitment to building an information infrastructure to support health care delivery, consumer health, quality measurement and improvement, public accountability, clinical and health services research, and clinical education. This commitment should lead to the elimination of most handwritten clinical data by the end of the decade.**

Aligning Payment Policies with Quality Improvement

Current payment methods do not adequately encourage or support the provision of quality health care. Although payment is not the only factor that influences provider and patient behavior, it is an important one.

All payment methods affect behavior and quality. For example, fee-for-service payment methods for physicians and hospitals raise concerns about potential overuse of services—the provision of services that may not be necessary or may expose the patient to greater potential harm than benefit. On the other hand, capitation and per case payment methods for physicians and hospitals raise questions about potential underuse—the failure to provide services from which the patient would likely benefit. Indeed, no payment method perfectly aligns financial incentives with the goal of quality improvement for all health care decision makers, including clinicians, hospitals, and patients. This is one reason for the widespread interest in blended methods of payment designed to counter the disadvantages of one payment method with the advantages of another.

Too little attention has been paid to the careful analysis and alignment of payment incentives with quality improvement. The current health care environment is replete with examples of payment policies that work against the efforts of clinicians, health care administrators, and others to improve quality. The following example, presented at an Institute of Medicine workshop on payment and quality held on April 24, 2000,[2] illustrates how payment policies can work against the efforts of clinicians, health care administrators, and others to improve quality:

> A physician group paid primarily on a fee-for-service basis instituted a new program to improve blood sugar control for diabetic patients. Specifically, pilot studies suggested that tighter diabetic management could decrease hemoglobin A1c levels by 2 percentage points for about 40 percent of all diabetic patients managed by the physician group. Data from two randomized controlled trials demonstrated that better sugar controls should translate into lower rates of retinopathy, nephropathy, peripheral neurological damage, and heart disease. The

---

[2] This case study has been excerpted from a paper prepared by and presented at the IOM workshop by Brent James, Intermountain Health Care, Salt Lake City, Utah, April 2000.

savings in direct health care costs (i.e., reduced visits and hospital episodes) from avoided complications have been estimated to generate a net savings of about $2,000 per patient per year, on average, over 15 years. Across the more than 13,000 diabetic patients managed by the physician group, the project had the potential to generate over $10 million in net savings each year. The project was costly to the medical group in two ways. First, expenses to conduct the project, including extra clinical time for tighter management, fell to the physician group. Second, over time, as diabetic complication rates fell, the project would reduce patient visits and, thus, revenues as well. But the savings from avoided complications would accrue to the insurer or a self-funded purchaser.

The committee believes that all purchasers, both public and private, should carefully reexamine their payment policies.

Recommendation 10: **Private and public purchasers should examine their current payment methods to remove barriers that currently impede quality improvement, and to build in stronger incentives for quality enhancement.**

Payment methods should:

• Provide fair payment for good clinical management of the types of patients seen. Clinicians should be adequately compensated for taking good care of all types of patients, neither gaining nor losing financially for caring for sicker patients or those with more complicated conditions. The risk of random incidence of disease in the population should reside with a larger risk pool, whether that be large groups of providers, health plans, or insurance companies.

• Provide an opportunity for providers to share in the benefits of quality improvement. Rewards should be located close to the level at which the re-engineering and process redesign needed to improve quality are likely to take place.

• Provide the opportunity for consumers and purchasers to recognize quality differences in health care and direct their decisions accordingly. In particular, consumers need to have good information on quality and the ability to use that information as they see fit to meet their needs.

• Align financial incentives with the implementation of care processes based on best practices and the achievement of better patient outcomes. Substantial improvements in quality are most likely to be obtained when providers are highly motivated and rewarded for carefully designing and fine-tuning care processes to achieve increasingly higher levels of safety, effectiveness, patient-centeredness, timeliness, efficiency, and equity.

• Reduce fragmentation of care. Payment methods should not pose a barrier to providers' ability to coordinate care for patients across settings and over time.

To assist purchasers in the redesign of payment policy based on these fundamental principles, a vigorous program of pilot testing and evaluating alternative design options should be pursued.

Recommendation 11: **The Health Care Financing Administration and the Agency for Healthcare Research and Quality, with input from private payers, health care organizations, and clinicians, should develop a research agenda to identify, pilot test, and evaluate various options for better aligning current payment methods with quality improvement goals.**

Examples of possible means of achieving this end include blended methods of payment for providers, multiyear contracts, payment modifications to encourage use of electronic interaction among clinicians and between clinicians and patients, risk adjustment, bundled payments for priority conditions, and alternative approaches for addressing the capital investments needed to improve quality.

Preparing the Workforce

A major challenge in transitioning to the health care system of the 21st century envisioned by the committee is preparing the workforce to acquire new skills and adopt new ways of relating to patients and each other. At least three approaches can be taken to support the workforce in this transition. One is to redesign the way health professionals are trained to emphasize the aims for improvement set forth earlier, including teaching evidence-based practice and using multidisciplinary approaches. Second is to modify the ways in which health professionals are regulated to facilitate the needed changes in care delivery. Scope-of-practice acts and other workforce regulations need to allow for innovation in the use of all types of clinicians to meet patient needs in the most effective and efficient way possible. Third is to examine how the liability system can constructively support changes in care delivery while remaining part of an overall approach to accountability for health care professionals and organizations. All three approaches are important and require additional study.

Recommendation 12: **A multidisciplinary summit of leaders within the health professions should be held to discuss and develop strategies for (1) restructuring clinical education to be consistent with the principles of the 21st-century health system throughout the continuum of undergraduate, graduate, and continuing education for medical, nursing, and other professional training programs; and (2) assessing the implications of these changes for provider credentialing programs, funding, and sponsorship of education programs for health professionals.**

Recommendation 13: The Agency for Healthcare Research and Quality should fund research to evaluate how the current regulatory and legal systems (1) facilitate or inhibit the changes needed for the 21st-century health care delivery system, and (2) can be modified to support health care professionals and organizations that seek to accomplish the six aims set forth in Chapter 2.

SUMMARY

The changes needed to realize a substantial improvement in health care involve the health care system as a whole. The new rules set forth in this report will affect the role, self-image, and work of front-line doctors, nurses, and all other staff. The needed new infrastructures will challenge today's health care leaders—both clinical leaders and management. The necessary environmental changes will require the interest and commitment of payers, health plans, government officials, and regulatory and accrediting bodies. New skills will require new approaches by professional educators. The 21st-century health care system envisioned by the committee—providing care that is evidence-based, patient-centered, and systems-oriented—also implies new roles and responsibilities for patients and their families, who must become more aware, more participative, and more demanding in a care system that should be meeting their needs. And all involved must be united by the overarching purpose of reducing the burden of illness, injury, and disability in our nation.

American health care is beset by serious problems, but they are not intractable. Perfect care may be a long way off, but much better care is within our grasp. The committee envisions a system that uses the best knowledge, that is focused intensely on patients, and that works across health care providers and settings. Taking advantage of new information technologies will be an important catalyst to moving us beyond where we are today. The committee believes that achieving such a system is both possible and necessary.

REFERENCES

Advisory Commission on Consumer Protection and Quality in the Health Care Industry. 1998. "Quality First: Better Health Care for All Americans." Online. Available at http://www.hcqualitycommission.gov/final/ [accessed Sept. 9, 2000].

Balas, E. Andrew and Suzanne A. Boren. Managing Clinical Knowledge for Health Care Improvement. *Yearbook of Medical Informatics* National Library of Medicine, Bethesda, MD:65–70, 2000.

Cain, Mary M., Robert Mittman, Jane Sarasohn-Kahn, and Jennifer C. Wayne. *Health e-People: The Online Consumer Experience*. Oakland, CA: Institute for the Future, California Health Care Foundation, 2000.

Centers for Disease Control and Prevention. 1999. "Chronic Diseases and Their Risk Factors: The Nation's Leading Causes of Death." Online. Available at http://www.cdc.gov/nccdphp/statbook/statbook.htm [accessed Dec. 7, 2000].

Chassin, Mark R. Is Health Care Ready for Six Sigma Quality? *Milbank Quarterly* 76(4):575–91, 1998.

Chassin, Mark R., Robert W. Galvin, and the National Roundtable on Health Care Quality. The Urgent Need to Improve Health Care Quality. *JAMA* 280(11):1000–5, 1998.

Colby, David C. Doctors and their Discontents. *Health Affairs* 16(6):112–4, 1997.

Copeland, C. Prescription Drugs: Issues of Cost, Coverage and Quality. *EBRI Issue Brief* April(208): 1–21, 1999.

Donelan, Karen, Robert J. Blendon, Cathy Schoen, et al. The Cost of Health System Change: Public Discontent In Five Nations. *Health Affairs* 18(3):206–16, 1999.

Egger, Ed. Nurse Shortage Worse Than You Think, But Sensitivity May Help Retain Nurses. *Health Care Strategic Management* 18(5):16–8, 2000.

Eisenberg, John M. Quality Research for Quality Healthcare: The Data Connection. *Health Services Research* 35:xii–xvii, 2000.

Goldman, Janlori. Protecting Privacy To Improve Health Care. *Health Affairs* 17(6):47–60, 1998.

Guterman, Stuart. The Balanced Budget Act of 1997: Will Hospitals Take A Hit On Their PPS Margins? *Health Affairs* 17(1):159–66, 1998.

Health Care Financing Administration. 1999. "1998 National Health Expenditures. Department of Health and Human Services. Washington, DC." Online. Available at http://www.hcfa.gov/stats/nhe-oact/hilites.htm [accessed Jan. 10, 2000].

Hoffman, A. Take 2 and E-mail Me in the Morning: Doctors Consult Patients Electronically. *New York Times.* June 3, 1997.

Hoffman, Catherine, Dorothy P. Rice, and Hai-Yen Sung. Persons With Chronic Conditions. Their Prevalence and Costs. *JAMA* 276(18): 1473–9, 1996.

Institute of Medicine *The Computer-Based Patient Record: An Essential Technology for Health Care.* Richard S. Dick and Elaine B. Steen, eds. Washington, D.C.: National Academy Press, 1991.

———— *Ensuring Quality Cancer Care.* Maria Hewitt and Joseph V. Simone, eds. Washington, D.C.: National Academy Press, 1999.

———— *America's Health Care Safety Net. Intact but Endangered.* Marion E. Lewin and Stuart Altman, eds. Washington, D.C.: National Academy Press, 2000a.

———— *To Err Is Human: Building a Safer Health System.* Linda T. Kohn, Janet M. Corrigan, and Molla S. Donaldson, eds. Washington, D.C: National Academy Press, 2000b.

Lindberg, Donald A. B. and Betsy L. Humphreys. A Time of Change for Medical Informatics in the USA. *Yearbook of Medical Informatics* National Library of Medicine, Bethesda, MD:53–7, 1999.

Medical Expenditure Panel Survey. 2000. "MEPS HC-006R: 1996 Medical Conditions." Online. Available at http://www.meps.ahrq.gov/catlist.htm [accessed Dec. 7, 2000].

National Institutes of Health. 2000. "An Overview." Online. Available at http://www.nih.gov/about/NIHoverview.html [accessed Aug. 11, 2000].

National Research Council. *Networking Health: Prescriptions for the Internet.* Washington, DC: National Academy Press, 2000.

Pharmaceutical Research and Manufacturers of America. 2000. "PhRMA Annual Report, 2000–2001." Online. Available at http://www.phrma.org/publications/publications/annual2000/ [accessed Nov. 11, 2000].

Picker Institute and American Hospital Association. *Eye on Patients Report.* 1996.

Ray, G. Thomas, Tracy Lieu, Bruce Fireman, et al. The Cost of Health Conditions in a Health Maintenance Organization. *Medical Care Research and Review* 57(1):92–109, 2000.

Reed, Marie C. and Robert F. St. Peter *Satisfaction and Quality: Patient and Physician Perspectives.* Washington, D.C.: Center for Studying Health System Change, 1997.

Schuster, Mark A., Elizabeth A. McGlynn, and Robert H Brook. How Good is the Quality of Health Care in the United States? *The Milbank Quarterly* 76(4):517–63, 1998.

Shindul-Rothschild, Judith, Diane Berry, and Ellen Long-Middleton. Where Have All The Nurses Gone? Final Results of Our Patient Care Survey. *American Journal of Nursing* 96(11):25–39, 1996.

Smith, Sheila, Mark Freeland, Stephen Heffler, et al. The Next Ten Years of Health Spending: What Does The Future Hold? *Health Affairs* 17(3):128–40, 1998.

Taylor, Humphrey. 2001. "Harris Poll #3, Most People Continue To Think Well Of Their Health Plans." Online. Available at http://www.harrisblackintl.com/harris_poll/index.asp [accessed Jan. 11, 2001].

The Robert Wood Johnson Foundation. *Chronic Care in America: A 21st Century Challenge.* Princeton, NJ: The Robert Wood Johnson Foundation, 1996. Online. Available at http://www.rwjf.org/library/chrcare/ [accessed Sept. 19, 2000].

U.S. Census Bureau. Health Insurance Coverage: 1999. *Current Population Survey.* by Robert J. Mills. Washington, D.C.: U.S. Census Bureau. September, 2000. Online. Available at: http://www.census.gov/hhes/www/hlthin99.html [accessed Jan. 22, 2001].

Wagner, Edward H., Brian T. Austin, and Michael Von Korff. Organizing Care for Patients with Chronic Illness. *Milbank Quarterly* 74(4):511–42, 1996.

Work Group on Computerization of Patient Records. *Toward a National Health Information Infrastructure: Report of the Work Group on Computerization of Patient Records.* Washington, D.C.: U.S. Department of Health and Human Services, 2000.

1

A New Health System for the 21st Century

Fundamental changes are needed in the organization and delivery of health care in the United States. The experiences of patients, their families, and health care clinicians, as well as a large body of evidence on the quality of care, have convinced the Committee on the Quality of Health Care in America that the time for major change has come. This chapter sets forth the evidence; the reasons underlying the inability of the health care system to meet patient needs; and the committee's framework for a new health system, which serves to structure the remaining chapters of this report.

THE QUALITY GAP

The year 1998 was a watershed in the quest for improvement in the quality of health care (Kizer, 2000). In that year, three major reports detailing serious quality-of-care concerns were issued. The Institute of Medicine's (IOM) National Roundtable on Health Care Quality documents three types of quality problems—overuse, underuse, and misuse. The report describes the problem as follows:

> The burden of harm conveyed by the collective impact of all of our health care quality problems is staggering. It requires the urgent attention of all the stakeholders: the health care professions, health care policymakers, consumer advocates and purchasers of care. The challenge is to bring the full potential benefit of effective health care to all Americans while avoiding unneeded and harmful interventions and eliminating preventable complications of care. Meeting this challenge demands a readiness to think in radically new ways about how to

deliver health care services and how to assess and improve their quality. Our present efforts resemble a team of engineers trying to break the sound barrier by tinkering with a Model T Ford. We need a new vehicle or perhaps, many new vehicles. The only unacceptable alternative is not to change. (Chassin et al., 1998)

The Advisory Commission on Consumer Protection and Quality also released a report on quality. That report calls for a national commitment to improve quality, concluding: "Exhaustive research documents the fact that today, in America, there is no guarantee that any individual will receive high-quality care for any particular health problem. The health care industry is plagued with overutilization of services, underutilization of services and errors in health care practice" (Advisory Commission on Consumer Protection and Quality in the Health Care Industry, 1998).

Finally, the reports of both of these national panels were supported by the results of an extensive literature review conducted by researchers at RAND Corporation and encompassing publications in leading peer-reviewed journals between 1993 and mid-1997 (Schuster et al., 1998). The report on those results substantiates the serious and pervasive nature of quality-of-care problems.

In the fall of 1998, the Committee on the Quality of Health Care in America established a Technical Advisory Panel on the State of Quality to review the most recent literature on quality. In collaboration with RAND, the earlier synthesis of the quality literature was updated to include work published between July 1997 and August 1998. The detailed results of this review, now covering 8 years and more than 70 publications, are included in Appendix A. The committee concurs with the findings of the panel that ". . . there is abundant evidence that serious and extensive quality problems exist throughout American medicine resulting in harm to many Americans."

The literature reviews conducted by RAND encompass studies categorized under the rubric of quality of care. Other reviews that probe more deeply in a specific clinical area (e.g., oncology) or focus on a particular type of quality problem (e.g., errors) provide further evidence of the systemic nature of quality-of-care problems.

One such study, an IOM report examining cancer care, reveals that quality problems occur across all types of cancer care and in all aspects of the process of care (Institute of Medicine, 1999). For example, problems with breast cancer care include underuse of mammography for early cancer detection, lack of adherence to standards for diagnosis (such as biopsies and pathology studies), inadequate patient counseling regarding treatment options, and underuse of radiation therapy and adjuvant chemotherapy following surgery.

In its first report, *To Err Is Human: Building a Safer Health System*, this committee reviewed the literature on a specific type of quality problem—medical errors. We found about 30 publications published during the last 10 to 12 years substantiating serious and widespread errors in health care delivery that resulted in frequent avoidable injuries to patients (Institute of Medicine, 2000).

These quality problems occur typically not because of a failure of goodwill, knowledge, effort, or resources devoted to health care, but because of fundamental shortcomings in the ways care is organized. The nation's current health care system often lacks the environment, the processes, and the capabilities needed to ensure that services are safe, effective, patient-centered, timely, efficient, and equitable.

UNDERLYING REASONS FOR INADEQUATE QUALITY OF CARE

Four key aspects of the current context for health care delivery help explain the quality problems outlined above: the growing complexity of science and technology, the increase in chronic conditions, a poorly organized delivery system, and constraints on exploiting the revolution in information technology. Each of these factors plays a role, and each exacerbates the effects of the others.

Growing Complexity of Science and Technology

Health care today is characterized by more to know, more to manage, more to watch, more to do, and more people involved in doing it than at any time in the nation's history. Our current methods of organizing and delivering care are unable to meet the expectations of patients and their families because the science and technologies involved in health care—the knowledge, skills, care interventions, devices, and drugs—have advanced more rapidly than our ability to deliver them safely, effectively, and efficiently (The Robert Wood Johnson Foundation, 1996).

For more than five decades, investments in biomedical research have increased steadily, resulting in an extraordinary expansion of medical knowledge and technology (Blumenthal, 1994). Between 1994 and 1999, the budget of the National Institutes of Health increased from $10.9 to $15.6 billion (National Institutes of Health, 2000), while the investment of pharmaceutical firms in research and development increased from about $13.5 to $24 billion (Pharmaceutical Research and Manufacturers of America, 2000). Spending on research and development in the medical device industry, most of which comes from private sources, totaled $8.9 billion in 1998 (The Lewin Group, 2000).

As suggested earlier, quality problems do not generally stem from a lack of knowledge, training, or effort by health professionals. Today, no one clinician can retain all the information necessary for sound, evidence-based practice. No unaided human being can read, recall, and act effectively on the volume of clinically relevant scientific literature. Since the results of the first randomized controlled trial were published more than 50 years ago (Cochrane, 1972; Daniels and Hill, 1952), health care practitioners have been increasingly inundated with information about what does and does not work to produce good outcomes in health care. Over the last 30 years, the increase in such trials has been stagger- ing—from just over 100 to nearly 10,000 annually. The first 5 years of this 30- year period accounts for only 1 percent of all the articles in the medical literature, while the last 5 years accounts for almost half (49 percent) (Chassin, 1998), and there is no indication that this rate is slowing. Studies on the effectiveness of medical practice have also become increasingly sophisticated, involving complex issues of patient selection and statistical procedures.

As the knowledge base has expanded, so too has the number of drugs, medi- cal devices, and other technological supports. For example, the average number of new drugs approved per year has doubled since the early 1980s, from 19 to 38 (The Henry J. Kaiser Family Foundation, 2000). Between 1990 and 1999, 311 new drugs were approved by the U.S. Food and Drug Administration (U.S. Food and Drug Administration, 2000). The cost of pharmaceuticals is the most rapidly growing component of health care expenditures. As clinical science continues to advance, the challenge of managing the use of existing and new pharmaceuticals and health technologies will intensify.

Without substantial changes in the ways health care is delivered, the prob- lems resulting from the growing complexity of health care science and technolo- gies are unlikely to abate; in fact, they will increase. For example, work being done in genomics offers significant promise for disease diagnosis and, eventu- ally, treatment. Engineering advances in miniaturization will place diagnostic, monitoring, and treatment tools directly into the hands of patients as science improves and costs are reduced. And the application of epidemiological knowl- edge to large populations and databases will enable us to understand more and more about the dynamics of wellness and disease.

Increase in Chronic Conditions

One of the consequences of advances in medical science and technology is that people are now living longer. Although health care is by no means the only factor that affects morbidity and mortality, innovations in medical science and technology have contributed greatly to increases in life expectancy. The average American born today can expect to live more than 76 years (National Center for Health Statistics, 2000). Roughly 1 additional year has been added to life expect- ancy every 5 years since 1965.

Because of changing mortality patterns, those age 65 and over constitute an increasingly large number and proportion of the U.S. population. Today, this age group accounts for approximately 1 in 8 persons, or 13 percent of the population (National Center for Health Statistics, 1999). In 2030, when the large baby boom cohort has entered old age, 1 in 5 persons (20 percent) is expected to be in this age group. These demographic changes have important implications for the organi- zation of the health care delivery system, but we have yet to address them in any serious way. One consequence of the aging of the population is an increase in the incidence and prevalence of chronic conditions.

Chronic conditions, defined as illnesses that last longer than 3 months and are not self-limiting, are now the leading cause of illness, disability, and death in this country, and affect almost half of the U.S. population (Hoffman et al., 1996). About 100 million Americans have one or more chronic conditions, and this number is estimated to grow to 134 million by 2020 (The Robert Wood Johnson Foundation, 1996). About 1 in 6 Americans is limited in daily activities in some way as a result of a chronic condition (The Robert Wood Johnson Foundation, 1996). Disabling chronic conditions affect all age groups; about two-thirds of those with such conditions are under age 65.

The majority of health care resources are now devoted to the treatment of chronic disease. In 1990, the direct medical costs for persons with chronic conditions was $425 billion, nearly 70 percent of all personal health care expenditures (The Robert Wood Johnson Foundation, 1996). The indirect costs—lost productivity due to premature death or inability to work—added another $234 billion to this figure.

Providing state-of-the-art health care to a population in which chronic conditions predominate is complicated by the fact that many of those afflicted have comorbid conditions. About 44 percent of those with a chronic illness have more than one such condition, and the likelihood of having two or more chronic conditions increases steadily with age. In 1987, annual medical costs per person were more than twice as high for those with one chronic condition ($1,829) as compared with those with acute conditions only ($817) (The Robert Wood Johnson Foundation, 1996). Annual medical costs per person increase much more for those with more than one chronic condition ($4,672).

Unlike much acute episodic care, effective care of the chronically ill is a collaborative process, involving the definition of clinical problems in terms that both patients and providers understand; joint development of a care plan with goals, targets, and implementation strategies; provision of self-management training and support services; and active, sustained follow-up using visits, telephone calls, e-mail, and Web-based monitoring and decision support programs (Von Korff et al., 1997). Much of the care provided to the chronically ill is given by patients and their families. Activities performed range from the provision of basic support care to active monitoring and management (e.g., self blood glucose monitoring by diabetics, use of peak flow meters by asthmatics). Although some degree of collaborative management is essential to achieve desired outcomes for many chronic conditions, patients vary a great deal in the amount of information they want to receive on their condition and their desire to participate in treatment decisions (Strull et al., 1984). Nonetheless, the collaboration involved in much of the care provided to the chronically ill adds another layer of complexity to the delivery of health care to this growing segment of the population.

Poorly Organized Delivery System

The current health care delivery system is highly decentralized. In a survey of physicians practicing in community settings, nearly 40 percent were in one-physician practices, and more than four of five practiced in settings with fewer than ten physicians (American Medical Association, 1998). Hospital consolidation is occurring in many markets; of the more than 5,000 community hospitals, 3,556 belong to some form of network or system (American Hospital Association, 2000). The formation of physician organizations is occurring much more slowly, however (Kohn, 2000).

The prevailing model of health care delivery is complicated, comprising layers of processes and handoffs that patients and families find bewildering and clinicians view as wasteful. Patients in a 1996 Picker Survey reported that the health care system is a "nightmare to navigate"—that it feels less like a system than a confusing, expensive, unreliable, and often impersonal disarray (Picker Institute and American Hospital Association, 1996). Care delivery processes are often overly complex, requiring steps and handoffs that slow down the care process and decrease rather than improve safety. These processes waste resources; leave unaccountable gaps in coverage; result in the loss of information; and fail to build on the strengths of all health professionals involved to ensure that care is timely, safe, and appropriate.

In a population increasingly afflicted by chronic conditions, the health care delivery system is poorly organized to provide care to those with such conditions. In a review of the literature on chronic care, Wagner et al. (1996) identified five elements required to improve patient outcomes for the chronically ill:

• *Evidence-based, planned care.* The literature is replete with evidence of the failure to provide care consistent with well-established guidelines for common chronic conditions such as hypertension (Stockwell et al., 1994), asthma (Legorreta et al., 1998; Starfield et al., 1994), and diabetes (Kenny et al., 1993). Successful chronic care programs tend to be ones that incorporate guidelines and protocols explicitly into practice.

• *Reorganization of practices to meet the needs of patients who require more time, a broad array of resources, and closer follow-up.* Such reorganization generally involves the delivery of care through a multidisciplinary team, the careful allocation of tasks among the team members, and the ongoing management of patient contact (appointments, follow-up) (Wagner et al., 1996).

• *Systematic attention to patients' need for information and behavioral change.* A review of 400 articles, randomized trials, and observational studies of self-management support interventions (Center for Advancement of Health, 1996), revealed substantial evidence that programs providing counseling, education, information feedback, and other supports to patients with common chronic conditions are associated with improved outcomes (Brown, 1990; DeBusk et al., 1994; Mullen et al., 1987).

• *Ready access to necessary clinical expertise.* Specialized clinical knowledge and expertise are important to improved outcomes. Evidence suggests that there are numerous ways to enhance access to such knowledge and expertise, including education of patients and primary care providers (Inui et al., 1976; Sawicki et al., 1993; Soumerai and Avorn, 1990), referrals to specialists, various consultation processes (e.g., teleconferencing, hot line to specialists) (Vinicor et al., 1987), collaborative care models whereby primary care providers and specialists practice together (Katon et al., 1995; McCulloch et al., 1994), and computer decision support systems (Barton and Schoenbaum, 1990; Litzelman et al., 1993; McDonald et al., 1988).

• *Supportive information systems.* Patient registries have been used effectively in many settings to issue reminders for preventive care and necessary follow-up, and to provide feedback to the provider practice on patient compliance and service use (Glanz and Scholl, 1982; Johnston et al., 1994; Macharia et al., 1992; Mugford et al., 1991; Stason et al., 1994). Mechanisms for sharing clinical and other information among all members of the care team, ranging from patient-carried medical records (Dickey and Petitti, 1992; Turner et al., 1990) to automated patient records, can also improve care.

Thus the American health care system does not have well-organized programs to provide the full complement of services needed by people with such chronic conditions as heart disease, cancer, diabetes, and asthma. Nor do we have mechanisms to coordinate the full range of services needed by those with multiple serious illnesses. And our current health system has only a rudimentary ability to collect and share patient information.

A growing body of evidence for some procedures and conditions suggests that higher volume is associated with better outcomes (Hewitt, 2000). We know little about the underlying factors that produce this relationship (e.g., more effective care processes, better processes for incorporating knowledge into practice, provider skill, effective multidisciplinary team, access to specialized resources). But the results are consistent with the conclusion that the growing complexity of health care necessitates more sophisticated and carefully designed care processes.

The application of engineering concepts to the design of care processes is a critical first step in improving patient safety. Yet few health care organizations have applied the lessons learned by other high-risk industries that have led to very low rates of injury. These lessons include organized approaches to collecting data on errors and analyzing their causes, minimizing reliance on human memory, and standardizing routine aspects of care processes (Chassin, 1998; Institute of Medicine, 2000). Patient safety emerges from systems that are skillfully designed to prevent harm (Cook, 1998). Although many, often simple, steps could be taken now and without great cost, knowledge about such actions has neither been disseminated among health care institutions nor widely implemented, probably because there are often no real penalties for failing to do so and no real rewards for effective improvements. Although Americans have come to expect high-technology care, they do not demand safety and reliability with the same insistence.

For the most part, health care organizations are only beginning to apply information technology to manage and improve patient care. A great deal of medical information is stored on paper. Communication among clinicians and with patients does not generally make use of the Internet or other contemporary information technology. Hospitals and physician groups operate independently of one another, often providing care without the benefit of complete information on the patient's condition or medical history, services provided in other settings, or medications prescribed by other providers.

Our attempts to deliver today's technologies with today's medical production capabilities are the medical equivalent of manufacturing microprocessors in a vacuum tube factory. The costs of waste, poor quality, and inefficiency are enormous. If the current delivery system is unable to utilize today's technologies effectively, it will be even less able to carry the weight of tomorrow's technologies and an aging population, raising the specter of even more variability in quality, more errors, less responsiveness, and greater costs associated with waste and poor quality.

The challenge before us is to move from today's highly decentralized, cottage industry to one that is capable of providing primary and preventive care, caring for the chronically ill, and coping with acute and catastrophic events. To meet this challenge, there must be a commitment to organizing services around common patient needs and applying information technology and engineering concepts to the design of care processes.

Constraints on Exploiting the Revolution in Information Technology

The advent of the Internet and the World Wide Web has placed us on the threshold of a change that is reshaping virtually all aspects of society, including health care delivery. The Internet supports a rising tide of consumerism, with greater demands for information and convenience in all areas of commerce. And Internet services are becoming cheaper and easier to access.

Four of ten U.S. households had Internet access as of August 2000 (U.S. Department of Commerce, 2000), and it is predicted that 90 percent will have access by 2010 or before (Rosenberg, 1999). Large increases in Internet access have occurred among most groups of Americans, regardless of income, education, race or ethnicity, location, age, or gender (U.S. Department of Commerce, 2000). Nonetheless, a "digital divide" remains, especially for the disabled and for African Americans and Hispanics.

Large numbers of patients are turning to the Internet for health care information and advice. An estimated 70 million Americans seek health information online (Cain et al., 2000). It is estimated that there are 10,000 or more health-related Web sites (Benton Foundation, 1999), allowing consumers to search for information on specific diseases and treatments, evaluate health plans and clinicians, pose questions to care providers, manage chronic conditions, participate in discussion groups, assess existing health risks, and purchase health-related products (National Research Council, 2000). There is however, much variability in the accuracy and completeness of health information found on the Web (Biermann et al., 1999).

The effect of these trends on health care will be a fundamental transformation in the ways services are organized and delivered and clinicians and patients interact. Individuals are making many of their own decisions about diagnosis and treatment. Increasingly, they are also bringing information to their physicians to obtain help in interpreting or judging its value for themselves.

To better understand how information technology can contribute to improving quality, the Committee on the Quality of Health Care in America held a workshop in September 1999 at which participants identified five key areas in which information technology could contribute to an improved health care delivery system:

• *Access to the medical knowledge-base.* Through use of the Web, it should be possible to help both providers and consumers gain better access to clinical evidence.

• *Computer-aided decision support systems.* Embedding knowledge in tools and training clinicians to use those tools to augment their own skills and experience can facilitate the consistent application of the expanding science base to patient care.

• *Collection and sharing of clinical information.* The automation of patient-specific clinical information is essential for many types of computer-aided decision support systems. Automation of clinical data offers the potential to improve coordination of care across clinicians and settings, which is critical to the effective management of chronic conditions.

• *Reduction in errors.* Information technology can contribute to a reduction in errors by standardizing and automating certain decisions and by aiding in the identification of possible errors, such as potential adverse drug interactions, before they occur.

• *Enhanced patient and clinician communication.* Information technology can change the way individuals receive care and interact with their clinicians. Instead of a $65 office visit and a half-day off work, a 2-minute e-mail communication could meet many patients' needs more responsively and at lower cost. Similarly, patients would be able to go online and obtain test results, inform their clinicians about how they are doing, send pictures and data, participate in interactive care management services, receive after-care instructions, and participate in support groups. Appropriately structured e-mail communication between patient and provider could also permit continuous monitoring of clinical conditions, especially for patients with chronic conditions that require self-management.

A recent report by the National Research Council of The National Academies, *Networking Health*, also concludes that "the Internet has great potential to improve Americans' health by enhancing communications and improving access to information for care providers, patients, health plan administrators, public health officials, biomedical researchers, and other health professionals" (National Research Council, 2000). In recent years, some applications have become commonplace, such as online searching for health information by patients and providers. Others, such as remote and virtual surgery and simulations of surgical procedures, are in early stages of development.

Although opportunities to improve access, quality, and service abound, the health care industry has been slow to invest in information technology. In 1996, the industry spent only $543 per worker on information technology, compared, for example, with $12,666 spent by securities brokers, and ranked 38th out of 53 industries surveyed (U.S. Department of Commerce, 1999). In a recent survey of 30 health plans, it was found that all had established Web sites to allow patients to obtain certain types of information and interact with the organization (e.g., online provider directory, search formulary, ability to query member services or file a complaint), and about one-half had the capability to conduct some types of transactions online (e.g., enrollment, referral processing, claims submission) (First Consulting Group, 2000). But none had automated entire service functions, such as online medical management, which would require significant changes in business strategy, involve many employees and/or partners, and entail sizable capital investments.

There are many technical, organizational, behavioral, and public policy challenges to greater use of information technology. Technical challenges include ensuring the security of personally identifiable information; making persistent, reliable broadband connectivity available to many locations, including rural clinics and patients' homes; establishing processes for authentication of the source and recipient of information; and making tools available for locating information of interest and for determining the quality of retrieved information (National Research Council, 2000).

Over the long run, however, organizational challenges may play the greatest role in constraining the adoption of various types of Internet applications. The diverse and highly decentralized structure of the health care industry, as discussed above, makes the business models for new applications complex and difficult, resulting in slow adoption of even highly successful pioneering applications. Efforts to introduce new applications also encounter resistance from health care professionals for a variety of reasons, including uncertainties about how such applications will alter relationships among and between clinicians, patients, and health care organizations (National Research Council, 2000).

Numerous public policy, payment, and legal issues also must be resolved. Many applications in the public health arena (e.g., videoconferencing during emergency situations, collection of information from local and state public health departments, incident reporting and disease surveillance) are within technical reach at relatively low cost, but are not widely used because of a lack of targeted public-sector funding and organizational barriers (e.g., shortage of adequately trained personnel). Fee-for-service payment, the most common method of payment for physicians, does not compensate clinicians for time spent on e-mail communication. State-based professional licensing requirements and restrictions on practice have stymied widespread use of other applications, such as remote medical consultations. Online access to and transfer of clinical information has also been slow to evolve, in part because of concerns about privacy and confidentiality. Chapter 7 reviews in greater detail the use of information technology to improve the quality of health care and some of the barriers to its more widespread adoption.

AGENDA FOR THE FUTURE AND ROAD MAP
FOR THE REPORT

Throughout the course of its work, the committee has been cognizant of the fact that the health care system has been in a rapid state of flux for more than 10 years and that this situation is likely to continue. Over the last decade, the primary impetus for change has been a desire to slow the rate of inflation of health care costs. During the coming decades, cost pressures will remain, but the health care system will also be shaped dramatically by broader forces transforming society in general, most notably the growth of the Internet and changing population needs for chronic care.

There is little doubt that the health care enterprise has been slow to change. Research documenting safety and quality concerns has been mounting for over a decade. Successful quality improvement initiatives are very slow to spread, and rarely adopted on a widespread basis. For these reasons, the committee believes that a more intense and far-reaching effort will be needed. Substantial improvement in quality over the coming decade can be achieved only by engaging the support of patients, clinicians, governing boards and managers of health care organizations, private and public purchasers, state and federal policy makers, regulators, researchers, and others. Change is needed at all levels, including the clinician and patient relationship; the structure, management, and operation of health care organizations; the purchasing and financing of health care; the regulatory and liability environment; and others.

This report offers general principles, not a detailed blueprint, for the building of a new system. In part, the committee cannot foresee all the new organizations, forces, technologies, needs, and relationships that will develop even in the early years of the 21st century. More than that, however, the committee has come to believe that a framework for a new health system should be based on systems that can organize themselves to achieve a shared purpose by adhering to a few well-thought-out general rules, adapting to local circumstances, and then examining their own performance (see Chapter 3 and Appendix B). In reshaping health care, local adaptation, innovation, and initiative will be essential ingredients for success.

With these precepts in mind, the committee proposes the following agenda designed to bridge the quality gap:

• That all health care constituencies, including policymakers, purchasers, regulators, health professionals, health care trustees and management, and consumers, commit to a national statement of purpose for the heath care system as a whole and to a shared agenda of six aims for improvement that can raise the quality of care to unprecedented levels.
• That clinicians and patients, and the health care organizations that support care delivery, adopt a new set of principles to guide the redesign of care processes.
• That the Department of Health and Human Services identify a set of priority conditions upon which to focus initial efforts, provide resources to stimulate innovation, and initiate the change process.
• That health care organizations design and implement more effective organization support processes to make change in the delivery of care possible.
• That purchasers, regulators, health professions, educational institutions, and the Department of Health and Human Services create an environment that fosters and rewards improvement by (1) creating an infrastructure to support evidence-based practice, (2) facilitating the use of information technology, (3) aligning payment incentives, and (4) preparing the workforce to better serve patients in a world of expanding knowledge and rapid change.

The succeeding chapters of this report detail in turn the elements of this agenda. Specifically, the report:

• Sets performance expectations or aims for improvement for the 21st-century health care system (Chapter 2).
• Explores the implications of these performance expectations for the interactions between patients and clinicians, and develops some simple rules to guide the actions of all stakeholders (Chapter 3).
• Encourages all stakeholders to focus immediate attention on the development of state-of-the-art care processes for common conditions, and calls for the establishment of a $1 billion innovation fund that can be used to invest in enhancing organizational capacity, building an information infrastructure, and training multidisciplinary teams, among other things (Chapter 4).

- Addresses the importance of building more effective organizational structures to (1) redesign care processes; (2) use information technologies; (3) manage knowledge and skills; (4) coordinate care across patient conditions, services, and settings over time; (5) develop effective teams, and (6) implement performance and outcome measurement for improvement and accountability (Chapter 5).
- Identifies critical steps that must be taken to support evidence-based practice, including making evidence more useful and accessible to support the clinical decisions of clinicians and patients, and constructing quality measures for improvement and accountability (Chapter 6).
- Explains why a more sophisticated information infrastructure is necessary to improve quality, and calls for a renewed national initiative to build such an infrastructure (Chapter 7).
- Illustrates some of the ways current payment policies impede efforts to improve quality, and explains the importance of better aligning payment incentives to encourage innovations and reward enhancements in quality (Chapter 8).
- Addresses critical issues related to the culture, education, and training of a health professional workforce prepared to succeed in the 21st-century delivery system (Chapter 9).

The committee's recommendations in these areas are presented in the respective chapters, highlighted in bold print.

In sum, health care is plagued today by a serious quality gap. The current health care delivery system is not robust enough to apply medical knowledge and technology consistently in ways that are safe, effective, patient-centered, timely, efficient, and equitable. As we strive to close this gap, we must seek health care solutions that are patient-centered, that is, humane and respectful of the needs and preferences of individuals. And, most important, we must build a 21st century health care system that is more equitable and meets the needs of all Americans without regard to race, ethnicity, place of residence, or socioeconomic status, including the nearly 43 million people who currently lack health insurance (U.S. Census Bureau, 2000).

REFERENCES

Advisory Commission on Consumer Protection and Quality in the Health Care Industry. 1998. "Quality First: Better Health Care for All Americans." Online. Available at http://www.hcqualitycommission.gov/final/ [accessed Sept. 9, 2000].

American Hospital Association. Resource Center Fact Sheet. Fast Facts on U.S. Hospitals. *Hospital Statistics, 2000.* Chicago, IL: Health Forum - An American Hospital Association Company, 2000.

American Medical Association. *Socioeconomic Characteristics of Medical Practice: 1997/98.* Chicago, Illinois: American Medical Association, 1998. Page 21.

Barton, Mary B. and Stephen C. Schoenbaum. Improving Influenza Vaccination Performance in an HMO Setting: The Use of Computer-Generated Reminders and Peer Comparison Feedback. *American Journal of Public Health* 80(5):534–6, 1990.

Benton Foundation. 1999. "Networking for Better Care: Health Care in the Information Age." Online. Available at http://www.benton.org/Library/health/ [accessed Sept. 18, 2000].

Biermann, J. Sybil, Gregory J. Golladay, Mary Lou V. H. Greenfield, and Laurence H. Baker. Evaluation of Cancer Information on the Internet. *Cancer* 86(3):381–90, 1999.

Blumenthal, David. Growing Pains for New Academic/Industry Relationships. *Health Affairs* 13(3): 176–93, 1994.

Brown, Sharon A. Studies of Educational Interventions and outcomes in Diabetic Adults: A Meta-Analysis Revisited. *Patient Education and Counseling* 16:189–215, 1990.

Cain, Mary M., Robert Mittman, Jane Sarasohn-Kahn, and Jennifer C. Wayne. *Health e-People: The Online Consumer Experience.* Oakland, CA: Institute for the Future, California Health Care Foundation, 2000.

Center for Advancement of Health. Indexed Bibliography of Behavioral Interventions of Chronic Disease. Washington, D.C., 1996.

Chassin, Mark R. Is Health Care Ready for Six Sigma Quality? *Milbank Quarterly* 76(4):575–91, 1998.

Chassin, Mark R., Robert W. Galvin, and the National Roundtable on Health Care Quality. The Urgent Need to Improve Health Care Quality. *JAMA* 280(11):1000–5, 1998.

Cochrane, A. L. Effectiveness and Efficiency, Random Reflections on Health Services. *The Nuffield Provincial Hospitals Trust,* 1972.

Cook, Richard I. *Two Years Before the Mast: Learning How to Learn About Safety.* 1998. Invited presentation. Annenberg Conference, "Enhancing Patient Safety and Reducing Errors in Health Care," Rancho Mirage, CA November 8–10, 1998.

Daniels, Marc and A. Bradford Hill. Chemotherapy of Pulmonary Tuberculosis in Young Adults. An Analysis of the Combined Results of Three Medical Research Council Trials. *BMJ* 31:1162–8, 1952.

DeBusk, Robert F., Nancy Houston Miller, H. Robert Superko, et al. A Case-Management System for Coronary Risk Factor Modification after Acute Myocardial Infarction. *Ann Int Med* 120: 721–9, 1994.

Dickey, Larry L. and Diana Petitti. A Patient-Held Minirecord to Promote Adult Preventive Care. *J Fam Pract* 34(4):457–63, 1992.

First Consulting Group. *Health Systems on the E-Health Path: A Survey of Scottsdale Institute Members.* Long Beach, CA: FCG, 2000. eHealth@FCG.com.

Glanz, Karen and Theresa O. Scholl. Intervention Strategies to Improve Adherence among Hypertensives: Review and Recommendations. *Patient Counselling and Health Education* 4(1):14–28, 1982.

Hewitt, Maria for the Committee on the Quality of Health Care in America and the National Cancer Policy Board. *Interpreting the Volume-Outcome Relationship in the Context of Health Care Quality.* Washington, D.C.: Institute of Medicine, National Academy Press, 2000. Online. Available at http://books.nap.edu/catalog/10005.html [accessed Jan. 29, 2001].

Hoffman, Catherine, Dorothy P. Rice, and Hai-Yen Sung. Persons With Chronic Conditions. Their Prevalence and Costs. *JAMA* 276(18): 1473–9, 1996.

Institute of Medicine. *Ensuring Quality Cancer Care.* Maria Hewitt and Joseph V. Simone, eds. Washington, D.C.: National Academy Press, 1999.

———. *To Err Is Human: Building a Safer Health System.* Linda T. Kohn, Janet M. Corrigan, and Molla S. Donaldson, eds. Washington, D.C: National Academy Press, 2000.

Inui, Thomas S., Edward L. Yourtee, and John W. Williamson. Improved Outcomes in Hypertension After Physician Tutorials: A Controlled Trial. *Ann Int Med* 84:646–51, 1976.

Johnston, Mary E., Karl B. Langton, R. Brian Haynes, and Alix Mathieu. Effects of Computer-Based Clinical Decision Support Systems on Clinician Performance and Patient Outcome: A Critical Appraisal of Research. *Ann Int Med* 120:135–42, 1994.

Katon, Wayne, Michael Von Korff, Edward Lin, et al. Collaborative Management to Achieve Treatment Guidelines: Impact on Depression in Primary Care. *JAMA* 273(13):1026–31, 1995.

Kenny, Susan J., Philip J. Smith, Merilyn G. Goldschmid, et al. Survey of Physician Practice Behaviors Related to Diabetes Mellitus in the U.S.: Physician Adherence to Consensus Recommendations. *Diabetes Care* 16(11):1507–10, 1993.

Kizer, Kenneth W. The National Quality Forum Enters the Game. *International Journal for Quality in Health Care* 12(2):85–7, 2000.

Kohn, Linda T. Organizing and Managing Care in a Changing Health System. *Health Services Research* 35(Part I):37–52, 2000.

Legorreta, Antonio P., Jennifer Christian-Herman, Richard D. O'Connor, et al. Compliance With National Asthma Management Guidelines and Specialty Care: A Health Maintenance Organization Experience. *Arch Int Med* 158:457–64, 1998.

Litzelman, Debra K., Robert S. Dittus, Michael E. Miller, and William M. Tierney. Requiring Physicians to Respond to Computerized Reminders Improves Their Compliance with Preventive Care Protocols. *J Gen Intern Med* 8:311–7, 1993.

Macharia, William M., Gladys Leon, Brian H. Rowe, et al. An Overview of Interventions to Improve Compliance with Appointment Keeping for Medical Services. *JAMA* 267(13):1813–7, 1992.

McCulloch, David K., Russell E. Glasgow, Sarah E. Hampson, and Ed Wagner. A Systematic Approach to Diabetes Management in the Post-DCCT Era. *Diabetes Care* 17(7):765–9, 1994.

McDonald, Clement J., Lonnie Blevins, William M. Tierney, and Douglas K. Martin. The Regenstrief Medical Records. *MD Computing* 5(5):34–47, 1988.

Mugford, Miranda, Philip Banfield, and Moira O'Hanlon. Effects of Feedback of Information on Clinical Practice: A Review. *BMJ* 303:398–402, 1991.

Mullen, Patricia D., Elizabeth A. Laville, Andrea K. Biddle, and Kate Lorig. Efficacy of Psycho-educational Interventions on Pain, Depression, and Disability in People with Arthritis: A Meta-Analysis. *Journal of Rheumatology* 14(suppl 15):33–9, 1987.

National Center for Health Statistics. *Health, United States, 1999. With Health and Aging Chartbook.* Hyattsville, MD: U.S. Government Printing Office, 1999.

——— *Health, United States, 2000. With Adolescent Health Chartbook.* Hyattsville, MD: U.S. Government Printing Office, 2000.

National Institutes of Health. 2000. "An Overview." Online. Available at http://www.nih.gov/about/NIHoverview.html [accessed Aug. 11, 2000].

National Research Council. *Networking Health: Prescriptions for the Internet.* Washington, DC: National Academy Press, 2000.

Pharmaceutical Research and Manufacturers of America. 2000. "PhRMA Annual Report, 2000–2001." Online. Available at http://www.phrma.org/publications/annual2000/ [accessed Nov. 11, 2000].

Picker Institute and American Hospital Association. *Eye on Patients Report.* 1996.

Rosenberg, Matt. Popularity of Internet Won't Peak for Years: Not until today's middle-schoolers reach adulthood will the technology really take off. *Puget Sound Business Journal.* May 24, 1999. Online. Available at http://www.bizjournals.com/seattle/stories/1999/05/24/focus9.html [accessed Jan. 22. 2001].

Sawicki, Peter T., Ingrid Muhlhauser, Ulrike Didjurgeit, and Michael Berger. Improvement of Hypertension Care by a Structured Treatment and Teaching Programme. *Journal of Human Hypertension* 7:571–3, 1993.

Schuster, Mark A., Elizabeth A. McGlynn, and Robert H Brook. How Good is the Quality of Health Care in the United States? *The Milbank Quarterly* 76(4):517–63, 1998.

Soumerai, Stephen B. and Jerry Avorn. Principles of Educational Outreach ('Academic Detailing') to Improve Clinical Decision Making. *JAMA* 263(4):549–55, 1990.

Starfield, Barbara, Neil R. Powe, Jonathan R. Weiner, et al. Costs vs. Quality in Different Types of Primary Care Settings. *JAMA* 272(24):1903–8, 1994.

Stason, William B., Donald S. Shepard, H. Mitchell Perry, Jr., et al. Effectiveness and Costs of Veterans Affairs Hypertension Clinic. *Medical Care* 32(12):1197–215, 1994.

Stockwell, David H., Shantha Madhavan, Hillel Cohen, Geoffrey Gibson, and Michael H. Alderman. The Determinants of Hypertension Awareness, Treatment, and Control in an Insured Population. *American Journal of Public Health* 84(11):1768–74, 1994.

Strull, William M., Bernard Lo, and Gerald Charles. Do Patients Want to Participate in Medical Decision Making? *JAMA* 252(21):2990–4, 1984.

The Henry J. Kaiser Family Foundation. *Prescription Drug Trends - A Chartbook.* Menlo Park, CA: The Henry J. Kaiser Family Foundation, 2000.

The Lewin Group, Inc. *Outlook for Medical Technology Innovation: Will Patients Get the Care They Need. Report #1: The State of the Industry.* Washington, DC: Health Insurance Manufacturers Association, 2000.

The Robert Wood Johnson Foundation. *Chronic Care in America: A 21ˢᵗ Century Challenge.* Princeton, NJ: The Robert Wood Johnson Foundation, 1996. Online. Available at http://www.rwjf.org/library/chrcare/ [accessed Sept. 19, 2000].

Turner, Robert C., Leo E. Waivers, and Kevin O'Brien. The Effect of Patient-Carried Reminder Cards on the Performance of Health Maintenance Measures. *Arch Int Med* 150:645–7, 1990.

U.S. Census Bureau. Health Insurance Coverage: 1999. *Current Population Survey.* by Robert J. Mills. Washington, D.C.: U.S. Census Bureau. September, 2000. Online. Available at: http://www.census.gov/hhes/www/hlthin99.html [accessed Jan. 22, 2001].

U.S. Department of Commerce. *The Emerging Digital Economy II.* Washington DC: Economic Statistics Administration, Office of Policy Development, 1999. Online. Available at: http://www.ecommerce.gov/eds/report.html [accessed Sept. 19, 2000].

———. *Falling Through the Net: Toward Digital Inclusion. A Report on American's Access to Technology Tools.* Washington DC: Economics and Statistics Administration; National Telecommunications and Information Administration, 2000. Online. Available at: http://www.ntia.doc.gov/ntiahome/digitaldivide/ [accessed Sept. 19, 2000].

U.S. Food and Drug Administration. Figure 3-2: Mean Approval Times for New Drugs, 1987–1999. *2000 Pharmaceutical Industry Profile.* Washington DC: Pharmaceutical Research and Manufacturing Association, 2000.

Vinicor, Frank, Stuart J. Cohen, Steven A. Mazzuca, et al. DIABEDS: A randomized trial of the effects of physician and/or patient education on diabetes patient outcomes. *Journal of Chronic Diseases* 40:234–56, 1987.

Von Korff, Michael, Jessie Gruman, Judith Schaefer, Susan J. Curry, and Edward H. Wagner. Collaborative Management of Chronic Illness. *Ann Int Med* 127(12):1097–102, 1997.

Wagner, Edward H., Brian T. Austin, and Michael Von Korff. Organizing Care for Patients with Chronic Illness. *Milbank Quarterly* 74(4):511–42, 1996.

2

Improving the 21st-Century
Health Care System

As discussed in Chapter 1, the American health care system is in need of major restructuring. This will not be an easy task, but the potential benefits are great. To cross the divide between today's system and the possibilities of tomorrow, strong leadership and clear direction will be necessary. As a statement of purpose for the health care system as a whole, the committee endorses and adopts the phrasing of the Advisory Commission on Consumer Protection and Quality in the Health Care Industry (1998).

Recommendation 1: All health care organizations, professional groups, and private and public purchasers should adopt as their explicit purpose to continually reduce the burden of illness, injury, and disability, and to improve the health and functioning of the people of the United States.

It is helpful to translate this general statement into a more specific agenda for improvement—a list of performance characteristics that, if addressed and improved, would lead to better achievement of that overarching purpose. To this end, the committee proposes six specific aims for improvement. Health care should be:

- *Safe*—avoiding injuries to patients from the care that is intended to help them.
- *Effective*—providing services based on scientific knowledge to all who could benefit and refraining from providing services to those not likely to benefit (avoiding underuse and overuse).

- *Patient-centered*—providing care that is respectful of and responsive to individual patient preferences, needs, and values and ensuring that patient values guide all clinical decisions.
- *Timely*—reducing waits and sometimes harmful delays for both those who receive and those who give care.
- *Efficient*—avoiding waste, in particular waste of equipment, supplies, ideas, and energy.
- *Equitable*—providing care that does not vary in quality because of personal characteristics such as gender, ethnicity, geographic location, and socioeconomic status.

Recommendation 2: All health care organizations, professional groups, and private and public purchasers should pursue six major aims; specifically, health care should be safe, effective, patient-centered, timely, efficient, and equitable.

The committee believes substantial improvements in safety, effectiveness, patient-centeredness, timeliness, efficiency, and equity are achievable throughout the health care sector. This opportunity for improvement is not confined to any sector, form of payment, type of organization, or clinical discipline. Problems in health care quality affect all Americans today, and all can benefit from a rededication to improving quality, regardless of where they receive their care.

The committee applauds the Administration and Congress for their current efforts to establish a mechanism for tracking the quality of care. Title IX of the Public Health Service Act (42 U.S.C. 299 et seq.; Agency for Healthcare Research and Quality Part A) provides support for the development of a National Quality Report, which is currently ongoing. Section 913(a)(2) of the act states: "Beginning in fiscal year 2003, the Secretary, acting through the Director, shall submit to Congress an annual report on national trends in the quality of health care provided to the American people."

Recommendation 3: Congress should continue to authorize and appropriate funds for, and the Department of Health and Human Services should move forward expeditiously with the establishment of, monitoring and tracking processes for use in evaluating the progress of the health system in pursuit of the above-cited aims of safety, effectiveness, patient-centeredness, timeliness, efficiency, and equity. The Secretary of the Department of Health and Human Services should report annually to Congress and the President on the quality of care provided to the American people.

Without ongoing tracking of quality to assess the country's progress in meeting the aims set forth in this chapter, interested parties—including patients, health care practitioners, policy makers, educators, and purchasers—cannot identify progress or understand where improvement efforts are most needed. Continued funding for this activity should be ensured.

SIX AIMS FOR IMPROVEMENT

Over the course of a lifetime, individuals have numerous encounters with the health system. Fortunately, many of these encounters are effective and result in good outcomes, but such is not always the case. The following scenario, based on the composite experience of a number of patients, illustrates some of the serious problems facing patients and clinicians, problems that persist despite the widespread dedication of clinicians to providing high-quality care.

Ms. Martinez, January 2000

Ms. Martinez, a divorced working mother in her early 50s with two children in junior high school, was new in town and had to choose an insurance plan. She had difficulty knowing which plan to select for her family, but she chose City-Care because its cost was comparable to that of other options, and it had pediatric as well as adult practices nearby.

Once she had joined CityCare, she was asked to choose a primary care physician. After receiving some recommendations from a neighbor and several co-workers, she called several of the offices to sign up. The first two she called were not accepting new patients. Although she knew nothing about the practice she finally found, she assumed it would be adequate.

Juggling repairs on their new apartment, finding the best route to work, getting the children's immunization records sent by mail, and making other arrangements to get them into a new school, Ms. Martinez delayed calling her new doctor's office for several months. When she called for an appointment, she was told that the first available nonurgent appointment was in 2 months; she hoped she would not run out of her blood pressure medication in the interim.

When she went for her first appointment, she was asked to complete a patient history form in the waiting room. She had difficulty remembering dates and significant past events and doses of her medications. After waiting for an hour, she met with Dr. McGonagle and had a physical exam. Although her breast exam appeared to be normal, Dr. McGonagle noted that she was due for a mammogram.

Ms. Martinez called a site listed in her provider directory and was given an appointment for a mammogram in 6 weeks. The staff suggested that she arrange to have her old films mailed to her. Somehow, the films were never sent, and distracted by other concerns, she forgot to follow up.

A week after the mammogram, she received a call from Dr. McGonagle's office notifying her of an abnormal finding and saying that she should make an appointment with a surgeon for a biopsy. The first opening with the surgeon was 9 weeks later. By now, she was very anxious. She hated even to think about having cancer in her body, especially because an older sister had died of the disease. For weeks she did not sleep, wondering what would happen to her children if she were debilitated or to her job if she had to have surgery and lengthy treatment. She was reluctant to call her mother, who was likely to imagine the worst, and did not know her new coworkers well enough to confide in them.

After numerous calls, she was finally able to track down her old mammograms. It turned out that a possible abnormal finding had been circled the previous year, but neither she nor her primary care physician had ever been notified.

Finally, Ms. Martinez had her appointment with the surgeon, and his office scheduled her for a biopsy. The biopsy showed that she had a fairly unusual form of cancer, and there was concern that it might have spread to her lymph nodes. She felt terrified, angry, sad, and helpless all at once, but needed to decide what kind of surgery to have. It was a difficult decision because only one small trial comparing lumpectomy and mastectomy for this type of breast cancer had been conducted. She finally decided on a mastectomy.

Before she could have surgery, Ms. Martinez needed to have bone and abdominal scans to rule out metastases to her bones or liver. When she arrived at the hospital for surgery, however, some of this important laboratory information was missing. The staff called and hours later finally tracked down the results of her scans, but for a while it looked as though she would have to reschedule the surgery.

During her mastectomy, several positive lymph nodes were found. This meant she had to see the surgeon, an oncologist, and a radiologist, as well as her primary care physician, to decide on the next steps. At last it was decided that she would have radiation therapy and chemotherapy. She was given the phone number for the American Cancer Society. Before 6 months had gone by, Ms. Martinez found another lump, this time under her arm. Cancer had spread to her lung as well. She was given more radiation, then more chemotherapy. Wherever she went for care, the walls were drab, the chairs uncomfortable, and sometimes she would wait hours for a scheduled appointment.

During her numerous procedures and tests, Ms. Martinez experienced many acts of consideration, empathy, and technical expertise for which she was grateful. Yet for Ms. Martinez, who had excellent health insurance and was seen by well-trained and capable clinicians, the system did not work and did not meet her needs. Her care failed on several accounts.

First, it was not *safe*. Neither she nor her previous primary care doctor had been notified of an abnormal finding on her earlier mammogram. As a result, at least a year elapsed before the abnormality was addressed. Ms. Martinez was never confident that those directing her care had all the information about her previous care and its results. Prior to her surgery, critical laboratory information was missing. She was repeatedly required to tell her story, which became longer and more complex as time passed. No one at the hospital followed her course of illness after her discharge.

Second, Ms. Martinez's care was not *effective*. She suffered preventable, long-lasting disability—and could have lost her life. It was not clear that her follow-up care consistently used the most up-to-date protocols. She needed consistent, reliable information, based on the best science available. Yet treatments tried and proven futile in one admission would be recommended in the next as if they were fresh ideas.

Third, her care was not *timely*. Repeated, extensive delays occurred between tests and follow-up care, delays that are not at all atypical in today's health system.

Fourth, her care was not *patient-centered*. She had little assistance or information to help her understand the implications of choices about her surgery, radiation therapy, or chemotherapy. Although office and hospital staff focused on immediate medical problems, her discomfort, fear, and uncertainty were never addressed, and she was offered few resources to help her.

Finally, her care was not *efficient* because much of its complexity and expense came from treating a tumor at a later stage than should have occurred.

Many other individuals experience systems of care that often do not work. This is true even for patients with excellent insurance, in fine institutions, cared for by conscientious and well-trained clinicians. Common, too, is frequent inability of patients to make their needs understood, to be treated with respect and compassion, to learn what to expect about their health condition and treatment, and to have caregivers and institutions they can trust. These patients tell stories of fragmented care in which relevant information is lost, overlooked, or ignored; of wasted resources; of frustrated efforts to obtain timely access to services; and of lost opportunities. When clinicians and their families and those steeped in health management become patients, they, too, find that there appears to be no one who can make the systems function safely and effectively (Berwick, 1996, 1999; Khan, 2000; Singer, 2000).

In this chapter, the committee puts forth six specific aims for improvement: health care should be safe, effective, patient-centered, timely, efficient, and equitable. These specific aims are intended to aid in achieving the overarching purpose stated in Recommendation 1 above. These aims are not new; they are familiar and have been valued, arguably for decades, among health care professionals, patients, policy makers, and communities. Yet American health care fails far too often with respect to these aims, despite its enormous cost and the dedication and good efforts of millions of American health care workers. After careful consideration, the committee has concluded that fundamental changes are necessary if our current health system is to achieve these aims. In its current forms, habits, and environment, American health care is incapable of providing the public with the quality health care it expects and deserves.

The call for such improvement is not an indictment of physicians, nurses, or, indeed, any of the people who give or lead care. The committee asserts, without reservation, that our health care can and should be far better than it is today, but it would be futile to seek that improvement by further burdening an overstressed health care workforce or by exhorting committed professionals to try harder. Instead, the improvements outlined here will require significant changes in the ways health care is organized, in the accessibility and usefulness of clinical evidence, in the environment of payment, and in other incentives that set the context for delivery of care. A redesigned care system can offer the health care workforce what it wants—a better opportunity to provide high-quality care.

The ultimate test of the quality of a health care system is whether it helps the people it intends to help. This rather simple statement, as expanded upon in the following detailed discussion of the six aims for improvement set forth earlier, represents a major shift in thinking about the purpose of health care—a shift in attention from what is done to patients to what is accomplished for them. The IOM has defined quality as "the degree to which health care services for individuals and populations increase the likelihood of desired outcomes and are consistent with current professional knowledge" (Institute of Medicine, 1990). The committee believes the health care system should define safety, effectiveness, patient-centeredness, timeliness, efficiency, and equity using measures determined by the outcomes patients desire, although clinicians should not be asked to compromise their ethical values. Desirable personal health outcomes include improvement (and prevention of deterioration) of health status and health-related quality of life, and management of physical and psychological symptoms. Desirable outcomes also include attention to interpersonal aspects of care, such as patients' concerns and expectations, their sense of dignity, their participation in decision making, and in some cases reduced burden on family and caregivers and spiritual well-being.

Such outcomes can be described at both the individual level (e.g., improvement in individual health status) and the population level (e.g., reduced aggregate burden of illness and injury in a population). The committee recognizes that the health of the public could be greatly improved by attention to and investment in a variety of areas, such as reducing violence and substance abuse and improving nutrition and transportation safety. This report, however, is focused specifically on the improvement of health care services to individuals. For this reason, we describe the six aims for improvement from the perspective of the individual's—usually a patient's—experience.

Safety

Patients should not be harmed by the care that is intended to help them, nor should harm come to those who work in health care. The earlier report by this committee, *To Err Is Human: Building a Safer Health System* (Institute of

Medicine, 2000b), addresses patient safety in detail. It defines patient safety as freedom from accidental injury. Although not all errors cause injury, accidental injury can be due to error, defined by the IOM (adapted from Reason, 1990) as either (1) the failure of a planned action to be completed as intended or (2) use of a wrong plan to achieve an aim. In health care these errors include, for example, administering the wrong drug or dosage to a patient, diagnosing pneumonia when the patient has congestive heart failure, and failing to operate when the obvious (as opposed to ambiguous) signs of appendicitis are present. Processes also should not harm patients through inadvertent exposure to chemicals, foreign bodies, trauma, or infectious agents.

The health care environment should be safe for all patients, in all of its processes, all the time. This standard of safety implies that organizations should not have different, lower standards of care on nights and weekends or during times of organizational change. In a safe system, patients need to tell caregivers something only once. To be safe, care must be seamless—supporting the ability of interdependent people and technologies to perform as a unified whole, especially at points of transition between and among caregivers, across sites of care, and through time. It is in inadequate handoffs that safety often fails first. Specifically, in a safe system, information is not lost, inaccessible, or forgotten in transitions. Knowledge about patients—such as their allergies, their medications, their diagnostic and treatment plans, and their specific needs—is available, with appropriate assurances of confidentiality, to all who need to know it, regardless of where and when they become involved in the process of giving care.

Ensuring patient safety also requires that patients be informed and participate as fully as they wish and are able. Patients and their families should not be excluded from learning about uncertainty, risks, and treatment choices. The committee believes an informed patient is a safer patient.

When complications occur, caregivers are ethically obligated to fully inform the patient of the event and its causes, assist recovery, and take appropriate action to prevent recurrences. For example, the Code of Ethics (E8.12) of the American Medical Association states, "It is a fundamental ethical requirement that a physician should at all times deal honestly and openly with patients . . . . Situations occasionally occur in which a patient suffers significant medical complications that may have resulted from the physician's mistake or judgment. In these situations, the physician is ethically required to inform the patient of all the facts necessary to ensure understanding of what has occurred" (American Medical Association, 2000).

In many cases, the best window on the safety and quality of care is through the eyes of the patient. For example, the Dana-Farber Cancer Institute in Boston, Massachusetts, includes patients on their review committees. Other approaches include inviting patients and health care workers to comment on the performance of the health system as they experience it, not solely for the purpose of generating satisfaction ratings, but also as a core way of learning about the system's performance and how to improve it.

Although Americans continue to trust health care clinicians, including doctors and nurses (The Gallup Organization, 2000; The Henry J. Kaiser Family Foundation, 2000), the committee is concerned about Americans' remarkably low level of confidence in the health care system overall. For example, in July 2000, only four in ten Americans surveyed for one poll reported having a lot or a great deal of confidence in "the medical system," though it is not clear who or what kinds of settings were encompassed by their answers (Chambers, 2000). Of the 15 major industries included in the poll, the medical system ranked in the bottom half along with public schools, television and print news, and big business; poll participants reported having greater confidence in banks, the President, and the police. A Harris Poll conducted at the end of 1999 found that only 39 percent of respondents reported having a great deal of confidence in the "people in charge of running medicine" (Taylor, 1999). In 1998, The American Customer Satisfaction Index placed hospitals between the U.S. Postal Service and the Internal Revenue Service in customer satisfaction (Lieber, 1998).

One important route to restoring trust is through a commitment to transparency by all health care systems. Organizations and clinicians that act as though they have nothing to hide become more trustworthy. The health care system should seek to earn renewed trust not by hiding its defects, but by revealing them, along with making a relentless commitment to improve. The transition to openness is a difficult one for our often-beleaguered health care organizations, but it is a journey worth making. In the longer run, access to information can inspire trust among patients and caregivers that the system is working effectively to advance health. Such trust involves patient confidence both that those who are responsible for care have the information they need—regardless of where that information was generated—and that those organizations and caregivers will act in patients' best interests and actively seek to advance their health.

Achieving a higher level of safety is an essential first step in improving the quality of care overall. Improving safety will in turn require systematic efforts from a broad array of stakeholders, including a commitment of clear and sustained leadership at the executive and board levels of organizations; a greatly changed culture of health care in which errors are tracked, analyzed, and interpreted for improvement rather than blame; extensive research on the factors leading to injury; and new systems of care designed to prevent error and minimize harm (Institute of Medicine, 2000b).

Effectiveness

Effectiveness refers to care that is based on the use of systematically acquired evidence to determine whether an intervention, such as a preventive service, diagnostic test, or therapy, produces better outcomes than alternatives—

including the alternative of doing nothing. Evidence-based practice requires that those who give care consistently avoid both underuse of effective care and overuse of ineffective care that is more likely to harm than help the patient (Chassin, 1997).

To say that a health care intervention is effective implies an evidence base. Such evidence-based practice has been defined by Sackett and colleagues and is adapted here (Sackett et al., 1996): evidence-based practice is the integration of best research evidence with clinical expertise and patient values. *Best research evidence* refers to clinically relevant research, often from the basic sciences of medicine, but especially from patient-centered clinical research into the accuracy and precision of diagnostic tests (including the clinical examination); the power of predictive markers; and the efficacy and safety of therapeutic, rehabilitative, and preventive regimens. *Clinical expertise* means the ability to use clinical skills and past experience to rapidly identify each patient's unique health state and diagnosis, individual risks and benefits of potential interventions, and personal values and expectations. *Patient values* refers to the unique preferences, concerns, and expectations that are brought by each patient to a clinical encounter and must be integrated into clinical decisions if the patient is to be served.

Effective care should ensure use of the available, relevant science base. Evidence comes from four main types of research: laboratory experiments, clinical trials, epidemiological research, and outcomes research, including analyses of systematically acquired and properly studied case reports involving one or a population of patients (Agency for Healthcare Research and Quality, 2000). Laboratory experiments—usually on cells or tissues in laboratory animals—are conducted to determine the cause of a disease or how a drug or treatment works. Randomized clinical trials compare outcomes among patients who are randomly assigned to control or treatment groups; other clinical trials compare populations that may be assigned by nonrandom methods. Epidemiological research examines the natural course of disease in particular groups of people; the relationships between people and their health habits, lifestyles, and environment; and risk factors for certain diseases. Outcomes research uses information about how well treatments work in everyday practice settings. The findings of this research sometimes serve as the basis for clinical practice guidelines.

Although the concept of evidence-based practice has come to be regarded by some as implying rigid (even mindless) adherence to the evidence drawn from randomized controlled trials (Grahame-Smith, 1995; *The Lancet*, 1995), we mean it here to encompass the use of best available clinical evidence from systematic research of many designs and integration of that evidence with clinical expertise—the proficiency and judgment that are acquired through experience and applied with knowledge about individual patients and consideration of their priorities and values. The committee is well aware that for many aspects of health care, scant or no evidence of either effectiveness or ineffectiveness exists. In other areas, evidence may be available only for certain patient groups or for the treatment of patients who do not have coexisting health problems. Thus, it is clearly not possible to base all care on sound scientific evidence, and certainly not exclusively on randomized controlled trials, which narrowly define study populations and exclude or control for factors that are inevitably relevant in real-world care settings. Nonetheless, the committee believes health care organizations and professionals could do a far better job than they do today in determining the most appropriate therapies on the basis of the strength of the scientific evidence; the stakes involved; clinical judgment; and, especially where the evidence is equivocal, shared patient and clinician decision making. In the ideal system of the future, the knowledge base about effective care and its use in health care settings will constantly expand through improved methods of accessing, summarizing, and assessing information and making it available at the point of care for the patient.

Knowing which services are likely to be effective also requires that health care systems continuously monitor the results of the care they provide and use that information to improve care for all patients. At a minimum, health care practitioners and organizations could be far more reflective and systematic than is generally the case today in studying their own patterns of care and outcomes, a vision that Codman (1914) had nearly a century ago when he recommended that all surgeons and hospitals carefully follow their patients after discharge from the hospital to learn whether the treatment they had received had been helpful.

Patient-Centeredness

This aim focuses on the patient's experience of illness and health care and on the systems that work or fail to work to meet individual patients' needs. Similar terms are *person-centered, consumer-centered, personalized,* and *individualized.* Like these terms, *patient-centered* encompasses qualities of compassion, empathy, and responsiveness to the needs, values, and expressed preferences of the individual patient.

Patients and their families are now better educated and informed about their health care than ever before. As noted earlier, the explosive growth in the use of the Internet by Americans of all ages (National Public Radio Online, 2000) includes intense interest in health information (Brown, 1998; Cyber Dialogue, 2000). In an October 1998 survey of Internet users, 27 percent of female and 15 percent of male Internet users said that they accessed medical information weekly or daily (Eysenbach et al., 1999; Georgia Tech Research Corporation, 1998). Increasingly, individuals make many of their own decisions about diagnosis and treatment and bring information to their physicians with the expectation of help in interpreting or judging its value for themselves. These new health care consumers represent new opportunities for responding to patient needs and reestablishing clinician–patient relationships that are at the heart of good health care.

Many patients have expressed frustration with their inability to participate in decision making, to obtain information they need, to be heard, and to participate in systems of care that are responsive to their needs. The Picker Institute in Boston, Massachusetts, has been tracking patients' experiences in hospitals, clinics, and other settings since 1988 (Cleary et al., 1991; Picker Institute and American Hospital Association, 1996). In a 1999 report, patients said that, for the most part, doctors, nurses, and medical staff were courteous, and that as patients they were treated with respect and received attention to their basic physical needs. They also reported, however, that hospital discharge often meant an abrupt transition without information on how they should care for themselves, when to resume activities, what side effects of medications should be monitored, or how to have their questions answered. Above all, patients cited difficulty in obtaining the information they wanted, whether in hospitals, clinics, or doctors' offices. In the scenario presented earlier, little consideration was given to satisfying Ms. Martinez' preferences or to ensuring that she had sufficient information to make informed decisions.

The evidence bears out these perceptions. The right of patients to be informed decision makers is well accepted, but not always well implemented. An analysis of audiotaped encounters between patients and their primary care physicians or general and orthopedic surgeons revealed that overall, only 9 percent met the authors' definition of completely informed decision making (Braddock et al., 1999). In another study of physician–patient interaction during visits to general internal medicine specialists, physicians listened to patients' concerns for an average of about 18 seconds before interrupting (Beckman and Frankel, 1984).

Gerteis et al. (1993) have identified several dimensions of patient-centered care: (1) respect for patients' values, preferences, and expressed needs; (2) coordination and integration of care; (3) information, communication, and education; (4) physical comfort; (5) emotional support—relieving fear and anxiety; and (6) involvement of family and friends. Each dimension is briefly discussed below.

- *Respect for patients' values, preferences, and expressed needs.* Patient-centered care responds precisely to each patient's wants, needs, and preferences. It gives patients abundant opportunities to be informed and involved in medical decision making, and guides and supports those providing care in attending to their patients' physical and emotional needs, and maintaining or improving their quality of life to the extent possible. Patient-centered care is highly customized and incorporates cultural competence. Some patients wish to avoid risk; others may choose a risky intervention despite a relatively low likelihood of benefit. Patients' preferences are likely to change over time and to depend on the clinical problems in question; therefore, the enterprise of shared decision making is a dynamic one, changing as patients and circumstances change.

- *Coordination and integration of care.* Because of the special vulnerability that accompanies illness or injury, coordination of care takes on special importance. Many patients depend on those who provide care to coordinate ser-vices—whether tests, consultations, or procedures—to ensure that accurate and timely information reaches those who need it at the appropriate time. Patient-centered care addresses the need to manage smooth transitions from one setting to another or from a health care to a self-care setting.

• *Information, communication, and education.* With respect to their health, people tend to want to know (1) what is wrong (diagnosis) or how to stay well, (2) what is likely to happen and how it will affect them (prognosis), and (3) what can be done to change or manage their prognosis. They need answers that are accurate and in a language they understand. Patients are diverse in the way they prefer to interact with caregivers: some seek ongoing personal face-to-face relationships; others prefer to interact with the health care system only when unavoidable and with no substantial interpersonal relationship, being comfortable with e-mail and other Web-based communication technologies. Common to all such interactions is the desire for trustworthy information (often from an indi-vidual clinician) that is attentive, responsive, and tailored to an individual's needs.

• *Physical comfort.* Among the committee's more disturbing findings is the frequency with which patients experience pain, shortness of breath, or some other discomfort. Especially at the end of life, they need not undergo such suffering. Sadly, many patients fail to receive state-of-the-art pain relief or respiratory management (Ingham and Foley, 1998; SUPPORT Principal Investi-gators, 1995). Attention to physical comfort implies timely, tailored, and expert management of such symptoms.

• *Emotional support—relieving fear and anxiety.* Suffering is more than just physical pain and other distressing symptoms; it also encompasses signifi-cant emotional and spiritual dimensions (Byock, 1998; Cassell, 1991). Patient-centered care attends to the anxiety that accompanies all injury and illness, whether due to uncertainty, fear of pain, disability or disfigurement, loneliness, financial impact, or the effect of illness on one's family.

• *Involvement of family and friends.* This dimension of patient-centered care focuses on accommodating family and friends on whom patients may rely, involving them as appropriate in decision making, supporting them as caregivers, making them welcome and comfortable in the care delivery setting, and recogniz-ing their needs and contributions.

Health care should cure when possible, but always help to relieve suffer-ing—both are encompassed by the notion of a healing relationship (Crawshaw et al., 1995; Quill, 1983). To accomplish these goals, both technical care and interpersonal interactions should be shaped to meet the needs and preferences of individual patients (Tressolini and The Pew-Fetzer Task Force, 1994; Veatch, 1991). Because patients are highly variable in their preferences, clinicians cannot assume that they alone can make the best decisions for their patients (Balint, 1993; Barry et al., 1995; Brock, 1991; Emanuel and Emanuel, 1992; Szasz and

Hollender, 1956; Wagner et al., 1995). Patients increasingly want to obtain information and to be involved in decision making (Deber et al., 1996; Degner and Russell, 1988; Guadagnoli and Ward, 1998; Mansell et al., 2000; Mazur and Hickam, 1997). Moreover, meeting the aim of patient-centeredness can improve the outcomes patients desire (Brown, 1990; DeBusk et al., 1994; Linden and Chambers, 1994; Mullen et al., 1987), at least in part, by increasing their participation in decision making (Greenfield et al., 1985, 1988; Kaplan et al., 1989; Mahler and Kulik, 1991; Orth et al., 1987; Stewart, 1995).

As with communication styles, patients differ in their views about how active they wish to be in decision making. In some cases, patients want a large role, and in other cases they may delegate most decision making to a clinician. The goal of patient-centeredness is to customize care to the specific needs and circumstances of each individual, that is, to modify the care to respond to the person, not the person to the care.

Timeliness

Timeliness is an important characteristic of any service and is a legitimate and valued focus of improvement in health care and other industries (Fishman, 1999; Fung and Magretta, 1998; Goldsmith, 1989; Kenagy et al., 1999; Maister, 1984; Roach, 1991; Sirkin and Stalk, 1990; van Biema and Greenwald, 1997; Womack et al., 1991). However, long waits are the norm in most doctors' offices, in emergency rooms, on the telephone, in responses to inquiries, in specialty care, on gurneys in hallways waiting for procedures, and awaiting test results, both in institutions and in the community. In addition to emotional distress, physical harm may result, for example, from a delay in diagnosis or treatment that results in preventable complications. The long waits for appointments described in the scenario presented earlier, which are common today, may have resulted in a much more advanced diagnosis for Ms. Martinez. Lack of timeliness also signals a lack of attention to flow and a lack of respect for the patient that are not tolerated in consumer-centered systems in other service industries. It suggests that care has not been designed with the welfare of the patient at the center.

Waits also plague those who give care. Surgeons know that operations rarely start on time; doctors and nurses wait "on hold" as they try to track down vital information, and delays and barriers involved in referrals eat up the time and energy of both referring doctors and consulting specialists. In the earlier scenario, Ms. Martinez' surgery was nearly cancelled because important information that should have been in her record was missing, and staff spent valuable time finding it and rearranging schedules to avoid having to cancel the operation.

Any high-quality process should flow smoothly. Delays should occur rarely. Waiting times should be continually reduced for both patients and those who give care. Much waiting today appears to result from the presumption that certain kinds of face-to-face encounters are required for patients to receive the help or interaction they require. Health systems must develop multiple ways of responding to patients' needs beyond patient visits, including the use of the Internet. Reducing waiting time does not have to increase expense. Experience has shown repeatedly that in many areas, improving access reduces costs in health care (Barry-Walker, 2000; Cohn et al., 1997; Fuss et al., 1998; Stewart et al., 1997; Tidikis and Strasen, 1994; Tunick et al., 1997) and in other industries (Heskett et al., 1997). Promising work in health care has begun to result in reduced delays by decreasing cycle time and by applying lessons from other industries on continuous rather than batch production (Nolan et al., 1996). These approaches are described further in Chapter 7.

Efficiency

In an efficient health care system, resources are used to get the best value for the money spent (Palmer and Torgerson, 1999). The opposite of efficiency is waste, the use of resources without benefit to the patients a system is intended to help. There are at least two ways to improve efficiency: (1) reduce quality waste, and (2) reduce administrative or production costs.

Not all but many types of quality improvements result in lower resource use. This is true for improvements in effectiveness that result from reductions in overuse. It is also true for most improvements in safety, which result in fewer injuries. Quality waste from both overuse (see Appendix A) and errors (Institute of Medicine, 2000b) is abundant in health care and contributes to excess costs.

Some researchers have attempted to quantify administrative costs that constitute waste (Woolhandler and Himmelstein, 1997; Woolhandler et al., 1993). Others have identified waste in the work of smaller health care units and sought systematically to reduce such waste through a variety of strategies, including eliminating processes that are not useful (such as tests), multiple entries (such as clerical reentry of physicians' prescriptions and laboratory orders), classifications that add complexity without adding value (such as types of appointments and job classifications), and layers of control (such as approvals and sign-offs). Waste can also be reduced by recycling and appropriate reuse of resources (such as data and water) and by wise substitutions (Kain et al., 1999; Klein et al., 2000; Langley et al., 1996; Luck and Peabody, 2000; Poplin, 2000; Skillman et al., 2000; Walczak, 2000; Zairi et al., 1999). Other approaches rely on matching supply to demand and using sampling for measurement instead of measuring 100 percent of events. Several of these approaches are described in greater detail in Chapter 7.

Because of the high levels of waste in the current system, the committee sees no immediate conflict in the simultaneous pursuit of lower costs through efficiency and better patient experiences through safety, effectiveness, patient-centeredness, and timeliness. There is little doubt that current resources can be spent more wisely to pursue the aims set forth in this chapter.

Equity

This chapter began with a statement of purpose for the health system: "to continually reduce the burden of illness, injury, and disability, and to improve the health and functioning of the people of the United States." The aim of equity is to secure these benefits for all the people of the United States. This aim has two dimensions: equity at the level of the population and equity at the level of the individual. At the population level, the goal of a health care system is to improve health status and to do so in a manner that reduces health disparities among particular subgroups. Equity in care implies universal access, a promise that has yet to be either made or kept. Lack of health insurance has a profound effect on access to appropriate services, and is directly associated with poor functioning, increased morbidity, and increased mortality (American College of Physicians–American Society of Internal Medicine, 2000; Baker et al., 2000; Franks et al., 1993; Haas and Goldman, 1994; Hafner-Eaton, 1993; Kasper et al., 2000). Institutions and health professionals that deliver uncompensated care to uninsured or underserved patients are at risk financially (Institute of Medicine, 2000a), and evidence suggests that the provision of uncompensated care is declining (Cunningham et al., 1999; Mann et al., 1997). The committee believes lack of access to care is a very powerful barrier to quality.

With regard to equity in care giving, all individuals rightly expect to be treated fairly by social institutions, including health care organizations. The availability of care and quality of services should be based on individuals' particular needs and not on personal characteristics unrelated to the patient's condition or to the reason for seeking care. In particular, the quality of care should not differ because of such characteristics as gender, race, age, ethnicity, income, education, disability, sexual orientation, or location of residence (Ayanian et al., 1999; Canto et al., 2000; Fiscella et al., 2000; Freeman and Payne, 2000; Kahn et al., 1994; Pearson et al., 1992; Philbin and DiSalvo, 1998; Ross et al., 2000; Yergan et al., 1987).

Conflicts Among the Aims

For the most part, the six aims are complementary and synergistic. At times, however, there will be tensions among them. Health care institutions, clinicians, and patients will sometimes need to work together to balance competing or conflicting objectives. Two examples are the potential conflict between the aims of patient-centeredness and effectiveness, and the need to balance the aim of equity as applied to the population with achievement of the other aims at the level of the individual.

Some readers might question whether a commitment to evidence-based care conflicts with an emphasis on patient-centered care. We emphasize that the commitment to patient-centered care is not intended to imply that clinicians have an obligation to provide unnecessary services merely because patients request them. All unneeded services have the potential to cause harm. For example, false-positive results on a test can lead to a cascade of testing and psychological distress. Because unnecessary services can do harm and offer no benefit, ethical principles dictate that a physician not recommend or prescribe requested treatment that is of no known benefit—whether, for example, the request is for antibiotics, diagnostic tests, or a wide variety of invasive procedures.

A VISION OF FUTURE CARE

The six aims for improvement described in this chapter define the tasks ahead for the health care system, for organizations, and for clinical practices that wish to contribute to the overarching social purpose set forth at the beginning of this chapter. These aims can lead us all to fundamentally better care. Having presented earlier in this chapter a scenario in which almost everything went wrong, we conclude the chapter with a scenario depicting care as it could be if the six aims were realized:

Maureen Waters, January 2002

Maureen Waters, a single working mother with teenage children, was new in town. When the family moved to Southcity, she had to select an insurance plan. She chose CityCare because its cost was comparable to that of other options, and it was associated with a major university-affiliated hospital.

When Ms. Waters joined CityCare, she was asked to choose a primary care physician. After talking with her neighbors and coworkers, she was pleased to confirm some of what she had learned from having online access to profiles and to information on office hours, credentials, patient satisfaction, and outcomes for each physician and group.

Again online, using a secure site, she chose a physician, completed background and health risk appraisal information for herself and her children, and never again had to supply this information. An hour later, her choice of a physician was confirmed by the plan. She also received a reply from her new physician's office that, on the basis of her health risk appraisal, she should made an appointment to meet with her primary care physician, have her hypertension assessed, and obtain medication refills. The reply also included information about blood tests that should be done before her first appointment.

Because she was due for a breast exam and mammogram, a referral to a breast care center was attached to the reply. Also online, she was able to schedule a time convenient for her (Sunday afternoon) at one of several locations in South-city.

Since the information for the appointment had already been completed, she went directly to a breast care center, where the exam and mammogram were completed without delay. Before leaving, she learned that a lump discovered during the breast exam had been confirmed by mammogram and sonography, and that she should have a biopsy to determine the nature of the finding. The radiographic results were available to her as digital images that could be e-mailed to her physician.

Because her health profile included hypertension, Ms. Waters needed to see her primary care physician to evaluate her hypertension control and discuss next steps before any further treatment that might include surgery could occur. Dr. Fine had an open scheduling system that allowed Ms. Waters to be seen the next morning.

Dr. Fine explained that although the breast lump was the first issue on the agenda, she was still concerned about Ms. Waters' other health issues and her preventive care. The doctor therefore suggested that Ms. Waters return after blood work had been done, using the same online open scheduling system that had made it easy for her to be seen that day. Ms. Waters was reassured not only by the process, but also, as a newcomer to the city, by Dr. Fine's concern about her well-being and role as her advocate, especially because of her concerns about the upcoming biopsy and what it might mean.

During the visit, Dr. Fine was able to give Ms. Waters profiles of surgeons, describe their interpersonal as well as technical skills, and coach her about questions or issues she might want to explore. Ms. Waters also had received information from the groups about their research efforts and the protocols they used. While she was in the primary care office, the staff arranged for her to have the biopsy done early that week by the surgeon she had selected. In a small room containing a computer, she consulted the CHESS database, a National Library of Medicine database for consumers, and Cancerfacts.com for information about treatment options, the meaning of test results, rates of recurrence, side effects, resources available to her locally, and the names of support groups. She forwarded to her own computer information that she wanted to read and follow up on later and took with her the addresses of several of the Web sites.

The biopsy showed an early-stage cancer. Ms. Waters was able to see her physician the next day to learn about and discuss her options for treatment. She was linked with other patients who had faced similar choices. She immediately began plans for treatment, which was completed without delay.

Throughout this process, Ms. Waters had information available to her in several ways. Although her style was to read as much as she could and ask when she was confused, she spoke with other women who were most comfortable accepting what their doctor recommended in terms of treatment, but sought resources for rehabilitation and advice about managing the side effects of their therapy.

When she felt the need to do so, she spoke with or e-mailed Dr. Fine. At other times she spoke with the nurse practitioner who worked with Dr. Fine. Throughout this process, she could examine her own records, including test results. Ms. Waters had no paperwork to complete, no duplicative questions, and no trouble reaching professionals when she had concerns or questions.

REFERENCES

Advisory Commission on Consumer Protection and Quality in the Health Care Industry. 1998. "Quality First: Better Health Care for All Americans." Online. Available at http://www.hcqualitycommission.gov/final/ [accessed Sept. 9, 2000].

Agency for Healthcare Research and Quality. 2000. "Now You Have a Diagnosis: What's Next? Using Health Care Information to Help Make Treatment Decisions." Online. Available at http://www.ahrq.gov/consumer/diaginfo.htm [accessed Dec. 5, 2000].

American College of Physicians–American Society of Internal Medicine. 2000. "No Health Insurance? It's Enough to Make You Sick - Scientific Research Linking the Lack of Health Coverage to Poor Health." Online. Available at http://www.acponline.org/uninsured/lack-contents.htm [accessed Dec. 6, 2000].

American Medical Association. E-8.12 Patient Information. *Code of Medical Ethics. Current Opinions of the Council on Ethical and Judicial Affairs.* Chicago, IL: American Medical Association, 2000.

Ayanian, John Z., Joel S. Weissman, Scott Chasan-Taber, and Arnold M. Epstein. Quality of Care by Race and Gender for Congestive Heart Failure and Pneumonia. *Medical Care* 37(12):1260–9, 1999.

Baker, David W., Martin F. Shapiro, and Claudia L. Schur. Health Insurance and Access to Care for Symptomatic Conditions. *Arch Int Med* 160(9):1269–74, 2000.

Balint, Enid. *The Doctor, the Patient, and the Group: Balint Revisited.* New York, NY: Routledge, 1993.

Barry, Michael J., Floyd J. Fowler, Jr., Albert G. Mulley, Jr., et al. Patient Reactions to a Program Designed to Facilitate Patient Participation in Treatment Decisions for Benign Prostatic Hyperplasia. *Medical Care* 33(8):771–82, 1995.

Barry-Walker, Jean. The Impact of Systems Redesign on Staff, Patient, and Financial Outcomes. *J Nurs Adm* 30(2):77–89, 2000.

Beckman, Howard B. and Richard M. Frankel. The Effect of Physician Behavior on the Collection of Information. *Ann Int Med* 101:692–6, 1984.

Berwick, Donald M. Quality Comes Home. *Ann Int Med* 125(10):839–43, 1996.

———. Escape Fire. Plenary Address, Institute for Healthcare Improvement Annual Forum. 1999.

Braddock, Clarence H. III, Kelly A. Edwards, Nicole M. Hasenberg, et al. Informed Decision Making in Outpatient Practice: Time to Get Back to Basics. *JAMA* 282(24):2313–20, 1999.

Brock, Dan W. The Ideal of Shared Decision Making Between Physicians and Patients. *Kennedy Inst Ethics J* 1(1):28–47, 1991.

Brown, M. *The HealthMed Retrievers: Profiles of Consumers Using Online Health and Medical Information.* New York, NY: Cyber dialogue, 1998. Cited in Ferguson, Tom. Digital Doctoring Opportunities and Challenges in Electronic Patient-Physician Communication. *JAMA* 280:1361–2, 1998.

Brown, Sharon A. Studies of Educational Interventions and Outcomes in Diabetic Adults: A Meta-Analysis Revisited. *Patient Education and Counseling* 16:189–215, 1990.

Byock, Ira. *Dying Well: The Prospect for Growth at the End of Life.* New York, NY: Riverhead Books, 1998.

Canto, John G., Jeroan J. Allison, Catarina I. Kiefe, et al. Relation of Race and Sex to the Use of Reperfusion Therapy in Medicare Beneficiaries with Acute Myocardial Infarction. *N Engl J Med* 342(15):1094–100, 2000.

Cassell, Eric J. *The Nature of Suffering: The Goals of Medicine.* New York, NY: Oxford University Press, 1991.

Chambers, Chris. 2000. "Gallup News Service. Military Number One in Public Confidence, HMOs Last. Poll Releases, July 10, 2000." Online. Available at http://www.gallup.com/poll/releases/pr000710.asp [accessed July 13, 2000].

Chassin, Mark R. Assessing Strategies for Quality Improvement. *Health Affairs* 16(3):151–61, 1997.

Cleary, Paul D., Susan Edgman-Levitan, Marc Roberts, et al. Patients Evaluate their Hospital Care: A National Survey. *Health Affairs* 10:254–67, 1991.

Codman, Ernest A. The Product of a Hospital. *Surgery, Gynecology and Obstetrics* 18:491–6, 1914.

Cohn, Lawrence H., Donna Rosborough, and John Fernandez. Reducing Costs and Length of Stay and Improving Efficiency and Quality of Care in Cardiac Surgery. *Ann Thorac Surg* 64(6 Suppl):S58–60; discussion S80–2, 1997.

Crawshaw, Ralph, David E. Rogers, Edmund D. Pellegrino, et al. Patient–Physician Covenant. *JAMA* 273(19):1553, 1995.

Cunningham, Peter J., Joy M. Grossman, Robert F. St. Peter, and Cara S. Lesser. Managed Care and Physicians' Provision of Charity Care. *JAMA* 282(12):1087–92, 1999.

Cyber Dialogue. 2000. "Cybercitizen Health." Online. Available at http://www.cyberdialogue.com/solutions/strategy/industry/cch.html [accessed Dec. 5, 2000].

Deber, Raisa B., Nancy Kraetschmer, and Jane Irvine. What Role Do Patients Wish to Play in Treatment Decision Making? *Arch Int Med* 156:1414–20, 1996.

DeBusk, Robert F., Nancy Houston Miller, H. Robert Superko, et al. A Case-Management System for Coronary Risk Factor Modification after Acute Myocardial Infarction. *Ann Int Med* 120:721–9, 1994.

Degner, Lesley F. and Catherine Aquino Russell. Preferences for Treatment Control Among Adults with Cancer. *Research in Nursing & Health* 11:367–74, 1988.

Emanuel, Ezekiel J. and Linda L. Emanuel. Four Models of the Physician–Patient Relationship. *JAMA* 267(16):2221–6, 1992.

Eysenbach, Gunther, Eun Ryoung Sa, and Thomas L. Diepgen. Shopping Around the Internet Today and Tomorrow: Towards the Millennium of Cybermedicine. *BMJ* 319:1294, 1999.

Fiscella, Kevin, Peter Franks, Marthe R. Gold, and Carolyn M. Clancy. Inequality in Quality. Addressing Socioeconomic, Racial, and Ethnic Disparities in Health Care. *JAMA* 283(19):2579–84, 2000.

Fishman, Charles. This is a Marketing Revolution. *Fast Company* 24:204, 1999.

Franks, Peter, Carolyn M. Clancy, and Marthe R. Gold. Health Insurance and Mortality: Evidence From a National Cohort. *JAMA* 270(6):737–41, 1993.

Freeman, Harold P. and Richard Payne. Racial Injustice in Health Care. *N Engl J Med* 342(14):1045–7, 2000.

Fung, Victor and Joan Magretta. Fast, Global, and Entrepreneurial: Supply Chain Management, Hong Kong style. An interview with Victor Fung. *Harvard Business Review* 76:102–14, 187, 1998.

Fuss, Mae Ann, Yvonne E. Bryan, Kim S. Hitchings, et al. Measuring Critical Care Redesign: Impact on Satisfaction and Quality. *Nursing Administration Quarterly* 23:1–14, 1998.

Georgia Tech Research Corporation. 1998. "GVU's Tenth WWW User Survey." Online. Available at http://www.cc.gatech.edu/gvu/user_surveys/survey-1998-10/graphs/use/q109.htm [accessed Dec. 5, 2000].

Gerteis, Margaret, Susan Edgman-Levitan, and Jennifer Daley. *Through the Patient's Eyes. Understanding and Promoting Patient-centered Care.* San Francisco, CA: Jossey-Bass, 1993.

Goldsmith, Jeff. A Radical Prescription for Hospitals. *Harvard Business Review* 67(3):104–11, 1989.

Grahame-Smith, David. Evidence Based Medicine: Socratic Dissent. *BMJ* 310:1126–7, 1995.

Greenfield, Sheldon, Sherrie H. Kaplan, and John E. Ware, Jr. Expanding Patient Involvement in Care: Effects on Patient Outcomes. *Ann Int Med* 102:520–8, 1985.

Greenfield, Sheldon, Sherrie H. Kaplan, John E. Ware, Jr., et al. Patients' Participation in Medical Care: Effects on Blood Sugar Control and Quality of Life in Diabetes. *J Gen Intern Med* 3:448–57, 1988.

Guadagnoli, Edward and Patricia Ward. Patient Participation in Decision-making. *Social Science & Medicine* 47(3):329–39, 1998.

Haas, Jennifer S. and Lee Goldman. Acutely Injured Patients with Trauma in Massachusetts: Differences in Care and Mortality, by Insurance Status. *American Journal of Public Health* 84(10):1605–8, 1994.

Hafner-Eaton, Chris. Physician Utilization Disparities Between the Uninsured and Insured. Comparisons of the Chronically Ill, Acutely Ill, and Well Nonelderly Populations. *JAMA* 269(6):787–92, 1993.

Heskett, James L., W. Earl Sasser, Leonard A. Schlesinger, et al. *The Service Profit Chain: How Leading Companies Link Profit and Grown to Loyalty, Satisfaction and Value.* New York, NY: Free Press, 1997.

Ingham, Jane M. and Kathleen M. Foley. Pain and the Barriers to Its Relief at the End of Life: A Lesson for Improving End of Life Care. *The Hospice Journal* 13(1–2):89–100, 1998.

Institute of Medicine *Medicare: A Strategy for Quality Assurance. Volume I.* K. N. Lohr, ed. Washington, D.C.: National Academy Press, 1990.

———— *America's Health Care Safety Net. Intact but Endangered.* Marion E. Lewin and Stuart Altman, eds. Washington, D.C.: National Academy Press, 2000a.

———— *To Err Is Human: Building a Safer Health System.* Linda T. Kohn, Janet M. Corrigan, and Molla S. Donaldson, eds. Washington, D.C.: National Academy Press, 2000b.

Kahn, Katherine L., Marjorie L. Pearson, Ellen R. Harrison, et al. Health Care for Black and Poor Hospitalized Medicare Patients. *JAMA* 271(15):1169–74, 1994.

Kain, Z. N., A. Fasulo, and S. Rimar. Establishment of a Pediatric Surgery Center: Increasing Anesthetic Efficiency. *J Clin Anesth* 11(7):540–4, 1999.

Kaplan, Sherrie H., Sheldon Greenfield, and John E. Ware, Jr. Assessing the Effects of Physician–Patient Interactions on Outcomes of Chronic Disease. *Medical Care* 27(3, Supplement):S110–27, 1989.

Kasper, Judith D., Terence A. Giovannini, and Catherine Hoffman. Gaining and Losing Health Insurance: Strengthening the Evidence for Effects on Access to Care and Health Outcomes. *Medical Care Research and Review* 57(3):298–318, 2000.

Kenagy, John W., Donald M. Berwick, and Miles F. Shore. Service Quality in Health Care. *JAMA* 281(7):661–5, 1999.

Khan, Muhammad Asim. Patient–Doctor. *Ann Int Med* 133(3):233–5, 2000.

Klein, Ben J., Richard T. Radecki, Michael P. Foris, et al. Bridging the Gap Between Science and Practice in Managing Low Back Pain. A Comprehensive Spine Care System in a Health Maintenance Organization Setting. *Spine* 25(6):738–40, 2000.

Langley, Gerald J., Kevin M. Nolan, Thomas W. Nolan, et al. *The Improvement Guide. A Practical Approach to Enhancing Organizational Performance.* San Francisco, CA: Jossey-Bass, 1996.

Lieber, Ronald B. Now Are You Satisfied? The 1998 American Customer Satisfaction Index. *Fortune* 137(3):161+Smart Managing, 1998.

Linden, Wolfgang and Laura Chambers. Clinical Effectiveness of Non-Drug Treatment for Hypertension: A Meta-Analysis. *Annals of Behavioral Medicine* 16 (1):35–45, 1994.

Luck, J. and J. W. Peabody. Improving the Public Sector: Can Reengineering Identify How to Boost Efficiency and Effectiveness at a VA Medical Center? *Health Care Manage Rev* 25(2):34–44, 2000.

Mahler, Heike I. M. and James A. Kulik. Health Care Involvement Preferences and Social-Emotional Recovery of Male Coronary-Artery-Bypass Patients. *Health Psychology* 10(6):399–408, 1991.

Maister, David H. *The Psychology of Waiting Lines. Case No. 9-684-064.* Boston, Mass: Harvard Business School Publishing, 1984.

Mann, Joyce M., Glenn A. Melnick, Anil Bamezai, and Jack Zwanziger. A Profile of Uncompensated Hospital Care, 1983–1995. A Look at Who Provides the Most Uncompensated Care and What Effect Market Conditions Have on Care for the Poor. *Health Affairs* 16(4):223–32, 1997.

Mansell, Dorcas, Roy M. Poses, Lewis Kazis, and Corey A. Duefield. Clinical Factors That Influence Patients' Desire for Participation in Decisions About Illness. *Arch Int Med* 160:2991–6, 2000.

Mazur, Dennis J. and David H. Hickam. Patients' Preferences for Risk Disclosure and Role in Decision Making for Invasive Medical Procedures. *J Gen Intern Med* 12:114–7, 1997.

Mullen, Patricia D., Elizabeth A. Laville, Andrea K. Biddle, and Kate Lorig. Efficacy of Psychoeducational Interventions on Pain, Depression, and Disability in People with Arthritis: A Meta-Analysis. *Journal of Rheumatology* 14(suppl 15):33–9, 1987.

National Public Radio Online. 2000. "Survey Shows Widespread Enthusiasm for High Technology. Poll by National Public Radio, the Henry J. Kaiser Family Foundation, and Harvard University's Kennedy School of Government." Online. Available at http://www.npr.org/programs/specials/poll/technology [accessed Apr. 5, 2000].

Nolan, Thomas W., Marie W. Schall, Donald M. Berwick, et al. *Reducing Delays and Waiting Times Throughout the Healthcare System.* Boston, MA: Institute for Healthcare Improvement, 1996.

Orth, James E., Stiles William B., Scherwitz Larry, et al. Patient Exposition and Provider Explanation in Routine Interviews and Hypertensive Patients' Blood Pressure Control. *Health Psychology* 6(1):29–42, 1987.

Palmer, Stephen and David J. Torgerson. Definition of Efficiency. *BMJ* 318:1136, 1999.

Pearson, Marjorie L., Katherine L. Kahn, Ellen R. Harrison, et al. Differences in Quality of Care for Hospitalized Elderly Men and Women. *JAMA* 268(14):1883–9, 1992.

Philbin, E. F. and T. G. DiSalvo. Influence of Race and Gender on Care Process, Resource Use, and Hospital-Based Outcomes in Congestive Heart Failure. *American Journal of Cardiology* 82(1): 76–81, 1998.

Picker Institute and American Hospital Association. *Eye on Patients Report.* 1996.

Poplin, Caroline. Productivity in Primary Care: Work Smarter, Not Harder. *Arch Int Med* 160(9): 1231–3, 2000.

Quill, Timothy E. Partnerships in Patient Care: A Contractual Approach. *Ann Int Med* 98(2):228–34, 1983.

Reason, James. *Human Error.* New York, NY: Cambridge University Press, 1990.

Roach, Stephen S. Services Under Siege—The Restructuring Imperative. *Harvard Business Review* 69:82–91, 1991.

Ross, Nancy A., Michael C. Wolfson, James R. Dunn, et al. Relation Between Income Inequality and Mortality in Canada and in the United States: Cross Sectional Assessment Using Census Data and Vital Statistics. *BMJ* 320:898–902, 2000.

Sackett, David L., William M. C. Rosenberg, J. A. Muir Gray, et al. Evidence Based Medicine: What It Is and What It Isn't. *BMJ* 312:71–2, 1996.

Singer, Sara J. What's Not to Like About HMOs: A Managed Care Maven Struggles with an HMO Runaround at a Vulnerable Time. *Health Affairs* 19(4):206–9, 2000.

Sirkin, Harold and George Stalk, Jr. Fix the Process, Not the Problem. *Harvard Business Review* 68:26–33, 1990.

Skillman, J. J., C. Paras, M. Rosen, et al. Improving Cost Efficiency on a Vascular Surgery Service. *Am J Surg* 179(3):197–200, 2000.

Stewart, Michael G., Edward J. Hillman, Donald T. Donovan, and Sarper H. Tanli. The Effects of a Practice Guideline on Endoscopic Sinus Surgery at an Academic Center. *American Journal of Rhinology* 11(2):161–5, 1997.

Stewart, Moira A. Effective Physician–Patient Communication and Health Outcomes: A Review. *Can Med Assoc J* 152(9):1423–33, 1995.

SUPPORT Principal Investigators. A Controlled Trial to Improve Care for Seriously Ill Hospitalized Patients: The Study to Understand Prognoses and Preferences for Outcomes and Risks of Treatments (SUPPORT). *JAMA* 274(20):1591–8, 1995.

Szasz, Thomas S. and Marc H. Hollender. The Basic Models of the Doctor-Patient Relationship. *Arch Int Med* 97:585–92, 1956.

Taylor, Humphrey. 1999. "Harris Poll #9: For the Second Year Running, There Has Been a Dramatic Increase in Confidence in Leadership of Nation's Major Institutions." Online. Available at http://www.harrisblackintl.com/harris_poll/index.asp?PID=32 [accessed July 13, 2000].

The Gallup Organization. 2000. "Gallup Poll Topics: A–Z. Honesty/Ethics in Professions." Online. Available at http://www.gallup.com/poll/indicators/indhnsty_ethcs.asp [accessed July 12, 2000].

The Henry J. Kaiser Family Foundation. 2000. "Kaiser/Harvard National Survey of Americans' View on Managed Care." Online. Available at http://www.kff.org/content/archive/1328/mcaretopb.html [accessed July 6, 2000].

The Lancet. Evidence-Based Medicine, In Its Place (editorial). *The Lancet* 346:785, 1995.

Tidikis, Frank and Leann Strasen. Patient-Focused Care Units Improve Services and Financial Outcomes. *Healthcare Financial Management* 48:38–44, 1994.

Tressolini, Carol P. and The Pew-Fetzer Task Force. *Health Professional Education and Relationship-Centered Care*. San Francisco, CA: Pew Health Professions Commission, 1994.

Tunick, P. A., S. Etkin, A. Horrocks, et al. Reengineering a cardiovascular surgery service. *Joint Commission Journal on Quality Improvement* 23(4):203–16, 1997.

van Biema, Michael and Bruce C. Greenwald. Managing Our Way to Higher Service-sector Productivity. *Harvard Business Review* 75:87–95, 1997.

Veatch, Robert M. *The Patient-Physician Relation. The Patient as Partner, Part 2*. Indianapolis, IN: Indiana University Press, 1991.

Wagner, Edward H., Paul Barrett, Michael J. Barry, et al. The Effect of a Shared Decisionmaking Program on Rates of Surgery for Beningn Prostatic Hyperplasia. Pilot Results. *Medical Care* 33(8):765–70, 1995.

Walczak, Steven. Redesigning the Medical Office for Improved Efficiency: An Object-Oriented Event-Driven Messaging System. *J Med Syst* 24(1):29–37, 2000.

Womack, James P., Daniel T Jones, and Daniel Roos. *The Machine That Changed the World*. New York, NY: Harpercollins, 1991.

Woolhandler, Steffie and David U. Himmelstein. Costs of Care and Administration at For-Profit and Other Hospitals in the United States. *N Engl J Med* 336(11):769–74, 1997. Erratum in *N Engl J Med* 337:1783, 1997.

Woolhandler, Steffie, David U. Himmelstein, and James P. Lewontin. Administrative Costs in U.S. Hospitals. *N Engl J Med* 329(6):400–3, 1993.

Yergan, J., A. B. Flood, J. P. LoGerfo, and P. Diehr. Relationship Between Patient Race and the Intensity of Hospital Services. *Medical Care* 25(7):592–603, 1987.

Zairi, M., J. Whymark, and M. Cooke. Best Practice Organisational Effectiveness in NHS Trusts. Allington NHS Trust Case Study. *J Manag Med* 13(4–5):298–307, 1999.

3

Formulating New Rules
to Redesign and Improve Care

Achieving the aims described in Chapter 2 will require profound changes, beginning with a new framework to guide those who undertake those changes. This chapter describes ten new rules to guide the transition to a health system that better meets patients' needs.

Recommendation 4: Private and public purchasers, health care organizations, clinicians, and patients should work together to redesign health care processes in accordance with the following rules:

1. *Care based on continuous healing relationships.* Patients should receive care whenever they need it and in many forms, not just face-to-face visits. This rule implies that the health care system should be responsive at all times (24 hours a day, every day) and that access to care should be provided over the Internet, by telephone, and by other means in addition to face-to-face visits.

2. *Customization based on patient needs and values.* The system of care should be designed to meet the most common types of needs, but have the capability to respond to individual patient choices and preferences.

3. *The patient as the source of control.* Patients should be given the necessary information and the opportunity to exercise the degree of control they choose over health care decisions that affect them. The health system should be able to accommodate differences in patient preferences and encourage shared decision making.

4. *Shared knowledge and the free flow of information.* Patients should have unfettered access to their own medical information and to clinical knowledge. Clinicians and patients should communicate effectively and share information.

5. *Evidence-based decision making.* Patients should receive care based on the best available scientific knowledge. Care should not vary illogically from clinician to clinician or from place to place.

6. *Safety as a system property.* Patients should be safe from injury caused by the care system. Reducing risk and ensuring safety require greater attention to systems that help prevent and mitigate errors.

7. *The need for transparency.* The health care system should make information available to patients and their families that allows them to make informed decisions when selecting a health plan, hospital, or clinical practice, or choosing among alternative treatments. This should include information describing the system's performance on safety, evidence-based practice, and patient satisfaction.

8. *Anticipation of needs.* The health system should anticipate patient needs, rather than simply reacting to events.

9. *Continuous decrease in waste.* The health system should not waste resources or patient time.

10. *Cooperation among clinicians.* Clinicians and institutions should actively collaborate and communicate to ensure an appropriate exchange of information and coordination of care.

These ten rules translate readily into a set of new patient expectations for health care (see Box 3-1). The committee believes these new expectations are consistent with and reinforce the steps that must be taken to achieve a significant improvement in quality. We also believe they are consistent with the kind of care most clinicians strive to provide each day, but without the support of well-designed care systems and absent an environment that nurtures innovation and excellence.

To create a new health care system that more closely matches the purpose and aims described in Chapter 2, it will be necessary, first, to examine old assumptions to understand why they have led to our current ineffective health care systems, and second, to consciously craft new operating assumptions embodied in the rules set forth above. As a guide in formulating its agenda for change, the committee used as a framework recent work in understanding complex adaptive systems (Kauffman, 1995; Stacey, 1996; Waldrop, 1992; Weick, 1995; Zimmerman et al., 1998) and its application to what have become known as "learning organizations" (Senge, 1990) (see Appendix B for an introduction to this field).

BOX 3-1   What Patients Should Expect
from Their Health Care

1. **Beyond patient visits:** You will have the care you need when you need it . . . *whenever* you need it. You will find help in many forms, not just in face-to-face visits. You will find help on the Internet, on the telephone, from many sources, by many routes, in the form you want it.
2. **Individualization:** You will be known and respected as an individual. Your choices and preferences will be sought and honored. The usual system of care will meet most of your needs. When your needs are special, the care will adapt to meet you on your own terms.
3. **Control:** The care system will take control only if and when you freely give permission.
4. **Information:** You can know what you wish to know, when you wish to know it. Your medical record is yours to keep, to read, and to understand. The rule is: "Nothing about you without you."
5. **Science:** You will have care based on the best available scientific knowledge. The system promises you excellence as its standard. Your care will not vary illogically from doctor to doctor or from place to place. The system will promise you all the care that can help you, and will help you avoid care that cannot help you.
6. **Safety:** Errors in care will not harm you. You will be safe in the care system.
7. **Transparency:** Your care will be confidential, but the care system will not keep secrets from you. You can know whatever you wish to know about the care that affects you and your loved ones.
8. **Anticipation:** Your care will anticipate your needs and will help you find the help you need. You will experience proactive help, not just reactions, to help you restore and maintain your health.
9. **Value:** Your care will not waste your time or money. You will benefit from constant innovations, which will increase the value of care to you.
10. **Cooperation:** Those who provide care will cooperate and coordinate their work fully with each other and with you. The walls between professions and institutions will crumble, so that your experiences will become seamless. You will never feel lost.

Following a brief review of this work, we describe in greater detail the ten rules outlined above.

HEALTH CARE ORGANIZATIONS
AS COMPLEX ADAPTIVE SYSTEMS

A health care system can be defined as a set of connected or interdependent parts or agents—including caregivers and patients—bound by a common purpose and acting on their knowledge. Health care is complex because of the great number of interconnections within and among small care systems. For example, office practices and critical care units in hospitals are linked to other units (such as laboratories and emergency departments) and are often embedded in even larger "umbrella" organizations such as hospitals, health plans, and integrated delivery systems.

Health care systems are adaptive because unlike mechanical systems, they are composed of individuals—patients and clinicians who have the capacity to learn and change as a result of experience. Their actions in delivering health care are not always predictable, and tend to change both their local and larger environments. The unpredictability of behavior in complex adaptive systems can be seen as contributing to huge variation in the delivery of health care. If such a system is to improve its performance—that is, improve the quality of care it provides— some of these actions need to be specified to the extent possible so they are predictable with a high level of reliability. Other actions are not specifiable because their relationship to outcomes is not well understood (see Figure B-1 in Appendix B).

The task for clinicians and managers, then, is not to treat all situations alike, but to understand when specification and standardization are appropriate and when they are not. The challenge of improving quality lies in understanding that in situations lacking high levels of certainty and clinical agreement, flexibility that results in variation based on patient needs is appropriate. The converse, overspecification, can result in too many handoffs, unnecessary steps, and a lack of the ability to customize.

On the other hand, variation should be minimal in situations in which the levels of certainty and clinical agreement are high and the science base is consistent. In health care today, many processes are underspecified and understandardized. Many irrational variations in practice cannot be justified as better meeting patients' needs, and they represent lost opportunities for benefit.

A surprising finding from research on complex adaptive systems is that relatively simple rules can lead to complex, innovative system behavior. An understanding of complex adaptive behavior has been advanced by studies of biological systems, such as the flocking of birds or schooling of fish to avoid predators. These studies and computer models have confirmed that a few simple rules can guide complex behavior toward a goal. Such systems move toward their goals by having (1) a common purpose (in this case, avoiding predators); (2) internal motivation (surviving another day); and (3) some simple rules that guide individual behavior (keeping up with the group, moving toward the center of mass of the group, and avoiding collisions). Two more familiar examples of simple rules that have given rise to great variety and complexity in social systems are the Ten Commandments and the Bill of Rights, both of which have been interpreted flexibly but remain remarkably robust over time. Good rules describe how the system should function, but do not need to specify this functioning in detail. This insight can help inform the work of redesigning health care as well.

Two particular social systems functioning today illustrate the diverse, creative, and complex actions that can arise from shared aims and general directions (what some writers in the field call a "good enough vision"). The first example is the Internet, which was built to share research data electronically using agreed-upon transfer protocols and conventions. Its explosive growth and adaptation since that time could not have been foreseen, controlled, or designed in detail because the complexity was too great, and individuals who might have wished to do so were unavoidably bound by their old experience. A few simple rules were enough for a functional complex system to emerge on its own.

A second example, the credit card company Visa International, illustrates the power of a few simple rules. As members of a for-profit corporation, banks that issue Visa cards agree to the graphic layout of the card and a common clearinghouse that allows any card to be used anywhere worldwide. Its members are otherwise free to compete intensively on all other aspects of business. This design has resulted in huge growth worldwide despite different currencies, customs, and banking systems.

The committee believes these important lessons about simple rules for complex adaptive systems can be applied to health care systems as well. In redesigning health care, the building blocks are the simple processes that make up the work of small systems of care and their interconnections.

Two preconditions are required to build a new health system that can achieve the aims set forth in Chapter 2: common purpose and simple rules. First, those in the system need a common purpose that builds on the good intentions and internal motivations of the people within the health care community. The statement of purpose and aims set forth in Chapter 2 lay out a common purpose for the health system.

Second, a new set of simple rules is needed to guide behavior in the 21st-century health care system. Identifying these rules is a key task in describing a health care system capable of dramatic changes in quality. To this end, the committee proposes a new set of simple rules to guide behavior in the 21st-century health care system. Each rule is contrasted with the current approach and associated assumption it supercedes. The descriptions of the approaches that are used today are not intended to be pejorative, but to capture common practices and contrast these with the committee's vision for the future. The descriptions of today's approaches should be easily recognizable by current clinicians and others in health care. The 21st-century rules we propose, on the other hand, will not be obvious to many of today's clinicians, leaders, or health care consumers. Rather, they represent the precepts the committee believes should guide the behavior and underlie the actions of health care professionals and others as they design new care systems. The committee believes such a change in the ways that patients and their families, clinicians, and others in health care organizations interact with the health care system can produce major improvements in the quality of care. We believe these rules provide broad latitude for innovative thinking that can move the health care system in the direction of being safe, effective, patient-centered, timely, efficient, and equitable.

Several cautions are in order, however. First, as is in the nature of complex adaptive systems, the rules are interrelated and are, therefore, intended to be applied as a set rather than viewed as a menu of choices. Second, to take any one rule to its extreme is likely to lead to a caricature of the intended performance. This is also true of the descriptions of today's approaches, which do not capture many of the good practices currently found in health care. The rules and descriptions are strong, but common sense must apply to their interpretation. Third, the rules provide guidance applicable to most clinical interactions, but they do not cover every possible clinical decision. Fourth, as with the six aims, rules will occasionally conflict with one another. The responsibility of the clinician is to try to resolve or mediate these conflicts most appropriately for a given patient at a particular time. In some cases, however, conflict among rules will remain. Notwithstanding, tension among rules is a property of a complex adaptive system that can represent an area of creativity and growth.

The rules do not need to be highly specific; as in any complex adaptive system, the workforce will translate the rules into wise local actions. But they do have to be powerful and logically related to the aims. Further, they should feel like changes from prevailing approaches.

TEN SIMPLE RULES FOR THE
21ST-CENTURY HEALTH CARE SYSTEM

Table 3-1 summarizes ten simple rules for the 21st-century health care system. In the following subsections, each rule is described and contrasted with the corresponding current approach. There is not in all cases a strong evidence base indicating that following a rule would result in better patient and population outcomes. Where such evidence is available, it is cited; where it is not, this is indicated, and the rationale for the committee's espousal of the rule is provided.

Rule 1: Care Based on Continuous Healing Relationships

In the 21st-century health care system, care should be organized and paid for so that all types of health care interactions that improve information transfer and strengthen the healing relationship are encouraged. What patients want and need from their care is relief from suffering and uncertainty—knowledge about what is wrong, what is likely to happen, and what can be done to change or manage that outcome. Sometimes, such relief can be provided only in a face-to-face visit. But many needs can and should be met through other forms of care, all centered on a relationship with the clinician. The current system often requires a visit as the only legitimate format for care, and more important, as the only form of professional work that is compensated and measured in the health care world as

TABLE 3-1   Simple Rules for the 21st-Century Health Care System

Current Approach	New Rule
Care is based primarily on visits.	Care is based on continuous healing relationships.
Professional autonomy drives variability.	Care is customized according to patient needs and values.
Professionals control care.	The patient is the source of control.
Information is a record.	Knowledge is shared and information flows freely.
Decision making is based on training and experience.	Decision making is evidence-based.
Do no harm is an individual responsibility.	Safety is a system property.
Secrecy is necessary.	Transparency is necessary.
The system reacts to needs.	Needs are anticipated.
Cost reduction is sought.	Waste is continuously decreased.
Preference is given to professional roles over the system.	Cooperation among clinicians is a priority.

"productivity." Under this new rule, care would be available through many new modes of communication, and would be accessible to patients exactly when they need it, any day at any time, not just between 8:00 a.m. and 5:00 p.m. weekdays. The Internet is likely to be a major platform for such communication.

Face-to-face visits will likely continue to be an important form of clinician and patient interaction; for many people, some direct human contact is critical to establish and maintain a strong healing relationship. Face-to-face visits also allow the clinician to physically examine the patient and observe the patient's demeanor. But in many cases, face-to-face visits are not wanted by either clinician or patient, nor are they truly needed. Substituting other forms of care, such as electronic communication, for some face-to-face visits presents an opportunity not only to improve care—make it safer, more effective, patient-centered, and timely—but also to make it more efficient.

Through the judicious use of electronic and other forms of communication, it may also be possible to make more clinician time available to improve the quality of the face-to-face visits that do occur. In today's health care system, necessary face-to-face visits are often delayed or rushed. There may be insufficient time during the visit to understand the psychological underpinnings of symptoms or their relationship to other ongoing health problems. And there may be little time to provide the patient and family with information about a health condition and adequate emotional support for the pain, loneliness, and grief that may accompany the illness (Branch, 2000).

The new rule asserts that the product of health care is not visits or "encounters" but healing relationships that allow patients to obtain the trustworthy information and support they need. A focus on the healing relationship emphasizes that this transfer of trustworthy information is the core product of health care, not something tacked onto a health care visit. In the 21st-century health care system, interaction should be understood in a fundamentally different way. Interaction is not the price of care; it *is* care (Berwick, 1999). A patient with a question represents an opportunity, not a burden. Time spent in building patients' skills in self-care is not a way of shifting care; it *is* care. And access to information is not desirable because it allows care to be completed more quickly or supports compliance; it *is* care.

The new rule calls for *continuous access* (24 hours a day, 7 days a week, 365 days a year. Three points are critical to understanding how this could be achieved by the 21st-century health care system. First, as suggested above, "access" does not necessarily mean face-to-face contact with a health care professional. Second, such access would not be a matter of extending the current system; rather, it would involve fundamental redesign, attention to human factors, and respect for the limits of human beings. Third, with information technology, continuous access is possible in health care just as it has become increasingly possible in so many other venues of American society through new forms of electronic communication.

A continuous flow of interactions can span evenings, nights, and weekends if information systems make scheduling, access to medical records, e-mail, and the like available directly to patients. Such interactions would also be more individualized, patient-centered, and timely than much of today's care. Much can be learned in this regard from the financial services industry. Just as banking customers have been freed from using teller lines that were open only from 9:00 a.m. to 3:00 p.m. on weekdays, information technology can liberate patient care from the confines of the face-to-face visit. The knowledge and technology now exist to provide many alternatives to visits, including self-care that is strongly supported and unequivocally encouraged (Hart, 1995; Lorig et al., 1993, 1999; Von Korff et al., 1997; Wagner et al., 1996); group visits for patients with like needs, with or without professionals being involved (Beck et al., 1997; Kane and Sands, 1998); use of the Internet for access to scientific information and well-managed discussion groups; and e-mail communication between patients and clinicians (Jadad, 1999; Plsek, 1999; Simon et al., 2000).

We emphasize that this rule cannot be accommodated by the current system working three shifts, nor does it mean that ambulatory settings would never close. Hospitals today rely on back-up double shifts for nursing staff and very long hours for resident physicians, an approach that ignores a large body of work on the effects of fatigue on human performance (Galinsky et al., 1993; Pilcher and

---

BOX 3-2 New Rule 1: Care Based on Continuous Healing Relationships

Henry L. is 24 years old and newly identified as HIV positive. He has an apartment in an urban area. Henry e-mails Dr. Sosa at 6:45 a.m.: "I am worried that a rash that just appeared on my left wrist is related to HIV status and may be an early sign that my disease is getting worse. What do you think? I have checked out the computer database, talked to some friends in my HIV chat room, and am still confused." Dr. Sosa replies at 8:00 a.m. that she would like to have a high-resolution, two-way interactive video–computer visit with Henry at 8:50 a.m. to look at the rash and talk with him.

At 8:50, this video–computer visit takes place. Dr. Sosa examines the rash (using high-resolution optics) and compares it with other dermatological images stored in a database. She prescribes a topical ointment, offers reassurance, and asks Henry to contact her in 3 days for a progress report. She asks whether he has any other questions and whether he has given any more thought to joining a support group.

Huffcutt, 1996; Samkoff and Jacques, 1991; Sawin and Scerbo, 1995). Through the application of sound design concepts (discussed in Chapter 5), a continuous-access system can be safer and more effective (Espinosa and Nolan, 2000; Womack and Jones, 1996; Womack et al., 1991).

Box 3-2 presents a scenario that illustrates this new rule.

Rule 2: Customization Based on Patient Needs and Values

In the current health system, autonomy of clinical decision making is a fundamental value. However, a system that holds to this value fails to make the best use of scientific knowledge. Variations in approaches today often reflect different local and individual styles of practice and training that may or may not be consistent with the current evidence base. The new rule states that variations in treatment should be based primarily on differing patient needs and preferences.

Doctors and other clinicians stand to gain a great deal from this change in perspective. The volume of scientific medical literature today far outpaces the capacity of any clinician—whether medical, nursing, or other health professional—to remain up to date. Weed (2000) has pointed out that to ask an individual practitioner to rely on his or her memory to store and retrieve all the facts relevant to patient care is like asking a travel agent to memorize airline schedules. Information technology can assist by combining probabilities and indicating the likelihood of benefit from myriad possible diagnostic and treatment approaches. The clinician's brain should be used only when less expensive, creative, and resourceful capacities are insufficient.

The new rule implies that *patient values drive variability*. Patients differ because of variations in personality, nationality, and ethnicity, and in the beliefs and expectations associated with various religions and cultures (Carrese and Rhodes, 1995; Carrillo et al., 1999; Lavizzo-Mourey, 1996; Smith, 1998). Clinicians can recognize such variations by sharing with patients the best available information about alternative ways to treat a given condition, what is known about the likely effects of treatment, and the uncertainty associated with different alternatives when applied to the patient's individual circumstances. For example, patients with prostate disease of a given severity have a choice among prostatectomy, other treatments, and watchful waiting. Some men weigh the possibility of adverse side effects from surgery more heavily than others, and this influences their choice of treatment. Other men weigh the likelihood of recurrence more heavily. Similarly, menopausal women may choose whether to take hormone replacement therapy based in part on how concerned they are about its risks as compared with its benefits. For patients with angina, there may be choices among bypass surgery, angioplasty, or medication. All such choices may be influenced by the extent to which patients are bothered by symptoms, as well as their willingness to risk unfavorable outcomes. Both are highly individual judgments for which patients need good information to make a decision and support after informed choices have been made (Barry et al., 1995; Mort, 1996; Wagner et al., 1995).

Rule 3: The Patient as the Source of Control

In the current system, control over decisions, access, and information is typically in the hands of caregivers and is ceded to patients only when caregivers choose to do so. For example, patients are often required to obtain permission to see their own medical records, to have visitors, or to participate in treatment decisions. A common practice today is that control over the time, type, and location of care and the information needed to make such decisions resides with professionals. The corresponding new rule asserts that, except in unusual circumstances, control should reside with patients.

This rule represents a significant change in how many clinicians would approach patient care, but it is very consistent with the direction in which the clinician–patient relationship has been evolving (Bastian and Richards, 1999; Harrison, 2000) and with widely understood concepts of informed consent (Taylor, 2000). In recent decades, there has been a steady transition from authoritarian models of care to approaches that encourage greater patient access to information and input into decision making, but this transition is far from complete (Emanuel and Emanuel, 1992). The latter approaches correspond to a growing scientific literature in which it is shown that informed patients participating actively in decisions about their own care appear to have better outcomes, lower costs, and higher functional status than those held to more passive roles (Gifford et al., 1998; Lorig et al., 1993, 1999; Superio-Cabuslay et al., 1996; Von Korff et al., 1998). Of 21 studies published between 1983 and 1993 that measured whether the quality of physician–patient communication affected patient health outcomes for conditions such as breast cancer, diabetes, peptic ulcer disease, hypertension, and headaches, 16 reported positive outcomes, 4 reported positive (but not significant) results, and 1 was inconclusive (Stewart, 1995).

A recent review of the literature (Guadagnoli and Ward, 1998) reveals that most patients want to be involved in treatment decisions and to know about available alternatives. In a study of more than 400 elderly veterans offered an invasive medical intervention (Mazur and Hickam, 1997), almost all (93.4 percent) wanted their physician to provide them with information about risks. In examining risk disclosure, Degner and Russell (1988) found in a small study of cancer patients that virtually all preferred a "shared control model." Similarly, among 300 patients presented with vignettes about decision making, the large majority wanted to be involved and supported in the decision-making process (Deber et al., 1996). Yet, physicians typically underestimate the extent to which patients want information about their care (Strull et al., 1984). Even today, patients rarely receive adequate information for informed decision making (Braddock et al., 1999), despite strong legal underpinnings and professional acknowledgment of its importance.

This new rule is not intended to imply, however, that patients should be forced to share decision making, only that they should be able to exercise the degree of control they wish. Indeed, patients vary in the extent to which they want to be involved in decision making. Arora and McHorney (2000) found that 69 percent of patients with chronic disease (hypertension, diabetes, myocardial infarction, congestive heart failure, and depression) preferred to delegate their medical decisions to their physicians. These and other researchers have found that the likelihood of preferring an active role increases with level of education, but decreases significantly with age (Stiggelbout and Kiebert, 1997). Evidence indicates further that patient preferences may be related to the nature of the decisions to be made, the type of illness, and its severity (Mansell et al., 2000). A 1989 study revealed, for example, that interest in shared decision making declined with increased severity of illness (Ende et al., 1989).

Work by Kaplan and others on patient empowerment (Greenfield et al., 1985, 1988; Kaplan et al., 1989) has demonstrated that it takes time for patients to be included as partners and that in many cases they need to be coached to assume such a role. In settings where this has occurred, however, research has demonstrated the value of the approach. Kaplan et al. (1989) found that patients who had been coached to ask questions during office visits reported fewer functional limitations and had better control of blood sugar and blood pressure than did patients in the control group. Investigators using interactive video to help patients with decision making reported that in a prospective cohort study, patients rated the program very positively in helping them make informed choices about surgical intervention for benign prostatic hypertrophy (Barry et al., 1995; Wagner et al., 1995).

Accomplishing the goal of shared decision making does not necessarily require a high-technology approach. Virginia Mason Medical Center in Seattle, Washington, for example, provides patients with a short form called "Doc Talk" to help them prepare for a visit to their doctor. By reviewing the list of suggested topics before the visit and making notes for themselves, patients are encouraged to ensure that their concerns are addressed (*Doc Talk*, 1999). A group of Australian investigators used a similar approach with cancer patients and concluded that a question prompt sheet is a simple, inexpensive, and effective means of promoting the asking of questions by cancer patients (Brown et al., 1999).

As noted earlier, patients are increasingly able to use the Internet and other interactive technologies to help them make informed decisions about their medical treatment. Examples of such information include (1) patients' access to their own health records, including laboratory results and diagnostic images; (2) interactive systems for shared decision making (Barry et al., 1995; Wagner et al., 1995) to help patients understand treatment options and the level of medical uncertainty of each, and integrate their own lifestyles and personal beliefs into their decision making; and (3) direct access by patients to information about clinical trials (such as the National Cancer Institute's PDQ database of clinical trials), the clinical research literature, and well-prepared syntheses.

Rule 4: Shared Knowledge and the Free Flow of Information

Transfer of information—both scientific and personal—is a key form of care. In the 21st-century health care system, patients should have access to both types of information without restriction, delay, or the need for anyone else's permission.

Under the current approach, in which the patient visit is the organizing principle, the record is an artifact of that visit. Information is treated as retrospective, archival, passive, and inert. It is used as a record of what has happened or as a tool to defend or prosecute a lawsuit. There is often some barrier to knowledge transfer—whether requiring that the patient call for an appointment or obtain permission—that increases cost without adding value and fails to meet the patient's need.

The new rule represents a change in this view of the nature of health care information. It treats information as interactive, real-time, and prospective, and holds that *information is key to the patient–clinician relationship.* This rule is related to Rule 1, which states that care should be understood as a healing relationship that rests primarily on the transfer of knowledge through face-to-face visits and various forms of electronic communication. Information is not inert; rather the transfer of knowledge is care. Patients' unrestricted access to their health-related information is a key implication of Rule 4. Ensuring such access can help make information part of a healing relationship. Patients should also be able to see an audit log, that is, a list of all others who have seen their identifiable data.

Several debates have revolved around issues related to patient access to health information. The question of who owns that information remains a difficult and unsettled question (Institute of Medicine, 1994; Waller and Alcantara, 1998). The clinician or organization (such as a hospital) that creates the record has an obligation to protect it from, for example, destruction, tampering, or disclosure. In many states, patients have the right to access or obtain copies of their records, and they sometimes have the right to correct the information. Generally, however, legislation and practice severely limit the conditions (and sometimes impose very high costs for violating those limits) under which these rights are granted. Even where patients have a clear legal right to access their records, the reluctance of some health care organizations and practices may make accessing or obtaining copies of one's records very difficult in reality.

Although patients should have unfettered access to their records and should be able to add comments regarding, for example, their accuracy, the committee believes patients should not be allowed to alter, block access to, or delete information entered in their records by clinicians or others. Medical records are legal as well as patient-care documents. Ensuring that health information is accurate and complete is critical to its use for patient care, research and quality improvement, and legal and financial accountability.

Beyond the generally acknowledged right of a patient to know his or her diagnosis and treatment, patients are sometimes given a summary of their care to help them in their self-care. In the current system, patients who request access to their personal medical information are generally given paper copies of either abbreviated or complete versions of their records (Chambers, 1998; Fischbach et al., 1980; Giglio et al., 1978; Shenkin and Warner, 1973; Weed, 1981). Medical records tend to be large, cumbersome, filled with medical jargon, poorly organized, dispersed among many record holders, incomplete, inaccurate, and/or out of date. Paper records make tracking and understanding longitudinal data and their relationship to various interventions quite difficult (Weed, 1991). Information about the results of care, patient preferences, and patients' own contributions to their health and health care is sparse or nonexistent.

With the advent of Internet-based applications, it is now possible for medical records to be held physically or digitally in a variety of locations, and to be accessed in whole or in part by the patient or anyone to whom he or she grants permission for purposes of reading only or for reading and entering information (Eysenbach, 2000; Larkin, 1999). It is also possible to store patient records on "smart" cards (Schoenfelt, 1998)—wallet-sized cards with embedded chips that can be accessed with a card reader. Other applications include storage of digital images (such as x-rays) on CD-ROM for patients to keep (Mehta et al., 1999).

Relatively little is known about patients' preferences and reactions with regard to having access to their records, but studies have generally shown positive results. Michael and Bordley (1982) found that a majority of patients they surveyed desired access to their medical records. Other studies have revealed that patients appreciate being given all details or a summary of their care (Bronson et al., 1986; Giglio et al., 1978; Gittens, 1986). For example, a pilot study of shared records for people with mental illness revealed enthusiastic acceptance by both patients and health staff (Essex et al., 1990).

Little is known about the extent to which patients understand the information in their medical records. In one study, chronically ill patients who had access to their records reported understanding about half or more of the information they contained (Gittens, 1986). In a study of stroke patients, those having access to their complete medical record reported understanding more about their condition than did control patients who had been given only relevant descriptive medical information (Banet and Felchlia, 1997).

There is some evidence indicating that giving patients greater access to clinical information and their own personal health information improves the process of care and health outcomes:

• Smokers who had access to their medical records were more likely to state that smoking was a major health concern than were control patients who did not have such access. After 6 months, significantly more patients in the former group had quit smoking (65 percent) compared with those in the latter (29 percent) (Bronson and O'Meara, 1986).

• College students who were given information from their medical record were more likely than controls to increase their adherence to treatment advice (Giglio et al., 1978).

• Elderly patients whose medical records were shared with them were more likely to know their medical problems and treatments (although not more likely to adhere to medication regimens) (Bronson et al., 1986).

• In Australia, Liaw et al. (1998) gave a small set of patients with chronic problems (29 experimental and 22 controls) a computer-generated health record. They found that doing so was practical and well received, and led to positive trends in improved awareness of issues, health promotion, and disease management.

• Patients with chronic medical conditions who received copies of the progress notes in their medical records reported significant increases in overall physical function and overall health status, greater satisfaction with their care, and more interest in seeing their medical records than patients in a control group who did not receive this information (Maly et al., 1999).

• In a randomized controlled trial of women attending an antenatal clinic, those given their entire record (experimental group) as opposed to a summary card (control group) were more likely to report feeling "in control" during pregnancy, less likely to report feeling anxious and helpless, and more likely to have information on their records explained to them (Homer et al., 1999).

One exception to the above findings is a recent randomized control trial of 650 cancer patients. In that study, no differences in outcomes (i.e., global health status, emotional functioning, cognitive functioning, or satisfaction) were found between the experimental group, which received a supplementary record designed to improve communication, and the control group (Drury et al., 2000).

Patients' full access to their records could, of course, have unwanted effects unless new ways to help them use and learn from the information are devised. Patients may misunderstand or be frightened by such information, as a clinician's being unsure of a diagnosis and wanting to rule out a serious condition. Clinicians' concerns about patients seeing their records could also result in the preparation of "shadow records" for the clinician's own use or in omission of information from the record, thus compromising care by others who are unaware of the omitted information. It is unclear, moreover, whether patient access to medical records would increase or decrease liability exposure. These and other unintended consequences deserve serious consideration. The committee believes, however, that such circumstances will be the exception rather than the rule (Golodetz et al., 1976) and are not sufficient reason to impede all patients' access to their records. The potential benefits of such access are illustrated in Box 3-3, which describes a practice that uses patients' access to their health information in an interactive context.

BOX 3-3   Rule 4: Shared Knowledge and the Free Flow of Information

Mary Chao is a nurse practitioner who works with patients newly diagnosed with diabetes. She explains, "People learn by experience—the more ways they experience something, the better they will learn and retain it. I give each new patient a diary. I tell them, 'Don't worry about anything. Just write down your meals and blood sugars. At the next visit we will look at it.' Pretty soon they are drawing connections between what they are eating and their blood sugars."

Mary relates that even patients who have little formal education are active participants. One patient describes his self-management as being like an athlete in training. Most of her elderly patients who have had trouble keeping their blood sugar under control for decades now successfully monitor and manage their diabetes using their own clinical information, which they generate routinely and is available to them and their clinician in graph, chart, and other forms at the patients' own Web sites.

Rule 5: Evidence-Based Decision Making

In today's health system, it is widely believed that the best care for individuals is based on the training and experience of professionals. The new rule, on the other hand, could be stated: *The best care results from the conscientious, explicit, and judicious use of current best evidence and knowledge of patient values by well-trained, experienced clinicians.*

At their best, health care services match knowledge and need. When care does not match knowledge, it may fail to help—either by omission (failing to do what would help) or by waste (doing what cannot help). The health system today is too tolerant of mismatches between knowledge and action; that is, it is too accepting of both omission and waste. As a result, care is too often unreliable, advice and answers are inconsistent, and clinical practice varies without well-founded rationale. The new rule calls for standardization around best practices as appropriate for a given patient or the subpopulation to which a patient belongs. Such evidence-based decision making can free clinicians to make choices that science cannot guide—decisions based on relationship; observation; and the other senses, including touch.

What the new rule calls for is the use of systematically acquired knowledge in all its forms for decision making. The rule does not require that all decisions be based on the results of randomized controlled trials because such results are not always available and because other forms of knowledge exist, such as that derived from epidemiological and population-based data. Neither does the new rule discount clinician experience or the integration of information about a patient's special circumstances. Rather, it argues that all of these sources of knowledge are relevant and valuable when choosing how to apply evidence. The latter process involves four steps that require training and experience (with organizational and other supports): (1) formulation of a clear clinical question, (2) search for the relevant information from the best possible sources, (3) evaluation of the evidence for its validity and usefulness, and (4) implementation of those findings (Davidoff, 1999).

An emphasis on the use of systematically acquired knowledge derives from a field of study known as *evidence-based medicine* or, more broadly, *evidence-based practice*, which evolved during the last decade (Evidence-Based Medicine Working Group, 1992; Muir Gray, 1997; Risdale, 1995; Sackett et al., 2000). The approach often involves systematic examinations of clinical questions that includes a comprehensive review of the literature, standard methods of presenting data, and emphasis on the validity of the research methods. Individual studies are assessed and scored on the basis of their design and execution, including, for example, the selection of patients, the size of the study, and how confounding variables were accounted for (Cook et al., 1997; Lohr and Carey, 1999). Evidence-based practice is described in greater detail in Chapter 6.

The availability of systematic reviews and the resulting clinical guidelines for practicing clinicians (O'Connor et al., 1999) is an essential adjunct to practice. A growing body of evidence demonstrates that the use of clinical practice guidelines with other supportive tools, such as reminder systems, can improve patient care (Cabana et al., 1999; East et al., 1999; Morris, 1993; Thomsen et al., 1994; Wells et al., 2000). Despite the best of intentions, clinicians cannot be expected to process unaided all the details, strengths, and limitations of scientific evidence under normal conditions of practice in which the number of variables to be considered is great, but resources, including time, are severely limited (Weed, 1999).

The commitment to standardizing to excellence—using the best available information—does not begin with a slavish adherence to simplistic practice guidelines. With today's information systems, protocols can incorporate variations based on the individual patient's condition, such as kidney function and the presence of other chronic problems. An example is adult respiratory distress symptom, an extremely serious condition that in the late 1970s resulted in death for nearly 90 percent of intensive care unit (ICU) patients for whom it was diagnosed. A group of investigators at LDS Hospital in Salt Lake City was able to generate computer-generated guidelines for concurrent management of the many complex physiological parameters involved in treating this illness, which had resulted in several thousand separate instructions (Thomsen et al., 1994). The new system of computer-generated protocols adapted continuously to the patient's condition. ICU staff were required to take actions in response to the guidelines, accepting or rejecting the instructions on the basis of their judgment. With use, the instructions become more accurate, and the ICU staff came to trust them more. As a result, in 1991 the ICU reported an unprecedented survival rate for the disease of 45 percent (Suchyta et al., 1991). More recently, other investigators have reported using such clinical algorithms to achieve survival rates as high as 75 percent (East et al., 1999; Lewandowski et al., 1997).

A commitment to evidence-based practice may appear to conflict with Rule 3, according to which patient values should drive variability. A simplistic way of stating the tension between the two is: *The patient is always right, but sometimes the doctor knows best.* When a patient seeks inappropriate health care services, the challenge for clinicians is to find ways of reducing this conflict and, to the extent possible, resolving it, guided always by efforts to understand and respond to patient needs. If a conflict cannot be resolved through counseling, the clinician should refuse to provide nonbeneficial services. If a patient decides not to accept services that are likely be beneficial, the clinician needs to ensure that the patient understands the implications of his or her choice and support the patient in that choice.

Rule 6: Safety as a System Property

Patients are injured frequently because of poor system designs. For this reason, a means of accountability that relies on blaming individuals stands little or no chance of achieving significant improvements. The health care system must be able to deliver appropriate care, reliably and without error. The assumption underlying the current rule can be stated as: *Careful and competent professionals do not, or should not, make errors.* If errors occur, the current rule assumes that the problem must be due to a lack of competence or carelessness. It would follow that the best response to error would be to ensure that individuals are trained better, are alerted to the need to attend to safety and follow rules, are motivated to be careful, and are punished if they err.

The assumption underlying the new rule is quite different. This rule might be stated as: *Threats to patient safety are the end result of complex causes such as faulty equipment; system design; and the interplay of human factors, including fatigue, limitations on memory, and distraction. The way to improve safety is to learn about causes of error and use this knowledge to design systems of care so as to prevent error when possible, to make visible those errors that do occur (so they can be intercepted), and to mitigate the harm done when an error does reach the patient.* Put simply, in the new health care system, procedures, job designs, equipment, communication, and information technology should be configured to respect human factors and to make errors less common and less harmful when they do occur.

Health care is composed of a large set of interacting systems—paramedic, emergency, ambulatory, inpatient, and home health care; testing and imaging laboratories; pharmacies; and so forth—that are connected in loosely coupled but intricate networks of individuals, teams, procedures, regulations, communications, equipment, and devices. These systems function within such diverse and diffuse management, accountability, and information structures that the overall term *health system* is today a misnomer. Further, despite contractual relationships with insurers, many physicians are so tenuously connected to organizations that they do not view themselves as part of a system of care (Freidson, 1975; Pauly, 1980). In these and many other ways, the distinct cultures of medicine (and other health professions) add to its idiosyncrasy among high-risk industries. Nevertheless, experience in other high-risk industries has provided well-understood methods for improving safety.

Patient safety emerges from safe designs used in systems that incorporate an understanding of human factors. Such an approach can improve performance, prevent harm when error does occur, help systems recover from error, and mitigate further harm. Knowledge about human factors must be applied in designing tasks, processes, equipment, rules, and environments. Safety also requires leadership—by governing boards and corporate executives and by leaders of clinical groups embedded in larger organizations. To create safety systems requires that clinical leaders and managers use and continually contribute to the best knowledge about safe designs for tasks, equipment, processes, rules, and environments.

The biggest challenge to moving toward a safer health system is changing the culture from one of blaming individuals for errors to one in which errors are treated not as personal failures, but as opportunities to improve the system and prevent harm. One of the most important barriers to increasing patient safety is a lack of awareness of the extent to which errors occur daily in all health care settings and organizations. In today's health systems, the vast majority of errors are not reported because personnel fear they will be punished.

The committee's earlier report (Institute of Medicine, 2000) recommends that health care organizations and the professionals affiliated with them make continually improved patient safety a declared and serious aim by establishing patient safety programs with a defined executive responsibility. That report further recommends that patient safety programs: (1) provide strong, clear, and visible attention to safety; (2) implement nonpunitive systems for reporting and analyzing errors within their organizations; (3) incorporate well-understood safety principles, such as standardizing and simplifying equipment, supplies, and processes; and (4) establish interdisciplinary team training programs, such as those involving simulation, that incorporate training designed to improve and maintain skills, as well as improve communication among team members. Chapter 5 of this report examines some design principles that organizations can apply to improve safety.

Rule 7: Need for Transparency

The health care system should be uncompromising in its defense of patient confidentiality, a matter of great national concern. But the pursuit of confidentiality is not a reason for hiding the system's performance from those who depend on the system for care. This new rule calls for health systems to be accountable to the public; to do their work openly; to make their results known to the public and professionals alike; and to build trust through disclosure, even of the systems' own problems.

At times, today's health care system appears to put a premium on secrecy. Although it is critical to safeguard patient confidentiality, poorly designed policies and procedures that limit the sharing of information may be perceived by patients as a series of closed doors, locked cabinets, and private meetings. In the current system, concern about the burden of reporting and oversight, litigation, and blame has generated conflict and mistrust and cast transparency in its most negative light, resulting in resistance to disclosure of all kinds.

In the future health care system, the rule should be: *Have no secrets. Make all information flow freely so that anyone involved in the system, including patients and families, can make the most informed choices and know at any time whatever facts may be relevant to a patient's decision making.* This new rule is expected to supplement trust in the good training and intentions of health care professionals with trust based on good information and well-designed systems of care.

Although changes in the tort system may be desirable, improving the health care system cannot wait for such change to occur. Some organizations have successfully implemented programs of increased transparency despite the liability risk (Peterkin, 1990). Indeed, some evidence shows that open disclosure of errors may *decrease* the likelihood of malpractice loss (Kraman and Hamm, 1999; Pietro et al., 2000; Witman et al., 1990; Wu, 1999).

In the future health care system envisioned by the committee, transparency is the route to accountability—the identification of who is responsible both financially and clinically for the actions of health care organizations and individuals. The committee believes trust will improve in a health care system that poses few barriers to the flow of information, including aggregate (non-personally identifiable) research data and information about the quality of care. A health care system that operates under a rule of transparency will be more patient-centered and safer because patients will be able to recognize outdated and wrong information and to share in information that affects their care, such as the results of laboratory tests, medications being taken, and the correct doses.

Rule 8: Anticipation of Needs

Under the current approach, health care resources are marshaled when they are needed. The system works largely in a reactive mode, awaiting complications and underinvesting in prevention. The new system would not wait for trouble. It would use patient registries to track patients and draw them into care. It would use predictive models to anticipate demand and allocate its resources according to those predictions, thereby smoothing workflow. The corresponding 21st-century rule would state: *Organize health care to predict and anticipate needs based on knowledge of patients, local conditions, and a thorough knowledge of the natural history of illness.* A system that adopted this new rule would be more patient-centered and more effective. It would make and use better predictions about the flow of need and demand, allowing for anticipation of the needs of both individuals and the patient population at risk. Box 3-4 illustrates the new rule and the current approach.

Scenarios similar to the current approach described in Box 3-4 are common today. Crises for older persons occur because anticipatory management of multiple problems is rare. When care hinges on scheduled office visits or emergency room visits, anticipatory management that can prevent acute hospitalization is difficult. Under the new rule, anticipation could include more and better linkages among care teams, linkages among health systems and community resources, and more frequent communication with patients through telephone consultations and

---

BOX 3-4   Rule 8: Anticipation of Needs

Current Approach: React to Needs

Pearl Clayton is 86 years old. She has been widowed for 5 years and lives alone. She has recently shown signs of forgetfulness and has had two recent falls, one of which resulted in a fractured wrist. Her adult daughter and son-in-law would like her to go to a doctor and get a thorough evaluation, particularly of her forgetfulness. They procrastinate and do not get around to taking her. It is difficult to get any advice over the telephone. Finally, Pearl falls, fractures her hip, and is hospitalized. Her fall is related to a combination of over-the-counter sleeping pills and the use of alcohol, begun during a prolonged period of grief after she became widowed.

During her hospitalization, she suffers hypertension and grand mal seizures during which she aspirates; she develops severe pneumonia and spends 2 weeks intubated in an intensive care unit. At the end of this time, her broken hip finally can be repaired, but she has become so frail and confused that she cannot be transferred home and must go to a nursing home. During her time at the nursing home, her family, caregivers, and those in the hospital where she has periodic acute admissions have no guidance about the use of life-sustaining measures.

New Rule: Anticipation of Needs

Under the new rule, anticipatory management results in a mental status evaluation and home visits that make it possible to identify Pearl's problems in time to prevent the fall that would have led to her hip fracture. Even if the hip fracture had not been completely prevented, clinicians would have had available to them a complete and accurate medical history during Pearl's hospitalization so that those caring for her would have known to anticipate withdrawal symptoms from her medication and alcohol use. She would have received appropriate medical management, avoided aspiration and intubation, and recovered sufficiently to return to her own home.

---

community services. Notable efforts to adopt this approach in the United States include the innovative On Lok Senior Health Services, first organized in San Francisco's Chinatown, and its replications in the Program of All-Inclusive Care for the Elderly (PACE) (Eng et al., 1997; Rich, 1999). Such programs of care for frail elderly persons in the community have brought together resources likely to be needed by many elderly patients. Other countries, including the United Kingdom and Finland, have also focused on such linkages designed to anticipate patient needs (The Ministry of Social Affairs and Health and The Association of Finnish Local and Regional Authorities, 1999).

Rule 9: Waste Continuously Decreased

The current system tries to conserve resources through restrictions and budget limits, withholding services and creating queues to drive costs down. This is a destructive, short-term approach. A more modern approach would build on a better understanding of the nature of waste itself, identifying expenditures of all types that add no value—unused supplies, rework and redundancy, unhelpful inspection, lost ideas, and unused information—and systematically eliminating that waste. The United States spends over 50 percent more per person on health care than many other Western nations. Yet it does not appear that these vast expenditures are buying reliable levels of quality. The care in some places for some conditions is superb, but such is not the case everywhere, for all people, all the time.

Many of the problems with the current health care system are related to the belief that reducing expenditures alone will increase value. The current rule appears to be: *The value of our health care investment is increased by cost reductions, often by rationing services.* As a result, systems attempt to continue what they are doing with fewer resources, for example, by stretching staff over larger and larger numbers of tasks and patients. Other efforts to reduce costs have led to arbitrary limits on services such as lengths of stay in a hospital; the kinds of settings that are allowed for care; and the numbers of encounters, such as home health visits.

The committee believes this is not the route to improved value. The new rule states that increased value will not be derived by stressing the current system, that is, by asking people to work harder, faster, and longer, and while doing so, not to make (or admit to) any errors. Rather, increased value will result from systematically developed strategies that focus on the aims of the health care system outlined in Chapter 2—safety, effectiveness, patient-centeredness, timeliness, efficiency, and equity—and reduce all forms of waste by eliminating activities or resources that do not add value (Dresser, 1997; Langley et al., 1996; Saphir, 1999). Waste has been described as comprising seven types: (1) overuse of services (see Appendix A); (2) waiting (for example, for a laboratory test to be performed or for its results); (3) transportation (for example, requiring a patient to go to another site or floor for care); (4) processing (more steps than are needed to accomplish results); (5) stock (using more materials than are needed, maintaining unused materials in inventory or unused workforce skills); (6) motion (wasting both energy and time); and (7) defects in production. The latter type of waste has its counterpart in health care delivery in the form of mistakes in execution or lack of proficiency in performing a procedure such that the patient does not receive full benefit.

Many smart cost reductions are achievable as the side effects of improving the process of care. Health care systems need to build on the experience of other industries and the reports that have begun to appear in the literature from groups able to demonstrate gains in efficiency and quality of care and reduced waste and costs (Barry-Walker, 2000; Cohn et al., 1997; Fuss et al., 1998; Stewart et al., 1997; Tidikis and Strasen, 1994; Tunick et al., 1997).

The committee does not intend to imply that all types of quality improvement efforts will result in reduced waste or cost or that only cost-reducing quality improvement efforts should be undertaken. Underuse of health services as a result of barriers to access (e.g., lack of insurance) or provision of care inconsistent with the evidence base (e.g., failure to prescribe beta blockers when indicated following an acute myocardial infarction) is also a serious quality problem that must be addressed by the 21st-century health system.

Rule 10: Cooperation Among Clinicians

In the current system, care is taken to protect professional prerogatives and separate roles. The current system shows too little cooperation and teamwork. Instead, each discipline and type of organization tends to defend its authority at the expense of the total system's function—a problem known as suboptimization. Patients suffer through lost continuity, redundancy, excess costs, and miscommunication. Patients and families commonly report that caregivers appear not to coordinate their work, or even to know what others are doing. Suboptimization is seen, for example, in operating rooms that must maintain multiple different surgical tray setups for different doctors performing the same procedure. Each doctor gets what he or she wants, but at the cost of introducing enormous complexity and possible error into the system. In the new system, people will understand the advantage of high levels of cooperation, coordination, and standardization to guarantee excellence, continuity, and reliability.

The current approach focuses on role definition, certification and licensure, or doing one's own work as the top priority, rather than helping others do their work. It is the basis of professional self-esteem and status and a criterion of competence. That approach also, however, makes defined roles preeminent rather than meeting patients' needs. It lets the role "trump" the system, and the system suffers as a consequence.

Under the new rule, cooperation in patient care is more important than professional prerogatives and roles. The new rule emphasizes a focus on good communication among members of a team, using all the expertise and knowledge of team members and, where appropriate, sensibly extending roles to meet patients' needs (Bulger, 2000). This topic is discussed in more detail in Chapter 5.

REFERENCES

Arora, Neeraj K. and Colleen A. McHorney. Patient Preferences for Medical Decision Making: Who Really Wants to Participate? *Medical Care* 38(3):325–41, 2000.

Banet, Gerald A. and Mark A. Felchlia. The Potential Utility of a Shared Medical Record in A "First-Time" Stroke Population. *Journal of Vascular Nursing* 15(1):29–33, 1997.

Barry, Michael J., Floyd J. Fowler, Jr., Albert G. Mulley, Jr., et al. Patient Reactions to a Program Designed to Facilitate Patient Participation in Treatment Decisions for Benign Prostatic Hyperplasia. *Medical Care* 33(8):771–82, 1995.

Barry-Walker, Jean. The Impact of Systems Redesign on Staff, Patient, and Financial Outcomes. *J Nurs Adm* 30(2):77–89, 2000.

Bastian, Hilda and Tessa Richards. Australia's Consumer Champion. *BMJ* 319:730, 1999.

Beck, Arne, John Scott, Patrick Williams, et al. A Randomized Trial of Group Outpatient Visits for Chronically Ill Older HMO Members: The Cooperative Health Care Clinic. *J Am Geriatr Soc* 45:543–9, 1997.

Berwick, Donald M. Escape Fire. Plenary Address, Institute for Healthcare Improvement Annual Forum. 1999.

Braddock, Clarence H. III, Kelly A. Edwards, Nicole M. Hasenberg, et al. Informed Decision Making in Outpatient Practice: Time to Get Back to Basics. *JAMA* 282(24):2313–20, 1999.

Branch, William T. Is the Therapeutic Nature of the Patient–Physician Relationship Being Undermined? A Primary Care Physician's Perspective. *Arch Int Med* 160:2257-60, 2000.

Bronson, David L., Michael C. Costanza, and Henry M. Tufo. Using Medical Records for Older Patient Education in Ambulatory Practice. *Medical Care* 24(4):332–9, 1986.

Bronson, David L. and Kathrine O'Meara. The Impact of Shared Medical Records on Smoking Awareness and Behavior in Ambulatory Care. *J Gen Intern Med* 1:34–7, 1986.

Brown, R., P. N. Butow, M. J. Boyer, and M. H. N. Tattersall. Promoting Patient Participation in the Cancer Consultation: Evaluation of a Prompt Sheet and Coaching in Question-Asking. *British Journal of Cancer* 80(1/2):242–8, 1999.

Bulger, Roger J. The Quest for the Therapeutic Organization. *JAMA* 283(18):2431–3, 2000.

Cabana, Michael D., Cynthia S. Rand, Neil R. Powe, et al. Why Don't Physicians Follow Clinical Practice Guidelines? A Framework for Improvement. *JAMA* 282(15):1458–65, 1999.

Carrese, Joseph A. and Lorna A. Rhodes. Western Bioethics on the Navajo Reservation: Benefit or Harm? *JAMA* 274(10):826–9, 1995.

Carrillo, J. Emilo, Alexander R. Green, and Joseph R. Betancourt. Cross-Cultural Primary Care: A Patient-based Approach. *Ann Int Med* 130:829–34, 1999.

Chambers, Jo. Terminally Ill Patients Treated in the Community Should Keep a Copy of their Records. *BMJ* 317:283, 1998.

Cohn, Lawrence H., Donna Rosborough, and John Fernandez. Reducing Costs and Length of Stay and Improving Efficiency and Quality of Care in Cardiac Surgery. *Ann Thorac Surg* 64(6 Suppl):S58–60; discussion S80–2, 1997.

Cook, Deborah J., Cynthia D. Mulrow, and R. Brian Haynes. Systematic Reviews: Synthesis of Best Evidence for Clinical Decisions. *Ann Int Med* 126(5):376–80, 1997.

Davidoff, Frank. In the Teeth of the Evidence. The Curious Case of Evidence-Based Medicine. *The Mount Sinai Journal of Medicine* 66(2):75–83, 1999.

Deber, Raisa B., Nancy Kraetschmer, and Jane Irvine. What Role Do Patients Wish to Play in Treatment Decision Making? *Arch Int Med* 156:1414–20, 1996.

Degner, Lesley F. and Catherine Aquino Russell. Preferences for Treatment Control Among Adults with Cancer. *Research in Nursing & Health* 11:367–74, 1988.

Doc Talk. 1999. Reproduced by permission of Virginia Mason Medical Center.

Dresser, Ric. A Pragmatic Look at Hospital Reengineering. Successful Reengineering Requires the Right Leadership. *Health Progress* 78:44–7, 1997.

Drury, Mark, Patricia Yudkin, Jean Harcourt, et al. Patients with Cancer Holding their own Records: A Randomised Controlled Trial. *British Journal of General Practice* 50:105–10, 2000.

East, Thomas D., Laura K. Heermann, Richard L. Bradshaw, et al. Efficacy of Computerized Decision Support for Mechanical Ventilation: Results of a Prospective Multi-Center Randomized Trial. *Proc AMIA Symp* 251–5, 1999.

Emanuel, Ezekiel J. and Linda L. Emanuel. Four Models of the Physician–Patient Relationship. *JAMA* 267(16):2221–6, 1992.

Ende, Jack, Lewis Kazis, Arlene Ash, and Mark A. Moskowitz. Measuring Patients' Desire for Autonomy: Decision Making and Information-Seeking Preferences Among Medical Patients. *J Gen Intern Med* 4:23–30, 1989.

Eng, C., J. Pedulla, G. P. Eleazer, et al. Program of All-inclusive Care for the Elderly (PACE): An Innovative Model of Integrated Geriatric Care and Financing. *J Am Geriatr Soc* 45(2):223–32, 1997.

Espinosa, James A. and Thomas W. Nolan. Reducing Errors Made by Emergency Physicians in Interpreting Radiographs: Longitudinal Study. *BMJ* 320:737–40, 2000.

Essex, B., R. Doig, and J. Renshaw. Pilot Study of Records of Shared Care for People with Mental Illnesses. *BMJ* 300:1442–6, 1990.

Evidence-Based Medicine Working Group. Evidence-Based Medicine: A New Approach to Teaching the Practice of Medicine. *JAMA* 268(17):2420–5, 1992.

Eysenbach, Gunther. Consumer Health Informatics. *BMJ* 320:1713–6, 2000.

Fischbach, Ruth L., Antonia Sionelo-Bayog, Annette Needle, and Thomas L. Delbanco. The Patient and Practitioner as Co-authors of the Medical Record. *Patient Counselling and Health Education*:1–5, 1980.

Freidson, Eliot. *Doctoring Together: A Study of Professional Social Control.* New York, NY: Elsevier Scientific Publishing Company, Inc., 1975.

Fuss, Mae Ann, Yvonne E. Bryan, Kim S. Hitchings, et al. Measuring Critical Care Redesign: Impact on Satisfaction and Quality. *Nursing Administration Quarterly* 23:1–14, 1998.

Galinsky, Traci L, Roger R. Rosa, Joel S. Warm, and William N. Dember. Psychophysical Determinants of Stress in Sustained Attention. *Human Factors* 35(4):603–14, 1993.

Gifford, A. L., Laurent D. D., V. M. Gonzales, et al. Pilot Randomized Trial of Education to Improve Self-Management Skills of Men With Symptomatic HIV/AIDS. *J Acquir Immune Defic Syndr Hum Retrovirol* 18(2):136–44, 1998.

Giglio, Richard J., B. Spears, David Rumpf, and Nancy Eddy. Encouraging Behavior Changes by Use of Client-Held Health Records. *Medical Care* 16(9):757–64, 1978.

Gittens, Mary. Patients' Access to Their Records. *Journal of the Royal College of General Practitioners*:290, 1986.

Golodetz, Arnold, Johanna Ruess, and Raymond L. Milhous. The Right to Know: Giving the Patient his Medical Record. *Arch Phys Med Rehabil* 57:78–81, 1976.

Greenfield, Sheldon, Sherrie H. Kaplan, and John E. Ware, Jr. Expanding Patient Involvement in Care: Effects on Patient Outcomes. *Ann Int Med* 102:520–8, 1985.

Greenfield, Sheldon, Sherrie H. Kaplan, John E. Ware, Jr., et al. Patients' Participation in Medical Care: Effects on Blood Sugar Control and Quality of Life in Diabetes. *J Gen Intern Med* 3:448–57, 1988.

Guadagnoli, Edward and Patricia Ward. Patient Participation in Decision-making. *Social Science & Medicine* 47(3):329–39, 1998.

Harrison, Ailsa. Choice is a Gift from the Patient to the Doctor, Not the Other Way Around. *BMJ* 320:874, 2000.

Hart, Julian Tudor. Clinical and Economic Consequences of Patients as Producers. *Journal of Public Health Medicine* 17(4):383–6, 1995.

Homer, Caroline S., Gregory K. Davis, and Louise S. Everitt. The Introduction of a Woman-Held Record Into a Hospital Antenatal Clinic: The Bring Your Own Records Study. *Aust NZ J Obstet Gynaecol* Feb;39(1):54–7, 1999.

Institute of Medicine. *Health Data in the Information Age: Use, Disclosure, and Privacy.* M. S. Donaldson and K. N. Lohr, eds. Washington, D.C.: National Academy Press, 1994.

———. *To Err Is Human: Building a Safer Health System.* Linda T. Kohn, Janet M. Corrigan, and Molla S. Donaldson, eds. Washington, D.C: National Academy Press, 2000.

Jadad, Alejandro R. Promoting Partnerships: Challenges for the Internet Age. *BMJ* 319:761–4, 1999.

Kane, Beverley and Daniel Z. Sands. Guidelines for the Clinical Use of Electronic Mail with Patients. *J Am Med Inform Assoc* 5:104–11, 1998.

Kaplan, Sherrie H., Sheldon Greenfield, and John E. Ware, Jr. Assessing the Effects of Physician–
Patient Interactions on Outcomes of Chronic Disease. *Medical Care* 27(3, Supplement):S110–
27, 1989.

Kauffman, S. *At Home in the Universe: The Search for the Laws of Self-Organization and Complexity.* New York, NY: Oxford University, 1995.

Kraman, Steve S. and G. Hamm. Risk Management: Extreme Honesty May be the Best Policy. *Ann
Int Med* 131(12):963–7, 1999.

Langley, Gerald J., Kevin M. Nolan, Thomas W. Nolan, et al. *The Improvement Guide. A Practical
Approach to Enhancing Organizational Performance.* San Francisco, CA: Jossey-Bass, 1996.

Larkin, Howard. Permanent Record: Allowing patients to post their own medical records on the
Internet is becoming big business. *American Medical News*:21–2, 1999.

Lavizzo-Mourey, Risa J. Cultural Competence: Essential Measurement of Quality for Managed
Care Organizations. *Ann Int Med* 124(10):919–21, 1996.

Lewandowski, K., R. Rossaint, D. Pappert, et al. High Survival Rate in 122 ARDS Patients Managed
According to a Clinical Algorithm Including Extracorporeal Membrane Oxygenation. *Intensive
Care Med* 23:819–35, 1997.

Liaw, S. Teng, Anthony J. Radford, and Ian Maddocks. The Impact of a Computer Generated Patient
Held Health Record. *Australian Family Physician* 27(suppl 1):S39–43, 1998.

Lohr, Kathleen N. and Tomothy S. Carey. Assessing "Best Evidence:" Issues in Grading the Quality
of Studies for Systematic Reviews. *Journal on Quality Improvement* 25(9):470–9, 1999.

Lorig, Kate R., Peter D. Mazonson, and Halsted R. Holman. Evidence Suggesting that Health Education for Self Management in Chronic Arthritis has Sustained Health Benefits While Reducing
Health Care Costs. *Arthritis Rheumatism* 36(4):439–46, 1993.

Lorig, Kate R., David S. Sobel, Anita L. Steward, et al. Evidence Suggesting that a Chronic Disease
Self-Management Program Can Improve Health Status While Reducing Hospitalization: A
Randomized Trial. *Medical Care* 37(1):5–14, 1999.

Maly, Rose C., Linda B. Bourque, and Rita F. Engelhardt. A Randomized Controlled Trial of Facilitating Information Giving to Patients with Chronic Medical Conditions. *J Fam Pract* 48(5):356–
63, 1999.

Mansell, Dorcas, Roy M. Poses, Lewis Kazis, and Corey A. Duefield. Clinical Factors That Influence Patients' Desire for Participation in Decisions About Illness. *Arch Int Med* 160:2991–6,
2000.

Mazur, Dennis J. and David H. Hickam. Patients' Preferences for Risk Disclosure and Role in
Decision Making for Invasive Medical Procedures. *J Gen Intern Med* 12:114–7, 1997.

Mehta, Amit, Keith Dreyer, and James Thrall. Enhancing Availability of the Electronic Image Record
for Patients and Caregivers During Follow-Up Care. *Journal of Digital Imagining* 12(2, Suppl
1):78–80, 1999.

Michael, Max and Clay Bordley. Do Patients Want Access to Their Medical Records? *Medical Care*
20(4):432–5, 1982.

Morris, Alan H. Protocol Management of Adult Respiratory Distress Syndrome. *New Horizons*
1(4):593–602, 1993.

Mort, Elizabeth A. Clinical Decision-Making in the Face of Scientific Uncertainty: Hormone Replacement Therapy as an Example. *J Fam Pract* 42(2):147–51, 1996.

Muir Gray, J A. *Evidence-based Healthcare: How to Make Health Policy and Management Decisions.* New York, NY: Churchill Livingstone, 1997.

O'Connor, Annette M., Alaa Rostom, Fiset Valerie, et al. Decision Aids for Patients Facing Health
Treatment or Screening Decisions: Systematic Review. *BMJ* 319:731–4, 1999.

Pauly, Mark V. *Doctors and their Workshops.* Chicago, IL: NBER, 1980.

Peterkin, Allan. Guidelines Covering Disclosure of Errors Now in Place at Montreal Hospital. *Can Med Assoc J* 142(9):984–5, 1990.

Pietro, Daniel A., Linda J. Shyavitz, Smith Richard A., et al. Detecting and Reporting Medical Errors: Why the Dilemma? *BMJ* 320:794–6, 2000.

Pilcher, June J. and Allen I. Huffcutt. Effects of Sleep Deprivation on Performance: A Meta-Analysis. *Sleep* 19(4):318–26, 1996.

Plsek, Paul. Innovative Thinking for the Improvement of Medical Systems. *Ann Int Med* 131:438–44, 1999.

Rich, Michael L. The PACE Model: Description and Impressions of a Capitated Model of Long-Term Care for the Elderly. *The Care Management Journal* 1(1):62–70, 1999.

Risdale, Leone. *Evidence Based General Practice*. Philadelphia, PA: W.B. Saunders Co., 1995.

Sackett, David L., Sharon E. Straus, W. Scott Richardson, et al. *Evidence-Based Medicine: How to Practice & Teach EBM*. 2nd edition. London, England: Churchill Livingstone, 2000.

Samkoff, Judith S. and C. H. M. Jacques. A Review of Studies Concerning Effects of Sleep Deprivation and Fatigue on Residents' Performance. *Academic Medicine* 66(11):687–93, 1991.

Saphir, Ann. Study Questions Home Efficiency. Nursing Homes Could Cut Costs by More Than a Third and Maintain Productivity, Study Says. *Modern Healthcare* 29:52, 1999.

Sawin, David A. and Mark W. Scerbo. Effects of Instruction Type and Boredom Proneness in Vigilance: Implications for Boredom and Workload. *Human Factors* 37(4):752–65, 1995.

Schoenfelt, Suzanne. New Possiblilities for Patient Information Storage in a Technological Age. *Journal of AHIMA* 69(8):50–4, 1998.

Senge, Peter M. *The Fifth Discipline: The Art and Practice of the Learning Organization*. New York, NY: Doubleday/Currency, 1990.

Shenkin, Budd N. and David C. Warner. Sounding Board. Giving the Patient His Medical Record: A Proposal to Improve the System. *N Engl J Med* 289(13):688–92, 1973.

Simon, Gregory E., Michael VonKorff, Carolyn Rutter, and Edward Wagner. Randomised Trial of Monitoring , Feedback, and Management of Care by Telephone to Improve Treatment of Depression in Primary Care. *BMJ* 320:550–4, 2000.

Smith, Linda S. Concept Analysis: Cultural Competence. *Journal of Cultural Diversity* 5(1):4–10, 1998.

Stacey, Ralph D. *Complexity and Creativity in Organizations*. San Francisco, CA: Berrett-Koehler, 1996.

Stewart, Michael G., Edward J. Hillman, Donald T. Donovan, and Sarper H. Tanli. The Effects of a Practice Guideline on Endoscopic Sinus Surgery at an Academic Center. *American Journal of Rhinology* 11(2):161–5, 1997.

Stewart, Moira A. Effective Physician–Patient Communication and Health Outcomes: A Review. *Can Med Assoc J* 152(9):1423–33, 1995.

Stiggelbout, Anne M. and Gwendoline M. Kiebert. A Role for the Sick Role. Patient Preferences Regarding Information and Participation in Clinical Decision-making. *Can Med Assoc J* 157(4): 383–9, 1997.

Strull, William M., Bernard Lo, and Gerald Charles. Do Patients Want to Participate in Medical Decision Making? *JAMA* 252(21):2990–4, 1984.

Suchyta, Mary R., Terry P. Clemmer, James F. Orme, Jr., et al. Increased Survival of ARDS Patients with Severe Hypoxemia (ECMO Criteria). *Chest* 99(4):951–5, 1991.

Superio-Cabuslay, E., M. M. Ward, and Kate R. Lorig. Patient Education Interventions in Osteoarthritis and Rheumatoid Arthritis: A Meta-Analytic Comparison with Nonsteroidal Antiinflammatory Drug Treatment. *Arthritis Care Res* 9(4):292–301, 1996.

Taylor, Ian. Some Patients Are Happy for Doctors to Make Decisions. *BMJ* 320:58, 2000.

The Ministry of Social Affairs and Health, the National Research and Development Center for Welfare and Health STAKES and The Association of Finnish Local and Regional Authorities. *Quality Management in Social Welfare and Health Care for the 21ˢᵗ Century, National Recommendations.* Sarrijärvi, Finland: Gummerus, 1999.

Thomsen, George E., Donna Pope, Thomas D. East, et al. Clinical Performance of a Rule-Based Decision Support System for Mechanical Ventilation of ARDS patients. *Proc Annu Symp Comput Appl Med Care*:339–43, 1994.

Tidikis, Frank and Leann Strasen. Patient-Focused Care Units Improve Services and Financial Outcomes. *Healthcare Financial Management* 48:38–44, 1994.

Tunick, P. A., S. Etkin, A. Horrocks, et al. Reengineering a cardiovascular surgery service. *Joint Commission Journal on Quality Improvement* 23(4):203–16, 1997.

Von Korff, Michael, Jessie Gruman, Judith Schaefer, Susan J. Curry, and Edward H. Wagner. Collaborative Management of Chronic Illness. *Ann Int Med* 127(12):1097–102, 1997.

Von Korff, Michael, J. E. Moore, Kate R. Lorig, et al. A Randomized Trial of a Lay Person-Led Self-Management Group Intervention for Back Pain Patients in Primary Care. *Spine* 23(23):2608–51, 1998.

Wagner, Edward H., Brian T. Austin, and Michael Von Korff. Organizing Care for Patients with Chronic Illness. *Milbank Quarterly* 74(4):511–42, 1996.

Wagner, Edward H., Paul Barrett, Michael J. Barry, et al. The Effect of a Shared Decisionmaking Program on Rates of Surgery for Benign Prostatic Hyperplasia. Pilot Results. *Medical Care* 33(8):765–70, 1995.

Waldrop, Malcom M. *Complexity: The Emerging Science at the Edge of Order and Chaos.* New York, NY: Simon and Schuster, 1992.

Waller, Adele A. and Oscar L. Alcantara. Ownership of Health Information in the Information Age. *Journal of AHIMA* 69(3):28–38, 1998.

Weed, Lawrence L. Physicians of the Future. *N Engl J Med* 304(15):903–7, 1981.

———. *Knowledge Coupling: New Premises and New Tools for Medical Care and Education.* New York, NY: Springer-Verlag, 1991.

———. Clinical Judgment Revisited. *Methods of Information in Medicine* 38:279–86, 1999.

———. April 2000. Personal communication: telephone conversation.

Weick, Karl E. *Sensemaking in Organizations.* Thousand Oaks, CA: Sage, 1995.

Wells, Kenneth B., Cathy Sherbourne, Michael Schoenbaum, et al. Impact of Disseminating Quality Improvement Programs for Depression in Managed Primary Care: A Randomized Controlled Trial. *JAMA* 283(2):212–20, 2000.

Witman, Amy B., Deric M. Park, and Steven B. Hardin. How Do Patients Want Physicians to Handle Mistakes? *Arch Int Med* 156:2565–9, 1990.

Womack, James P. and Daniel T. Jones. *Lean Thinking: Banish Waste and Create Wealth in Your Corporation.* New York, NY: Simon & Schuster, 1996.

Womack, James P., Daniel T Jones, and Daniel. Roos. *The Machine That Changed the World.* New York, NY: Harpercollins, 1991.

Wu, Albert. Handling Hospital Errors: Is Disclosure the Best Defense? *Ann Int Med* 131(12):970–2, 1999.

Zimmerman, Brenda J., Curt Lindberg, and Paul E. Plsek. *Edgeware: Complexity Resources for Healthcare Leaders.* Irving, TX: VHA Inc., 1998.

4

Taking the First Steps

The committee recognizes the enormity of the change that is required to achieve substantial improvements in the six major aims set forth in Chapter 2—that health care be safe, effective, patient-centered, timely, efficient, and equitable. The ten simple rules described in Chapter 3, designed to help guide the actions of clinicians, patients, and others in ways that will lead to such improvements, also characterize a fundamental cultural transformation taking place today in the health care sector. This nascent cultural transformation embodies a more explicit commitment to evidence-based practice and patient-centered care, and reflects recognition of the importance of well-designed systems of care.

To achieve the six aims, there must also be a very strong commitment to redesign. The current system will not work. New information technology should be embraced and new systems of care developed. Methods of payment must be modified to encourage and reward quality care. This chapter provides an approach for achieving better alignment of the evidence base, the organization of care, information, payment methods, and quality measurement around patients' health care needs.

Common chronic conditions should serve as a starting point for the restructuring of health care delivery because, as noted in Chapter 1, chronic conditions are now the leading cause of illness, disability, and death in the United States, affecting almost half of the population and accounting for the majority of health care resources used (Hoffman et al., 1996). Chronic conditions affect people of all ages. Although older people are more likely to have a chronic condition, people over age 65 account for only one-quarter of those living in the community with such a condition (The Robert Wood Johnson Foundation, 1996).

Today's health care system is not well designed to meet the needs of patients with common chronic conditions. Some patients receive good-quality care that is well coordinated, with good communication among the various clinicians involved. For too many others, however, care for even a single condition is fragmented across many clinicians and settings with little coordination or communication, and some needs remain undetected and/or unmet.

Given the magnitude of the change that is required, the committee believes that leadership at the national level is required to initiate the process of change by taking two important steps. First, a short list of priority conditions should be promulgated by the Department of Health and Human Services, and all health care stakeholders should then focus attention on making substantial progress toward the establishment of state-of-the-art processes for these conditions in the next 5 years. Second, resources should be provided to seed innovative projects at the delivery system level, especially those projects that have a high likelihood of producing knowledge and tools that can be applied on a widespread basis throughout the health care sector.

The committee believes such a focus on specific common clinical conditions is the best way to achieve the substantial improvement in quality that is required. Such conditions represent the needs around which patients have the greatest interaction with the system and make the most choices about cost and quality (and other issues). This is also the level at which care processes can be designed and refined. Thus, priority conditions offer the best opportunity for undertaking the development of the evidence base for practice; the reorganization of care; the development of supportive information technologies; and the design and refinement of quality measures and reporting processes, as well as payment incentives and rewards.

Recommendation 5: The Agency for Healthcare Research and Quality should identify not fewer than 15 priority conditions, taking into account frequency of occurrence, health burden, and resource use. In collaboration with the National Quality Forum, the agency should convene stakeholders, including purchasers, consumers, health care organizations, professional groups, and others, to develop strategies, goals, and action plans for achieving substantial improvements in quality in the next 5 years for each of the priority conditions.

Identifying priority conditions represents a starting point to support the organization of care, bring the evidence base into practice, develop information technology and infrastructure to support care, and develop mechanisms to measure and pay for quality care. Instead of defining care by where it is delivered or who delivers it, the system should be designed to optimize care for patients' needs across the entire continuum of care in the most effective and efficient way possible.

In identifying priority conditions, the Agency for Healthcare Research and Quality (AHRQ) should consider using the list of conditions identified through the Medical Expenditure Panel Survey (MEPS), a nationally representative household survey of health care use, expenditures, sources of payment, and insurance coverage conducted by AHRQ and the National Center for Health Statistics that includes information on health conditions (Medical Expenditure Panel Survey, 2000). MEPS identifies 15 "priority conditions" based on their prevalence, expense, or policy relevance: cancer, diabetes, emphysema, high cholesterol, HIV/AIDS, hypertension, ischemic heart disease, stroke, arthritis, asthma, gall bladder disease, stomach ulcers, back problems, Alzheimer's disease and other dementias, and depression and anxiety disorders.

The action plan for each priority condition should include strategies for designing and maintaining evidence-based processes; promoting primary, secondary and tertiary prevention; building the necessary information technology infrastructure to support delivery and coordination of care, system design and ongoing management, payment, and accountability; and aligning the incentives inherent in payment and accountability processes with the goals of quality improvement. AHRQ should also ensure that each action plan is supported by key stakeholders. In identifying and convening stakeholders, AHRQ should work with the National Quality Forum, a public–private partnership charged with development of a comprehensive quality measurement and public reporting strategy. Input should also be obtained from organizations that have made significant efforts to improve quality, such as the Institute for Healthcare Improvement, the Quality Center at the Bureau of Primary Health Care in the Health Resources Services Administration, the Veterans Health Administration, local delivery systems, and others.

Since the identification of priority conditions is a starting point toward achieving the six aims, AHRQ should conduct this work expeditiously. The number of priority conditions identified should grow over time to eventually cover the majority (e.g., 80 percent) of the care provided to patients.

Recommendation 6: Congress should establish a Health Care Quality Innovation Fund to support projects targeted at (1) achieving the six aims of safety, effectiveness, patient-centeredness, timeliness, efficiency, and equity; and/or (2) producing substantial improvements in quality for the priority conditions. The fund's resources should be invested in projects that will produce a public-domain portfolio of programs, tools, and technologies of widespread applicability.

Policies, incentives, tools, and technologies will be needed to support the changes required to achieve the six aims and redesign the health care system in accordance with the new rules set forth in Chapter 3. The formation of an innovation fund is one mechanism that can be used to seed projects aimed at redesigning care and developing programs to support the other recommendations presented in this report. For example, purchasers and delivery systems should work together to develop innovative programs that integrate the new rules for patient–clinician relationships (Chapter 3) and to redesign care processes for the priority conditions, making best use of information technology and engineering design concepts (Chapters 5 and 7). There must be a strong commitment to evaluating the impact and cost-effectiveness of innovative programs, and to the rapid diffusion of programs proven successful throughout the field. Although an innovation fund should support projects related to the priority conditions, it could also support other redesign projects, especially those relating to greater use of information technology.

The committee is not recommending a specific dollar amount for the proposed fund, but believes a sizable commitment, on the order of $1 billion over 3 to 5 years, is necessary given the magnitude of change needed. Just as a vigorous public commitment and an expenditure of approximately $1 billion over a 4-year period has led to the mapping of the human genome, a similar commitment is needed to retool the health care delivery system, or society will never reap the full value of the trillion dollars spent annually on health care services.

THE VALUE OF ORGANIZING AROUND
PRIORITY CONDITIONS

Identifying priority conditions can benefit all those involved in using, delivering, planning, or paying for health care. Patients and their families today must try to navigate a fragmented, complex health care system with insufficient information and an unclear understanding of how to find the best-quality care for their specific needs. Similarly, health professionals face pressures to improve quality and measurable outcomes without having systems in place that can help them easily identify the best practices for a given case or means of arranging for follow-up on a patient's needs across the entire continuum of care. Purchasers appear to focus more on cost than on quality, but have little outcome or quality information available to them. They may be willing to buy on the basis of quality, but see a health system that produces care inefficiently and is characterized by errors (or "defects") that would not be tolerated in their own industries. Regulators struggle with how best to provide oversight in a rapidly changing environment. Many people have an interest in ensuring quality care, but do not have a framework or tools for doing so.

A focus on priority conditions can align the efforts of diverse participants in the health care system, offer a meaningful level of organization to patients, and provide a starting point on which health care professionals and organizations can focus their efforts. Improved alignment between patient needs and the ways care is organized, delivered, measured, and paid for is important because fragmentation and misalignment in the current system inhibit systematic quality improvement. For example, patients need information, support, and reassurance to manage a chronic condition independently on a day-to-day basis and to recognize when help is needed from a clinician. However, the current health care system is organized around acute care needs. It does not facilitate the flow of information over time; offers little recognition or reward for coordinating care; and pays mainly for face-to-face (office) visits, not for information and/or reassurance that may be needed at other times. The aims described in Chapter 2 cannot be achieved without better alignment of organization, payment, and measurement with patients' needs.

A focus on specific conditions may also be more meaningful to patients. Prior research suggests that when people have a health care need, they are interested in comprehensive sets of services provided to people with similar conditions (Cleary and Edgman-Levitan, 1997; Fennell and Flood, 1998). Instead of describing their health experiences with one service or one provider, patients describe an episode of care (Cleary and Edgman-Levitan, 1997). For example, a patient who has had a heart attack will describe all components of his or her care, including the emergency room, medical service, surgical service, specialty physician office visit, generalist physician office visit, and rehabilitation care. Although the performance of each individual unit is important, simply aggregating the individual units is not sufficient for understanding the quality of health care provided when care involves many people and facilities, as is often the case today (Fennell and Flood, 1998). Additionally, people want information about people "like themselves." That is, they are seeking information that will tell them how well a health plan or clinical group cares for others with similar conditions (Cleary and Edgman-Levitan, 1997). An approach that facilitates the measurement and release of information around specific conditions can provide patients with such information. Also, with appropriately designed incentives and support systems, such an approach can provide an organizing framework for care so that providers have the flexibility to match services along the entire continuum of care to the needs of a specific patient and support continuous care relationships.

Defining care processes around specific conditions can also establish a suitable level of focus for significant quality improvement in health care. To achieve such improvement, it will be necessary to develop information about the processes and outcomes of care for specific population groups (Friedman, 1995). Meaningful groupings are required because the quality of care for one set of conditions cannot be generalized to patients with different conditions (Brook et al., 1996). The tasks of examining processes of care, linking those processes to outcomes for populations, comparing the effectiveness of alternative approaches, bringing the evidence base into practice, forming the teams that deliver complex care, and accurately adjusting for differences among patients to permit valid comparisons are difficult to accomplish simply by looking at patients in general. Rather, these tasks can best be accomplished for people with comparable needs. Once care has been defined around people's needs, meeting those needs becomes the ultimate target for these basic steps of quality improvement.

It is expected that most priority conditions will be strongly related to chronic conditions. As discussed in Chapter 1, care for people with chronic conditions represents an increasing portion of health care resources in the United States. Four chronic conditions (cardiovascular disease, cancer, chronic obstructive pulmonary disease, and diabetes) account for almost three-quarters of all deaths in the United States (Centers for Disease Control and Prevention, 1999). Compared with people with acute conditions, the annual medical costs per person were more than double for people with one chronic condition and almost six times higher for people with two or more chronic conditions[1] (The Robert Wood Johnson Foundation, 1996). A study in one health maintenance organization found that 38 percent of enrollees had at least one chronic condition, and their costs averaged twice those of people with no chronic condition (Fishman et al., 1997). A study at another health maintenance organization found that 78 percent of direct medical costs were attributable to just 25 acute and chronic conditions and that three cardiovascular conditions (ischemic heart disease, hypertension, and congestive heart failure) accounted for 17 percent of those costs (Ray et al., 2000). It has been estimated that the top 1 percent of spenders account for 30 percent of health spending, whereas the bottom 50 percent account for only 3 percent of spending (Berk and Monheit, 1992). Given this concentration, the majority of health services utilized can potentially be associated with a definable list of conditions.

Yet the health care system is not well designed to meet the needs of the chronically ill. The current delivery system responds primarily to acute and urgent health problems, emphasizing diagnosis, ruling out serious conditions, and relieving symptoms (Wagner et al., 1996b). Those with chronic conditions are better served by a systematic approach that emphasizes self-management, care planning with a multidisciplinary team, and ongoing assessment and follow-up (Wagner et al., 1996a). As noted in Chapter 1, successful chronic disease management programs:

• Use a protocol or plan that provides an explicit statement of what needs to be done for patients, at what intervals, and by whom, and that considers the needs of all patients with specific clinical features and how their needs can be met. The care plan is a tool that links the multiple visits and contacts that characterize care for chronic illness.
• Redesign practice to incorporate regular patient contact, collection of critical data on health and disease status, and strategies to meet the educational and psychosocial needs of patients who may need to make lifestyle and other changes to manage their disease. Regular follow-up is a hallmark of the design of successful programs.

---

[1]Direct medical costs included hospital care, physician services, dental services, other professional services, home health care, prescriptions, medical equipment, emergency services, and nursing home care.

• Include a strong focus on patient information and self-management so patients and their families acquire skills in self-management and can make needed lifestyle changes. Structured self-management and behavioral change programs improve patient outcomes.

• Ensure the availability of specialized expertise to the primary care practices that frequently have responsibility for managing patients with chronic illness. The traditional mechanism for accessing expertise is through a consultation or referral, which runs the risk of fragmenting care. Alternative approaches for making expertise available include teams with specialized knowledge (e.g., a diabetologist and nurse specialist working with general practitioners who care for diabetic patients); collaborative care arrangements (e.g., where specialists and generalists manage patients together); and, eventually, well-designed computer decision support systems.

• Rely on having good information about patients, their care, and outcomes in order to improve outcomes. Registries inform providers which patients have certain conditions to permit proactive clinical management. Use of reminder systems supports patient participation in explicit plans of care.

Wagner (2000) also notes the implications of such a model for how teams of clinicians work together. Successful teams should bring in new disciplines in medicine, but also nonmedical personnel. Establishment of care plans, good patient involvement, and a strong information base permit members of a care team to work together beyond organizational and practice boundaries.

Although good coordination and communication are essential for all care, they are especially important for chronic care. Patients may move through many settings of care, from home, to clinician office, to hospital, to nursing home, and back. Patients and their families often provide a sizable proportion of routine care, including the administration of medications, performance of some diagnostic tests, and compliance with physical therapy and nutritional plans. While the current health care system is built around visits, people with chronic illness need flexible models that provide more time and alternative contacts with the system. Although there are many basic, simple techniques that can be employed today (e.g., telephone follow-up rather than e-mail, or reminder systems that use flags on a chart rather than computerized reminder systems), the committee believes these simple techniques have been available for many years and have not been sufficient to achieve broad-based quality improvements. While any type of progress is welcome, at some point the health care system will need to embrace more automated methods and greater use of information technology to make significant progress.

Unfortunately, there are very few well-tested integrated models of chronic care management (Wagner et al., 1996a). While research may focus on specific components of care, it is more difficult to understand the interrelationship between the components and the influence of the organizational environment. For example, the Diabetes Control and Complications Trial demonstrated how to improve clinical management of patients with insulin-dependent diabetes. But the trial required special skills of both patients and clinicians, services that many insurance policies do not cover, and delivery of care by patient-centered teams (Lasker, 1993).

APPLICATIONS OF PRIORITY CONDITIONS

Figure 4-1 illustrates the multiple ways in which the priority conditions, once identified, can be applied. First, they can be used to synthesize the evidence base and delineate practice guidelines. This application is closely linked to and should guide the organization of care and coordination of care around patient needs. The priority conditions can also be applied in developing information systems, reducing suboptimization in payment for services, and simplifying the measurement

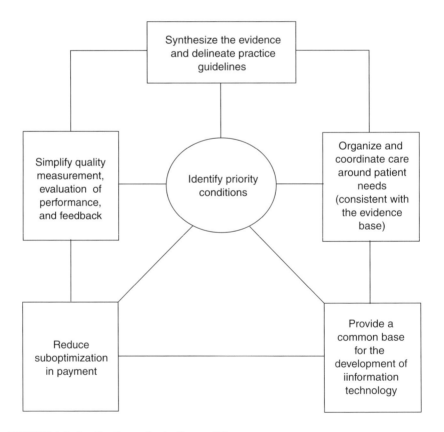

FIGURE 4-1 Applications of priority conditions.

and evaluation of care. Each of these applications is described below. Although some applications may occur more quickly than others, Figure 4-1 is not meant to imply a linear order to their accomplishment. Rather, the priority conditions can be used for any of these applications as soon as they have been identified.

Synthesize the Evidence Base and Delineate Practice Guidelines

The identification of priority conditions provides a framework for synthesizing the evidence, developing practice guidelines, and delineating best practices for clinical care. There is a significant lag between the discovery of better forms of treatment and their incorporation into actual care. The identification of priority conditions supports a well-thought-out organization of information to improve its accessibility and utility for both patients and health professionals (see Chapter 6). Identification of these conditions can guide the prioritization of issues for analysis and synthesis of evidence, delineation of practice guidelines, and development and application of automated decision support tools. It can also provide direction for stronger dissemination efforts aimed at communicating this information to clinicians and consumers. Even in clinical areas characterized by strong evidence and general consensus on practice, variability in practice suggests that current dissemination efforts could be improved. The Internet offers the opportunity to achieve such improvement by reaching sizable proportions of both consumers and clinicians in a timely manner.

One of the strongest examples of synthesizing the evidence base and applying it to clinical care is offered by the Veterans Health Administration (VHA). The VHA's Quality Enhancement Research Initiative (QUERI) is a quality improvement program that focuses on eight priority conditions: chronic heart failure, diabetes, HIV/AIDS, ischemic heart disease, mental health (depression and schizophrenia), spinal cord injury, stroke, and substance abuse (Demakis et al., 2000). These conditions were selected on the basis of the number of veterans affected, the burden of illness, and known health risks among the veteran population. Specific conditions were selected as the focus in the belief that quality improvement is most likely to occur when viewed in the context of the overall care of a patient and population, rather than the individual components of care (Demakis and McQueen, 2000).

The process implemented at the VHA involves defining best practices by reviewing currently available information and literature. For some conditions, such as diabetes, a great deal of information is available; for others, the information must be developed by a planning team. Once the evidence has been reviewed and best practice defined, the latter is compared with current practice to identify gaps in performance. Policies, procedures, and programs are then developed to organize care around the best practice, which also guides the evaluation of impact and feedback to enable learning from experience and continuously improving care. Thus, best practice affects how care is delivered, but evaluation of its impact also informs the continued development of best practice. The process used by the VHA also emphasizes the broad dissemination of information about best practice throughout their system, from large academic centers to smaller, community-based centers.

The VHA's approach is consistent with the concept of focusing on priority conditions in that it provides a framework for organizing and continually updating the evidence base, bringing it to the direct delivery of care, and evaluating its effect on improving care for patients. Synthesis and application of the evidence base, therefore, forces the reexamination of how care is organized to affect quality. By examining where current practice departs from the evidence base and best practice, suggestions for improving care may emerge that can direct changes in provider actions, patient responsibilities, or organizational approaches. It would be difficult to use this multifaceted, comprehensive care approach except at the level of a specific condition.

Organize and Coordinate Care Around Patient Needs

The primary purpose of identifying priority conditions is to facilitate the organization of care around the patient's perspective and needs rather than, as in the current system, around types of professionals and organizations. For example, the current system may require patients to travel to multiple locations to receive care (usually Monday through Friday, between 8:00 a.m. and 5:00 p.m.) instead of using modern technologies to facilitate access even for patients with mobility problems or those living in rural areas. Most hospitals are organized around physician specialties (such as thoracic surgery or internal medicine), not around common clinical needs of patients, which may cross departmental boundaries. (An example is diabetes care, which may require general medicine, endocrinology, ophthalmology, and vascular services.) Organizing care around priority conditions emphasizes meeting the needs of patients with those conditions, regardless of who provides their care or where. Attention must be paid to how care is coordinated across settings and provider types. A surgical procedure may be performed perfectly, but if there is inadequate postoperative care, follow-up care, home care, or other supports, the patient may encounter complications that compromise the quality of the episode of care. It is also important to recognize that patients may have to manage multiple conditions simultaneously, because they either have more than one chronic condition or have one chronic condition and an unrelated acute event. Indeed, there is evidence that patients actively receiving care for one chronic condition may not receive treatment for other, unrelated conditions (Redelmeier et al., 1998). Thus, one of the challenges of designing care around specific conditions is to avoid defining patients solely by their disease or condition.

There are several mechanisms for coordinating care across priority conditions. First, coordination could be performed by a health professional acting as a liaison across patients' multiple needs, ensuring the exchange of information and any necessary follow-up[2] (Bodenheimer et al., 1999). This individual could be a physician, nurse, case manager, or other type of professional working in the care delivery system. Second, some consumers might choose to actively coordinate their own care. This is a growing possibility as consumers and patients have access to more health information and are able to make use of the evidence base and practice guidelines for their specific conditions. Third, as information technology becomes more sophisticated, computer algorithms can be used to coordinate many activities, for example, sending reminders of needed follow-up or identifying missing information, such as test results. Finally, coordination could occur through a combination of all these methods, involving a health professional, the patient, and technological support.

Various approaches in practice today offer insight that can be applied in organizing care around specific conditions or types of needs, including disease management programs and centers of excellence. Each is briefly reviewed below.

Disease Management Programs

Multiple definitions of disease management programs have been put forth (Blumenthal and Buntin, 1998; Ellrodt et al., 1997; Homer, 1997). In general, they describe a systematic and comprehensive approach to improving the management of a condition. This approach involves improving coordination of care and controlling costs through the integration of components across the entire delivery system and the application of appropriate tools (e.g., guidelines, protocols, information systems) specifically designed for the population in question.

Disease management programs share some of the features envisioned for organization around priority conditions as described above, but also differ in important ways. The two are similar in that disease management represents a systematic approach to designing care, uses multidisciplinary teams to deliver care, and potentially includes services across the entire continuum of care. However, disease management programs differ in that they are frequently perceived primarily as a method for controlling costs (Bodenheimer, 2000; Homer, 1997; Ketner, 1999). They are often applied only to the most severely ill patients (generally categorized by historical costs) instead of to the entire population with a specific condition (Hunter, 2000; Ketner, 1999). This means not all patients with a condition are able to benefit from such programs. Although the programs are developed to improve care for patients, patients may not have much say in whether they receive care through such programs. Finally, there are no clear

---

[2]It should be noted that this discussion of coordination of care is not meant to imply support for or opposition to a gate-keeping function used by many groups to ensure appropriate access. Coordination can be provided with or without a gate-keeping role.

definitions of what is included or excluded from such programs, making it difficult to compare their effectiveness in treating similar populations.

One of the main concerns associated with disease management programs is the potential for fragmenting care, especially if the patient's primary care physician is not involved in the program. Again, this concern highlights the importance of coordination across conditions and the need to design such coordination systematically into care processes. Primary care models offer one approach to coordination, in which the primary care practitioner is both provider and coordinator of care. Alternatively, programs can be designed specifically to include or link an individual's primary care practitioners in care planning and assessment. The committee does not recommend one approach over another, but emphasizes the importance of designing coordination into care to avoid fragmentation.

Centers of Excellence

There is a growing body of evidence on the relationship between volume of service and outcomes. The IOM conducted a workshop in May 2000 to explore the volume–outcome relationship (Hewitt, 2000). A systematic review of the literature conducted for the workshop encompassed 88 studies concerning eight conditions and procedures.[3] This review led to the conclusion that for a wide variety of procedures, higher volume (by either the hospital or physician) is associated with better health outcomes. Statistically significant associations between higher volume and better outcomes were found in 79 percent of studies of hospital volume and 77 percent of studies of physician volume. None of the studies showed a negative effect of volume.

The Health Care Financing Administration has pursued Centers of Excellence as a way of operationalizing the volume–outcome relationship. Centers of Excellence are hospitals and physician groups that meet high quality standards, for which they are paid a single bundled fee for all services related to specific, complex procedures (Health Care Financing Administration, 1999). Evaluation of the experience with cardiac surgery has indicated that the approach can offer cost savings without compromising quality, measured as mortality rates (Cromwell et al., 1997). Although developed as a payment policy, the approach bears some similarity to organizing around priority conditions in that it gives health care organizations and professionals the flexibility to organize care appropriately for a specific population group. The approach is dissimilar in that it is focused primarily on selected complex procedures with a strong emphasis on costs, rather than being solely a quality-driven strategy (Cromwell et al., 1997; Health Care Financing Administration, 1999).

---

[3]Coronary artery bypass graft surgery, pediatric cardiac surgery, carotid endarterectomy, abdominal aortic aneurysm repair, cancer surgery, percutaneous transluminal coronary angioplasty, acute myocardial infarction, and acquired immunodeficiency syndrome (AIDS).

Provide a Common Base for the Development of Information Technology

Priority conditions can provide a framework for the development of an information infrastructure that is aligned around the clinical conditions frequently faced by patients. The absence of well-designed care processes is currently an impediment to the development and application of effective information technology systems. To be most useful, information technology must be designed to support the work of the care team. Consciously and skillfully designed care processes for priority conditions are an important step in establishing a foundation from which to design supportive information technology applications.

Common information technology systems are needed to effectively measure outcomes and processes of care and to provide benchmarks for continuous improvement. Currently, each provider group may implement its own information system, but incompatibilities inhibit communication among the many people caring for an individual patient. Priority conditions can provide a focus for the development of standards and terminology for use in managing and using information technology to improve care for patients. Best practices can help define standard information needs and guide the development of information technologies that can be used to implement best practices (e.g., decision support systems).

A significantly enhanced information infrastructure is critical to achieving the aims set forth in Chapter 2 and the other potential applications of the priority conditions. Synthesizing the evidence base, linking it to clinical practice, and making it accessible to a variety of potential users will require good information systems and, most likely, greater use of the Internet. Greater use of the Internet and telemedicine should in turn facilitate access to clinical expertise and support care for patients in their own communities, especially in rural areas. Better flows of information are also necessary to improve the ways care is organized and coordinated, especially across settings and over time. Using payment methods to reward quality will require stronger information systems to track costs and link them to processes of care. Finally, measurement and evaluation cannot be advanced without better technology for data collection and management (see Chapter 7 for further discussion on using information technology).

Reduce Suboptimization in Payment

A major barrier to quality improvement is the lack of reward that characterizes the most common payment methods used today (see Chapter 8). The current payment system often reinforces fragmentation by paying separately according to the setting of care and provider type, and by not giving providers the flexibility needed to customize care for individual patients. Furthermore, common payment methods can inhibit quality improvement to the extent that organizations that improve certain aspects of quality (e.g., by reducing readmission rates or office visits) can experience a reduction in their revenues, which serves as a disincentive for continuous improvement.

Priority conditions offer a framework for linking payment with patient needs and for designing incentives to reward quality. Alternative payment methods (e.g., fee for service or capitation) could be adapted to facilitate the delivery of care around priority conditions, consistent with the evidence base. Priority conditions could also provide a framework for purchasers to use in assessing the value of their purchases. See Chapter 8 for a detailed discussion on the relationship between payment and quality improvement.

Simplify Quality Measurement, Evaluation of Performance, and Feedback

Priority conditions improve the feasibility of quality measurement by offering a framework for the development of standards to guide the necessary data collection. At present, quality measurement for external accountability tends to focus on institutions or discrete services; there is little comparative information available for patients seeking specific care or physicians referring care. For example, a patient can obtain information on mammogram rates, but will find little information on methods of treatment or outcomes for breast care programs. Priority conditions can offer a framework for the development of core measures that address both processes and outcomes of care.

Part of the difficulty involved in obtaining such information is due to methodological barriers in measurement. The services of an individual physician are usually too small a unit for measurement of many aspects of clinical care processes and outcomes (Hofer et al., 1999). Even the typically sized medical group may be too small to provide reliable information on outcomes. Health plans may aggregate information, but clinicians are often affiliated with multiple plans. The delineation of priority conditions, the organization of services around these conditions, and the development of core sets of measures may help overcome some of these barriers to measurement.

Public- and private-sector oversight organizations are already organizing some of their activities around particular conditions. For example, the Foundation for Accountability has developed population- or condition-specific quality measurement guides related to adult asthma, alcohol misuse, breast cancer, diabetes, health status under age 65, and major depressive disorders (Foundation for Accountability, 1999a) and continues to work on quality measurement and consumer reporting approaches in the areas of child and adolescent health, coronary artery disease, end of life, and HIV/AIDS (Foundation for Accountability, 1999b). The Foundation's model organizes comparative information about quality performance into five categories based on how consumers think about their care: the basics, staying healthy, getting better, living with illness, and changing needs.

The Joint Commission on Accreditation of Healthcare Organizations (2000) has identified five specific areas for the development of indicators to assess hospital care: acute myocardial infarction, heart failure, pneumonia, surgical procedures and complications, and pregnancy and related conditions. Accreditation by the National Committee for Quality Assurance includes measures related to how well a health plan cares for people when they have a chronic illness in such areas as cardiovascular disease, cancer, asthma, pneumonia and influenza, and diabetes (National Committee for Quality Assurance, 1999). Peer Review Organizations focus their national quality improvement efforts on six clinical priority areas: acute myocardial infarction, breast cancer, diabetes, heart failure, pneumonia, and stroke (Health Care Financing Administration, 2000). Finally, the National Quality Forum is developing a comprehensive quality measurement and reporting strategy that will address priorities for quality measurement that are consistent with the national aims for quality improvement in health care set forth in this report (National Quality Forum for Health Care Quality Measurement and Reporting, 2000).

CRITERIA FOR IDENTIFYING
PRIORITY CONDITIONS

Various criteria can be used to identify the priority conditions. Two IOM committees have suggested criteria for setting priorities among conditions: one committee focused on how to set priorities for guideline development, the other on how to set priorities for technology assessment. The common criteria from both processes included prevalence, burden of illness, cost, variability in practice, and the potential to improve outcomes or reduce costs (Institute of Medicine, 1992, 1995).

As noted earlier, this committee suggests starting with the priority conditions identified in the MEPS. Some are long-term life-threatening conditions, such as cancer, diabetes, emphysema, high cholesterol, HIV/AIDS, hypertension, ischemic heart disease, and stroke. Others, such as arthritis, asthma, gall bladder disease, stomach ulcers, and back problems of any kind, are categorized as chronic manageable conditions. The list also includes Alzheimer's disease, depression, and anxiety disorders. MEPS obtains a larger sample size for seven of the conditions—hypertension, ischemic heart disease, asthma, diabetes, stroke, emphysema, and arthritis—to make population estimates. Although other sources are also available, the advantage of starting with the MEPS listing is its representative population sample, as opposed to claims data that rely on services having been used.

PROVIDING THE RESOURCES NEEDED
TO INITIATE CHANGE

The health care system in the United States needs significant redesign. Given the magnitude of the change required, the innovation fund recommended earlier is needed to seed projects that can help apply the concepts described in this report. A Health Care Quality Innovation Fund should finance the demonstration and evaluation of programs designed to implement the types of changes recommended in this report. Although a specific agenda should be established, the areas of interest for funding should address one or more of the issues covered in this report: techniques for implementing the rules for redesigning care set forth in Chapter 3, applying evidence to health care delivery, using information technology, aligning payment policies for quality, and preparing the workforce.

Emphasis should be placed on funding projects that will integrate the resulting innovations into processes of care. The goal is not simply to fund "good ideas," but rather to fund the implementation of good ideas in real-life settings, focusing on innovations that have a good likelihood of broad applicability to other sites. Evaluations will need to be carefully structured to be able to assess the programmatic features that contributed to a project's successful implementation, including how technical, cultural, and economic factors were addressed. Barriers encountered should also be identified, as well as how they were overcome or whether they presented too great an obstacle.

Funding may be provided to individual local health care organizations, private partnerships (e.g., those between purchasers and delivery systems), or public–private partnerships (e.g., those among delivery systems, local public health agencies, and consumer groups). Possible projects may relate to the direct delivery of health care for a specific population or to the development of an infrastructure that facilitates needed change (e.g., approaches for sharing data).

A portion of the Health Care Quality Innovation Fund should be set aside to provide resources to answer critical research questions. Implementation and evaluation of innovative projects are important, but some areas may require additional understanding to guide demonstrations and their implementation. For example, the change to using relative value units as a payment approach for physicians was legislated in 1989 for implementation in 1992, following about 10 years of research, testing, and evaluation (Hsaio and Stason, 1979). Possible areas requiring additional organizational research include understanding how financial and other types of incentives relate to organizational setting, how physician and nonphysician members of the care team can optimally interact and complement each other, what components and interactions of systems of care are most important for improving quality, and how to organize care for people with chronic conditions.

The committee views public support as important for catalyzing the needed changes for several reasons. First, a commitment of funds over several years can ensure a sustained and stable funding source. Projects funded by health care organizations through operating revenues represent a valuable contribution, but the stability and level of funding can be unpredictable, and perhaps unsustainable, in a rapidly changing marketplace.

Second, public support can provide partial funding for the up-front costs that health care organizations face in undertaking the changes recommended in this report. Organizations should be prepared to support the continuing costs of any initiatives, but public funding for some portion of up-front costs can be a valuable resource for an organization that is interested, willing, and ready to redesign the delivery of health care to improve quality. Thus, the Health Care Quality Innovation Fund represents a public–private approach to change, with the public sector providing seed money and the private sector using operating revenue to fund some of the up-front costs and any ongoing costs.

Third, rather than trying to identify large programs aimed at reforming the entire system, smaller applied projects of varying size and focus should be permitted to flourish. Public funding for a mix of projects would permit midcourse corrections to be made as greater understanding is gained on what types of projects work or fail. Use of public seed money can also require an objective evaluation of demonstration projects and public access to the tools and techniques used. Rather than remaining in the private domain, the information becomes a public good for use by all to learn how to improve health care quality.

Research and demonstrations for organizational redesign in health care occur today in both the private and public sectors, although the level of effort appears to be modest given the size of the task ahead. In the private sector, one of the main sources of funds for organizational design research is foundations. The Robert Wood Johnson Foundation has sponsored the Changes in Health Care Financing and Organization Program since 1988. It has provided over $50 million to stimulate research into new strategies in the financing and organization of health care and the impact of changes in the delivery system on quality, access, and costs. The program funds research, policy analysis, demonstrations, and evaluations to provide timely information to policy makers, purchasers, providers, and researchers.

Some health care organizations also devote a portion of their revenues to research and development projects. For example, Kaiser-Permanente has conducted work on risk adjustment methods for payment policy; Group Health Cooperative of Puget Sound has conducted extensive work on improving care for populations with chronic illness; and Intermountain Health Care in Salt Lake City has developed data systems for evaluating and improving process of care. Organizational design research is also being conducted at universities across the country.

On the public side, the primary source of funds for organizational design research is AHRQ. The Center for Organization and Delivery Studies was created in 1996 to provide leadership for research on health care markets, delivery systems and organizations (Agency for Healthcare Research and Quality, 2000a). The Integrated Delivery System Research Network is a new model of field-based research that partners health services researchers with large health care systems to develop and disseminate evidence on data and measurement systems and organizational best practices (Agency for Healthcare Research and Quality, 2000b). Approximately $4 million has been allocated over a 3-year period. Other AHRQ projects also contribute to innovation in health care delivery, such as work in medical informatics and patient safety. Other investments in organizational redesign in the public sector include those of the VHA, whose Quality Enhancement Research Initiative effort was described earlier in this chapter, and the Health Care Financing Administration's Office of Research and Development, funded at approximately $55 million in fiscal year 2001 (a decline of 11 percent from the prior year) (U.S. Department of Health and Human Services, 2000a). A portion of those funds supports projects that are consistent with redesigning health care delivery, including work related to competitive pricing, coordinated care for the chronically ill, and Centers of Excellence.

A great many resources are devoted to technological innovation in health care in the areas of pharmaceuticals, medical devices, and biotechnology. Investment in research and development was estimated at almost $36 billion in 1995, or about 3.5 percent of total health care spending (Neumann and Sandberg, 1998). Over $30 billion has been invested each year since 1993. Just over half of the investments were made in the private sector; the remainder of the spending was in the public sector, primarily the National Institutes of Health.

Although such investments have produced great advances in technological innovation, however, they have produced little innovation in the organization and delivery of care. The irony is that the current health care system cannot ensure that the new technologies are delivered effectively, efficiently, and safely to the people that can most appropriately benefit from them. This dilemma will likely worsen in the future with expected advances in genome research, tissue reengineering, pharmacogenetics, and other areas.

As noted earlier, the committee has not recommended a specific amount for a Health Care Quality Innovation Fund, but believes that an amount on the order of $1 billion over 3 to 5 years is needed. This amount represents one-quarter of 1 percent of the almost $400 billion the federal government currently spends on health care. By comparison, the top ten funded diseases at the National Institutes of Health were funded at $3.6 billion *just for the year 1996* (Gross et al., 1999), while approximately $1 billion was devoted to the human genome project over the last 4 years (U.S. Department of Health and Human Services, 2000b). There is no central source for determining the extent of public and private investments in innovation in health care organization and delivery; however, the public- and private-sector initiatives identified above may total $100 million annually. This is far short of the amount needed for the magnitude of changes required and far less than the $36 billion expended annually for technology research.

The following are examples of the types of projects that might be supported through the recommended fund.[4]

---

[4]These examples draw on some of the approaches to redesign being pursued by clinical leaders who were interviewed as part of an Institute of Medicine study aimed at identifying exemplary practices (Donaldson and Mohr, 2000).

Example 1—Using Information Technology to Improve the Timeliness of Services in a Hospital Emergency Department

An emergency department sought to redesign the process of care by reducing the time required to provide complete care to a patient—the cycle time. Reducing cycle times improves both patient satisfaction and productivity. The staff identified key processes of care, such as x-ray cycle time, time between arrival at the emergency department and seeing a physician, and time needed to get a patient admitted to a bed. They introduced the concept of parallel processing and designed algorithms to permit the simultaneous performance of multiple tasks. Additionally, they developed their own tracking system (since nothing acceptable for the purpose was available from vendors) to track where patients are in the process of care, as well as the status of the system, in 15-minute increments (almost real time). A touch screen informs staff instantly of any problems in specific care processes so they can intervene quickly. These efforts have reduced total cycle time for less urgent patients from 92 to 47 minutes, time between arrival and seeing a physician from 32 to 18 minutes, time between decision to admit and getting the patient to the floor from 210 to 60 minutes, and x-ray cycle time from 92 to 32 minutes. If supported by an innovation fund, this project would share its algorithms and tracking system, along with pitfalls encountered during the redesign, so that the improved process would be disseminated to other emergency departments.

Example 2—A Partnership to Improve Chronic Care

A hospital, two small primary care practices, and an endocrinologist decided to collaborate on the development of a state-of-the-art diabetic care program. They began by reviewing the practice guidelines and agreeing on the key elements of preventive, acute, and chronic care. In an attempt to identify best practices, they visited two of the leading diabetic care programs. They then reached agreement on the key elements of a care process, and on the quality measures to be collected and used in assessing the care process and patient outcomes. They also worked to establish an interactive patient education program, which could be used online or viewed on video in the office. A diabetic care team was formed, consisting of two primary care physicians, a nurse practitioner, and an endocrinologist. Relying heavily on e-mail, they were able to establish procedures for ongoing communication and management of diabetic patients.

Example 3—Reorganizing Staff for Patient-Centered Primary Care

A primary care center with multiple offices served 270,000 patients with 110 full-time equivalents (FTEs). The center had a 55-day waiting period for appointments, resulting in packed schedules for staff, a chaotic office environment, an overused urgent care clinic, and unhappy patients. The center decided to develop an open-access system so that patients could get an appointment either the same day they called or the next day, with their own physician whenever possible. Under the old system, patients calling for appointments would be sorted according to need: wellness care, acute illness, or chronic care. This approach was ineffective because patients might have two or three needs simultaneously; thus, they would make multiple appointments to meet different needs or go to the urgent care clinic, which further stressed the system.

In the redesigned system, the staff was organized into 15 teams, each with 7 to 9 physicians and nurse practitioners; the urgent care clinic was closed, and that staff was reassigned to the regular offices. Patients were no longer categorized according to the nurse's or receptionist's assessment of their need, but were seen based on their own perception of need. Whereas the number of visits was expected to increase because of "patients' insatiable demands," the total number of patient visits declined by 7 percent, and the no-show rate went from 20 percent to being "too small to show up in the statistics." Patients could meet all their needs in one visit with their regular doctor (rather than in one visit to the urgent care clinic and another visit to their regular doctor). The rate of patients able to see their own physician increased from 47 to 75 percent. The provision of preventive services also increased. Additionally, fewer patient charts were lost because they were pulled the day the patients came in, and with fewer lost charts, clinicians were more likely to have the information they needed when seeing a patient. Overall costs decreased because of fewer visits and the closure of the urgent care clinic. Additionally, the center thought it would be necessary to hire additional staff, but when the operational system was improved, this was not the case, so cost increases were avoided. If such a project were funded by an innovation fund, the primary care center would share its tools for appointment scheduling and staffing design.

The above examples illustrate the range and depth of redesign efforts that should occur. Because such efforts can be disruptive to current operations and take extended periods of time to accomplish, health care professionals and organizations need extra support and incentive to undertake them. An innovation fund should support the implementation of projects that could not otherwise be conducted during the routine course of business because they would be too disruptive for the patients and staff. As suggested in Example 1 above, use of a new information technology can be quite disruptive to the provision of services and staff functioning. In some cases, redesign may be so fundamental that temporary closure of a service may be required. For example, in another case that was part of an IOM study of exemplary practices (Donaldson and Mohr, 2000), one medical group had to close its offices for a short period of time to make the changes they deemed necessary. Few health care professionals and organizations can undertake such drastic steps to substantially reorganize their care processes without special (and temporary) assistance. Additional examples of reengineering and redesign projects are provided in Chapter 5.

REFERENCES

Agency for Healthcare Research and Quality. 2000a. "Overview: Center for Organization and Delivery Studies." Online. Available at http://www.ahrq.gov/about/cods/codsover.htm [accessed Jan. 29, 2001].

————. 2000b. "Integrated Delivery System Research Network (ISDRN): Field Partnerships to Conduct and Use Research, Fact Sheet. AHRQ Publication No. 01-P004." Online. Available at http://www.ahrq.gov/research/idsrn.htm [accessed Jan. 29, 2001].

Berk, Marc L. and Alan C. Monheit. The Concentration of Health Expenditures: An Update. *Health Affairs* 11(4):145–9, 1992.

Blumenthal, David and Melinda Beeuwkes Buntin. Carve Outs: Definition, Experience, and Choice Among Candidate Conditions. *American Journal of Managed Care* 4(Suppl):SP45–57, 1998.

Bodenheimer, Thomas. Disease Management in the American Market. *BMJ* 320:563–6, 2000.

Bodenheimer, Thomas, Bernard Lo, and Lawrence Casalino. Primary Care Physicians Should Be Coordinators, Not Gatekeepers. *JAMA* 281(21):2045–9, 1999.

Brook, Robert H., Elizabeth A. McGlynn, and Paul D. Cleary. Part 2: Measuring Quality of Care. *N Engl J Med* 335(13):966–70, 1996.

Centers for Disease Control and Prevention. 1999. "Chronic Diseases and Their Risk Factors: The Nation's Leading Causes of Death." Online. Available at http://www.cdc.gov/nccdphp/statbook/statbook.htm [accessed Dec. 7, 2000].

Cleary, Paul D. and Susan Edgman-Levitan. Health Care Quality: Incorporating Consumer Perspectives. *JAMA* 278(19):1608–12, 1997.

Cromwell, Jerry, Debra A. Dayhoff, and Armen H. Thoumaian. Cost Savings and Physician Responses to Global Bundled Payments for Medicare Heart Bypass Surgery. *Health Care Financing Review* 19(1):41–57, 1997.

Demakis, John G. and Lynn McQueen, July 11, 2000. Office of Health Services Research and Development Services, Veterans Administration. Personal communication: telephone conversation.

Demakis, John G., Lynn McQueen, Kenneth W. Kizer, and John R. Feussner. Quality Enhancement Research Initiative (QUERI): A collaboration between research and clinical practice. *Medical Care* 38(6, Suppl 1):I17–25, 2000.

Donaldson, Molla S. and Julie J. Mohr. *Exploring Innovation and Quality Improvement in Health Care Micro-Systems: A Cross-Case Analysis.* Washington, D.C.: Institute of Medicine, National Academy Press, 2000.

Ellrodt, Gray, Deborah J. Cook, Jean Lee, et al. Evidence-Based Disease Management. *JAMA* 278(20):1687–92, 1997.

Fennell, Mary L. and Ann B. Flood. Key Challenges in Studying Organizational Issues in Delivery of Healthcare to Older Americans. *Health Services Research* 33(June;Part II):424–33, 1998.

Fishman, Paul, Michael Von Korff, Paula Lozano, and Julia Hecht. Chronic Care Costs In Managed Care. The first single-plan comparison of chronic care costs shows why cost-effective clinical approaches are critical to managed care success. *Health Affairs* 16(3):239–47, 1997.

Foundation for Accountability. *Accountability Action* 3(2), 1999a.

————. 1999b. "Foundation for Accountability (FACCT) homepage." Online. Available at http://www.facct.org [accessed Dec. 7, 2000].

Friedman, Maria A. Issues in Measuring and Improving Health Care Quality. *Health Care Financing Review* 16(4):1–13, 1995.

Gross, Cary P., Gerard F. Anderson, and Neil R. Powe. The Relation between Funding by the National Institutes of Health and the Burden of Disease. *N Engl J Med* 340(24):1881–7, 1999.

Health Care Financing Administration. 1999. "Fact Sheet: Medicare's Prudent Purchasing Initiative." Online. Available at http://www.hcfa.gov/facts/fsprud.htm [accessed Dec. 7, 2000].

————. 2000. "Peer Review Organizations (PROs). Medicare's Health Care Quality Improvement Program v5-2." Online. Available at http://www.hcfa.gov/quality/5b1.htm [accessed Dec. 7, 2000].

Hewitt, Maria for the Committee on the Quality of Health Care in America and the National Cancer Policy Board. *Interpreting the Volume–Outcome Relationship in the Context of Health Care Quality.* Washington, D.C.: Institute of Medicine, National Academy Press, 2000. Online. Available at http://books.nap.edu/catalog/10005.html [accessed Jan. 29, 2001].

Hofer, Timothy P., Rodney A. Hayward, Sheldon Greenfield, et al. The Unreliability of Individual Physician "Report Cards" for Assessing the Costs and Quality of Care of a Chronic Disease. *JAMA* 281(22):2098–105, 1999.

Hoffman, Catherine, Dorothy P. Rice, and Hai-Yen Sung. Persons with Chronic Conditions. Their Prevalence and Costs. *JAMA* 276(18): 1473–9, 1996.

Homer, Charles J. Asthma Disease Management. *N Engl J Med* 337(20):1461–3, 1997.

Hsaio, W. C. and W. B. Stason. Toward Developing a Relative Value Scale for Medical and Surgical Services. *Health Care Financing Review* 1(23):23–38, 1979.

Hunter, David J. Disease Management: Has it a Future? *BMJ* 320:530, 2000.

Institute of Medicine *Setting Priorities for Health Technologies Assessment: A Model Process.* Molla S. Donaldson and Harold C. Sox, Jr., Eds. Washington, D.C.: National Academy Press, 1992.

―――. *Setting Priorities for Clinical Practice Guidelines.* Marilyn J. Field, ed. Washington, D.C.: National Academy Press, 1995.

Joint Commission on Accreditation of Healthcare Organizations. 2000. "ORYX: The Next Evolution in Accreditation. Questions and Answers about the Joint Commission's Planned Integration of Performance Measures into the Accreditation Process." Online. Available at http://www.jcaho.org/perfmeas/oryx%5Fqa.html [accessed Dec. 7, 2000].

Ketner, Lisa. Population Management Takes Disease Management to the Next Level. *Healthcare Financial Management* 53(8):36–9, 1999.

Lasker, Roz D. The Diabetes Control and Complications Trial, Implications for Policy and Practice. *N Engl J Med* 329(14):1035–6, 1993.

Medical Expenditure Panel Survey. 2000. "MEPS HC-006R: 1996 Medical Conditions." Online. Available at http://www.meps.ahrq.gov/catlist.htm [accessed Dec. 7, 2000].

National Committee for Quality Assurance. 1999. "NCQA Releases Final HEDIS 2000 Measures; Focus is on Heart Disease, Asthma, Women's Health." Online. Available at http://www.ncqa.org/Pages/Communications/news/H2KFINREL.html [accessed Dec. 7, 2000].

National Quality Forum for Health Care Quality Measurement and Reporting. 2000. "National Quality Forum Mission." Online. Available at http://www.qualityforum.org/mission/home.htm [accessed Dec. 7, 2000].

Neumann, Peter J. and Eileen A. Sandberg. Trends in Health Care R&D and Technology Innovation. *Health Affairs* 17(6):111–9, 1998.

Ray, G. Thomas, Tracy Lieu, Bruce Fireman, et al. The Cost of Health Conditions in a Health Maintenance Organization. *Medical Care Research and Review* 57(1):92–109, 2000.

Redelmeier, Donald A., Siew H. Tan, and Gillian L. Booth. The Treatment of Unrelated Disorders in Patients with Chronic Medical Diseases. *N Engl J Med* 338(21):1516–20, 1998.

The Robert Wood Johnson Foundation. *Chronic Care in America: A 21ˢᵗ Century Challenge.* Princeton, NJ: The Robert Wood Johnson Foundation, 1996. Online. Available at http://www.rwjf.org/library/chrcare/ [accessed Sept. 19, 2000].

U.S. Department of Health and Human Services. 2000a. "Fiscal Year 2001 Budget Request, Health Care Financing Administration." Online. Available at http://www.hcfa.gov/testimony/2000/000208.htm [accessed Jan. 29, 2001].

U.S. Department of Health and Human Services, National Institutes of Health National Human Genome Research Institute. 2000b. "FY 2001 Budget." Online. Available at http://www.nhgri.nih.gov/NEWS/fy2001.pdf [accessed Dec. 7, 2000].

Wagner, Edward H. The Role of Patient Care Teams in Chronic Disease Management. *BMJ* 320:569–72, 2000.

Wagner, Edward H., Brian T. Austin, and Michael Von Korff. Improving Outcomes in Chronic Illness. *Managed Care Quarterly* 42(2):12–25, 1996a.

―――. Organizing Care for Patients with Chronic Illness. *Milbank Quarterly* 74(4):511–42, 1996b.

5

Building Organizational
Supports for Change

Between front-line clinical care teams and the health care environment lies an array of health care organizations, including hospitals, managed care organizations, medical groups, multispeciality clinics, integrated delivery systems, and others. Leaders of today's health care organizations face a daunting challenge in redesigning the organization and delivery of care to meet the aims set forth in this report. They face pressures from employees and medical staff, as well as from the local community, including residents, business and service organizations, regulators, and other agencies. It is difficult enough to balance the needs of those many constituencies under ordinary circumstances. It is especially difficult when one is trying to change routine processes and procedures to alter how people conduct their everyday work, individually and collectively.

This chapter describes a general process of organizational development and then offers a set of tools and techniques, drawing heavily from engineering concepts, as a starting point for identifying how organizations might redesign care. Chapter 3 offered a set of rules that would redesign the nature of interactions between a clinician and a patient to improve the quality of care. This chapter describes how organizations can redesign care to systematically improve the quality of care for patients. This is not an exhaustive list of possible approaches, but a sampling of techniques used in other fields that might have applicability in health care. The broad areas discussed in this chapter apply to all health care organizations; the specific tools and techniques used would need to be adapted to an organization's local environment and patients.

Recommendation 7: The Agency for Healthcare Research and Quality and private foundations should convene a series of workshops involving representatives from health care and other industries and the research community to identify, adapt, and implement state-of-the-art approaches to addressing the following challenges:

- **Redesign of care processes based on best practices**
- **Use of information technologies to improve access to clinical information and support clinical decision making**
- **Knowledge and skills management**
- **Development of effective teams**
- **Coordination of care across patient conditions, services, and settings over time**
- **Incorporation of performance and outcome measurements for improvement and accountability**

To achieve the six aims identified in Chapter 2, board members, chief executive officers, chief information officers, chief financial officers, and clinical managers of all types of health care organizations will need to take steps to redesign care processes. The recommended series of workshops is intended to serve multiple purposes: (1) to help communicate the recommendations and findings of this report and engage leaders and managers of health care organizations in the pursuit of the aims, (2) to provide knowledge and tools that will be helpful to these individuals, and (3) to encourage the development of formal and informal networks of individuals involved in innovation and improvement.

STAGES OF ORGANIZATIONAL DEVELOPMENT

The design of health care organizations can be conceptualized as progressing through three stages of development to a final stage that embodies the committee's vision for the 21st-century health care system, as represented by the six aims set forth in Chapter 2 (see Table 5-1). Although settings and practices vary, the committee believes much of the health sector has been working at Stages 2 and 3 over the last decade or more. As knowledge and technologies continue to advance and the complexity of care delivery grows, the evolution to Stage 4 will require that Stage 3 organizations accelerate efforts to redesign their approaches to interacting with patients, organizing services, providing training, and utilizing the health care workforce.

Stage 1

Stage 1 is characterized by a highly fragmented delivery system, with physicians, hospitals, and other health care organizations functioning autonomously.

The scope of practice for many physicians is very broad. Patients rely on physician training, experience, and good intentions for guidance. Individual clinicians do their best to stay abreast of the literature and rely on their own practice experience to make the best decisions for their patients. Journals, conferences, and informal consultation with peers are the usual means of staying current. Information technology tools are almost entirely absent. Norman (1988) has characterized this approach to work as based on "knowledge in the head," with heavy dependence on learning and memory. The patient's role tends to be passive, with care being organized for the benefit of the professional and/or institution.

Stage 2

Stage 2 is characterized by the formation of well-defined referral networks, greater use of informal mechanisms to increase patient involvement in clinical decision making, and the formation of loosely structured multidisciplinary teams. For the most part, health care is organized around areas of physician specialization and institutional settings. Patients have more access to health information through print, video, and Internet-based materials than in Stage 1, and more formal mechanisms exist for patient input. However, these tend to be generic mechanisms, such as consent forms and satisfaction surveys. Patients have informal mechanisms for input on their care.

Most health data are paper based. Little patient information is shared among settings or practices; the result is often gaps, redundancy of data gathering, and a lack of relevant information. In this stage, institutions and specialty groups, for example, try to help practitioners apply science to practice by developing tools for knowledge management, such as practice guidelines.

Stage 3

In Stage 3, care is still organized in a way that is oriented to the interests of professionals and institutions, but there is some movement toward a patient-centered system and recognition that individual patients differ in their preferences and needs. Team practice is common, but changes in roles are often slowed or stymied by institutional, labor, and financial structures, as well as by law and custom. Some training for team practice occurs, but that training is typically fragmented and isolated by health discipline, such as medicine, nursing, or physical therapy.

Clinicians and managers recognize the increasing complexity of health care and the opportunities presented by information technology. Some real-time decision support tools are available, but information technology capability is modest, and stand-alone applications are the rule. Computer-based applications for laboratory data, ordering of medications, and records of patient encounters typically

TABLE 5-1 Stages of Evolution of the Design of Health Organizations

Stage	The Patient Experience	Knowledge and Skills Management	Care Delivery
1	• The physician determines what is in the best interest of the patient and controls care. The patient's role tends to be passive, with care being organized for the benefit of the professional and/or institution.	• There is heavy reliance on human memory and knowledge without significant real-time aids and tools. Information technology is almost entirely absent.	• Individual physicians craft solutions for individual patients.
2	• Members of the professional team informally share control among themselves, but physician autonomy predominates. Care is organized for the benefit of the professional and/or institution. • Patients have informal mechanisms for input on their care.	• Clinicians have some protocols and knowledge assistance available, but still rely on memory and basic knowledge management tools (journals, conferences, consultation with peers, general Internet information sites). Very little information technology is in use. • Patients receive some information from clinicians (generally stock print material and verbal information).	• Recognition of the variability in treatment may lead to interest in protocols and guidelines. • Traditional professional roles define working relationships.

3	• Formal mechanisms for patient input exist. • Care is organized for the benefit of the professional and/or institution, but there is some movement toward a patient-centered system.	• Clinicians and patients have ready access to clinical knowledge. There is significant reliance on best practices, guidelines, and disease management pathways for clinicians and patients. Some real-time decisionsupport tools are available, but information technology capability is modest. • Some training for team practice occurs.	• The professional team formally shares roles and responsibilities among its members. The physician as responsible leader emerges. Practices recognize the need for changing professional roles, but change is slowed or stymied by institutional and financial structures, law, and custom. • A small number of practices apply system design principles and incorporate information systems in their daily work. Many conditions are managed through special care management programs.
4	• Care processes and transactions are based on the new rules set forth in Chapter 3. Care is patient-centered, with patient and family being part of the health care team. Patients have access to as much information as they wish to have and opportunities to exercise as much control over their care as they desire.	• The environment is rich in clinical information for patients and clinicians. • Automated decision support systems incorporating patient-specific data are used at the point of patient care. • Skill development, training, and leadership support the multidisciplinary character of clinical practice.	• The delivery of services is coordinated across practices, settings, and patient conditions over time. Information technology is used as the basic building block for making systems work, tracking performance, and increasing learning. Practices use measures and information about outcomes and information technology to continually refine advanced engineering principles and to improve their care processes. The health workforce is used efficiently and flexibly to implement change.

cannot exchange data at all or are not based on common definitions. Practice groups—particularly those that are community based—typically lack information systems to make such decision support tools available at the point of patient care, or to integrate guidelines with information about specific patients. Clinical leaders recognize the need for what has been called "knowledge in the world" (Norman, 1988)—information that is retrievable when needed, replaces the need for detailed memory recall, and is continuously updated on the basis of new information. More organized groups rely on best practices, guidelines, and disease management pathways for clinicians and patients, but these are not integrated with workflow.

Stage 4

Stage 4 is the health care system of the 21st century envisioned by the committee. This system supports continued improvement in the six aims of safety, effectiveness, patient-centeredness, timeliness, efficiency, and equity. Health care organizations in this stage have the characteristics of other high-performing organizations. They draw on the experiences of other sectors and adapt tools to the unique characteristics of the health care field.

Patients have the opportunity to exercise as much or as little control over treatment decisions as they choose (as long as their preferences fall within the boundaries of evidence-based practice). Services are coordinated across practices, settings, and patient conditions over time using increasingly sophisticated information systems.

Whatever their form, health care organizations can be characterized as "learning organizations" (Senge, 1990) that explicitly measure their performance along a variety of dimensions, including outcomes of care, and use that information to change or redesign and continually improve their work using advanced engineering principles. They make efficient and flexible use of the health workforce to implement change, matching and enhancing skill levels to enable less expensive professionals and patients to do progressively more sophisticated tasks (Christensen et al., 2000).

The committee does not advocate any particular organizational forms for the 21st-century health care system. The forms that emerge might comprise corporate management and ownership structures, strategic alliances, and other contractual arrangements ("virtual" organizations) (COR Healthcare Resources, 2000; Robinson and Casalino, 1996; Shortell et al., 2000a). New information and delivery structures might be located in a particular city or region or might be the basis for collaborative networks or consortia (COR Health LLC, 2000). Whatever the organizational arrangement, it should promote innovation and quality improvement. Every organization should be held accountable to its patients, the populations it serves, and the public for its clinical and financial performance.

In some respects, such as economies of scale, workforce training and deployment, and access to capital, larger organizations will have a comparative advantage. In other cases, small systems will evolve to take on functions now performed by larger organizations. The use of intranet- or Internet-based applications and information systems may enable the development of an infrastructure to accomplish certain functions. New forms might include, for example, Web-based knowledge servers or broker-mediated, consumer-directed health care purchasing programs.

KEY CHALLENGES FOR THE REDESIGN OF HEALTH CARE ORGANIZATIONS

Health care services need to be organized and financed in ways that make sense to patients and clinicians and that foster coordination of care and collaborative work. They should be based on sound design principles and make use of information technologies that can integrate data for multiple uses (Kibbe and Bard, 1997a; Rosenstein, 1997). Whatever their form, organizations will need to meet six challenges, see Figure 5-1, that cut across different health conditions, types of care (such as preventive, acute, or chronic), and care settings:

- redesigning care processes;
- making effective use of information technologies;
- managing clinical knowledge and skills;
- developing effective teams;
- coordinating care across patient conditions, services, and settings over time; and
- incorporating performance and outcome measurements for improvement and accountability.

The following discussion of these six challenges includes excerpts from interviews with clinical leaders conducted as a part of an IOM study aimed at identifying exemplary practices (Donaldson and Mohr, 2000).

Redesigning Care Processes

I try to help people understand that we can "work smarter." You can feel rotten about how you are practicing. I tell them, "You are right—and it's going to get worse." But change is possible. We don't need a billion-dollar solution.

We need a billion $1 solutions. You have to create the will to change. There's the will to change, then execution.—Hospital-based endoscopy unit

Like any complex system, health care organizations require sophisticated tools and building blocks that allow them to function with purpose, direction, and high

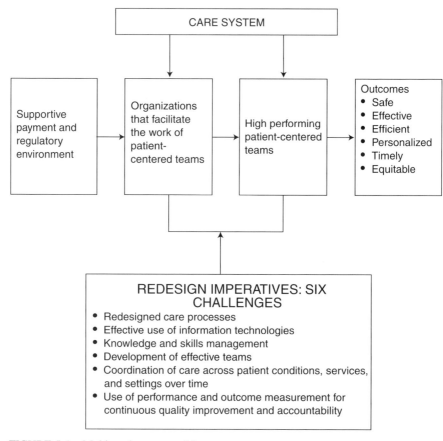

FIGURE 5-1   Making change possible.

reliability. Effective and reliable care processes—whether registering patients who come to the emergency room, ensuring complete immunizations for children, managing medication administration, ensuring that accurate laboratory tests are completed and returned to the requesting clinician, or ensuring that discharge from hospital to home after a disabling injury is safe and well coordinated—can be created only by using well-understood engineering principles. Not only must care processes be reliable, but they must also be focused on creating a relationship with a caregiver that meets the expectations of both the patient and the family. Redesign can transform the use of capital and human resources to achieve these ends.

Redesign may well challenge existing practices, data structures, roles, and management practices, and it results in continuing change. It involves conceptualizing, mapping, testing, refining, and continuing to improve the many processes of health care. Redesign aimed at increasing an organization's agility in responding to changing demand may be accomplished through a variety of approaches, such as simplifying, standardizing, reducing waste, and implementing methods of continuous flow (Bennis and Mische, 1995; Goldsmith, 1998).

Students of organizational theory have learned a great deal through careful examination of the work of organizations that use very complex and often hazardous technologies. The committee's earlier report, *To Err Is Human*, outlines the achievements of several manufacturing companies and the U.S. Navy's aircraft carriers in using replicable strategies to achieve great consistency and reliability (Institute of Medicine, 2000). Other world-class businesses, notably those that have received the prestigious Malcolm Baldrige National Quality Award, have embraced many of the tenets of quality improvement described by Deming, Juran, and others (Anderson et al., 1994), which include the need to improve constantly the system of production and services. Yet few health care organizations have developed successful models of production that reliably deliver basic effective services, much less today's increasingly advanced and complex technologies. Nor have most been able to continually assess and meet changing patient requirements and expectations.

Some health care organizations have dedicated considerable energy and resources to changing the way they deliver care. Although these organizations have recognized the need for leadership to provide the necessary commitment to and investment in change, they have also recognized that change needs to come from the bottom up as front-line health care teams recognize opportunities for redesigning care processes and acquire the skill to implement those new approaches successfully (National Committee for Quality Health Care, 1999; Washington Business Group on Health, 1998). Many other organizations have taken steps toward redesigning processes, but have found replication and deployment difficult or short-lived (Blumenthal and Kilo, 1998; Shortell et al., 1998). The committee recognizes these efforts and the difficulties that stem from, among other things, restructuring and economic pressure, misaligned incentives, professional entrenchment, competing priorities, organizational inertia, and lack of adequate information systems (Shortell et al., 1998).

A growing body of literature in health care indicates that well-designed care processes result in better quality (Desai et al., 1997; Griffin and Kinmouth, 1998). Some have argued that health care is not amenable to quality improvement approaches derived from other industries because inputs (patients) are so variable; outputs, such as health-related outcomes, so ill-defined; and the need for expert judgment and improvisation so demanding. Similar arguments have been made, but not substantiated, in other service industries and by those in the specialized departments (e.g., legal) of manufacturing industries that have subsequently experienced success in embracing principles of quality improvement (Galvin, 1998).

Fortunately, useful redesign principles that are now used widely in other industries can be (and in some cases have been) adapted to health care.

Engineering principles have been widely applied by other industries and in some health care organizations to design processes that improve quality and safety (Collins and Porras, 1997; Donaldson and Mohr, 2000; Hodgetts, 1998; Kegan, 1994; Peters and Waterman, 1982). The following subsections describe five such principles and their use by health care professionals to improve patients' experiences and safety, the flow of care processes, and coordination and communication among health professionals and with patients (Langley et al., 1996).

System Design Using the 80/20 Principle

> The nurse assesses the patient demographics, risk factors, support available, medication, lifestyle, and barriers to making changes. The first visit is usually 45 minutes to an hour long. Preventive screening visits are done yearly—assess vital signs, behavior, willingness to make changes. We take retinal photos, which are sent directly to the ophthalmologist, instead of sending the patient there. We learned that we need to risk stratify and fit the level of services to the level of risk. Services are less or more intense based on risk. We use protocols to identify risk level: primary—those with diabetes, secondary—those with diabetes and any other risk factors, tertiary—those who have already had a stroke, myocardial infarction, or renal failure.—Diabetic management group

This engineering principle can be restated: *Design for the usual, but recognize and plan for the unusual.* Process design should be explicit for the usual case—for 80 percent of the work. For the remaining 20 percent, contingency plans should be assembled as needed. This concept is useful both for designing systems of care and as an approach to acculturating new trainees. Also referred to as the Pareto Principle, the 80/20 principle is based on the recognition that a small number of causes (20 percent) is responsible for a large percentage (80 percent) of an effect (Juran, 1989; Transit Cooperative Research Program, 1995). In health care, for example, 20 percent of patients in a defined population may account for 80 percent of the work and incur 80 percent of costs. Similarly, 20 percent (or fewer) of common diagnoses may account for 80 percent of patients' health problems.

A fundamental approach in health care has been to build care systems to accommodate all possible occurrences. This approach is cumbersome and often the source of delays when, for example, laboratory tests are done in case a rare disease is present, or certain procedures must be followed in case an unusual event should happen. System design based on the 80/20 approach exploits the existence of routine work, often a large proportion of the total work load, that is involved in an assortment of patient problems. One determines what work is routine and designs a simple, standard, and low-cost process for performing this work efficiently and reliably. This leaves the more complex work to be performed employing processes that appropriately use higher-skilled personnel or more advanced technologies.

In accordance with this principle, approaches to planning care are designed to reflect the different sorts of clinical problems encountered in practice. Level 1 represents the most predictable needs. In a pediatric practice, well-child health supervision, immunization, and middle-ear infections represent a large portion of the work and very predictable needs. In an obstetrics–gynecology practice, prenatal care and contraceptive counseling are examples of Level 1. In adult primary care, examples include management of hypertension, acute sprains, low back pain, and sinusitis. For newly diagnosed patients with asthma, instruction in the use of an inhaler is an example of predictable work. The more predictable the work, the more it makes sense to standardize care so that it can be performed by a variety of workers in a consistent fashion.

When needs are predictable, standardization encompasses the key dimensions of work that should be performed the same way each time using a defined process and is a key element of the principle of mass customization discussed later in this section. For example, variation in the care of patients with community-acquired pneumonia can be reduced by identifying and standardizing the key dimensions of care. Standardization may involve very complex or very simple technologies and processes. An example of the latter is a nursing assistant stamping on a patient's chart, "Immunization up to date?" and circling "Yes" or "No" for a clinician to see as he or she enters the exam room. Focused standardization often entails simplifying processes. For example, instead of each clinician on staff having a different protocol, clinicians might agree to use a single chemotherapy protocol for most patients, or a single dose, route, or frequency for a commonly administered medication. Although it might be permissible to use other protocols, clinicians would have to agree to evaluate the outcomes for patients under both the standard and nonstandard protocols to determine which was best (Institute of Medicine, 2000). In another example, Duke University's pediatric emergency department uses a color-coded tape to measure a child's length and an approximate weight range. Color-coded supplies (e.g., IV tubing, airway masks, syringes) correspond to the four weight ranges. Standardizing equipment for each color zone ensures that dosages and equipment are appropriate and safe for children in that range (Glymph, 2000).

Level 2 represents health care needs of medium predictability. At this level, it is important for practice settings to triage patients accurately to determine their needs. Examples are patients with chronic illnesses, such as asthma or diabetes, whose condition is not under control and who need special services to help them. Some patients might best be served by group visits with a diabetic counselor, others might need individual support, and others might need hospitalization. Appropriate triage based on needs could include working out a care plan with patients in terms of exercise, weight loss, and insulin control and providing them with materials and resources to help them meet their objectives.

Level 3 represents patients with rare or complex health care health conditions for which special resources must be assembled. In such cases, applying excellent listening skills, assembling resources, and managing the clinician–patient relationship are especially important. Examples are a patient with an infectious disease that is rare and difficult to identify, or the need to assemble a multidisciplinary team for health supervision of children with special needs, such as those with cystic fibrosis, meningomyelocele, or craniofacial syndromes (Carey, 1992).

The assembling of these resources can sometimes be accomplished within a single office practice. In other cases, a relationship with another system—another critical care unit or an individual such as a subspecialist, for example—may be required. Recent evidence indicates that for ambulatory care, nurses and nurse practitioners can manage a substantial proportion of the work (Mundinger et al., 2000; Shum et al., 2000). The remaining 20 percent of the work would correspond to the third level, which requires the most highly trained practitioners.

Design for Safety

> When lab results are returned by e-mail, they come back by provider, and I can attach them to the patient's chart. When I open the patient record, the "desktop" flags alert me to abnormal results.—Primary care practice

> The doctor–patient relationship is important, but perhaps more important is how much [doctors] can rely on the system not to let [the patient] slip through the cracks. —Primary care practice

The prevention, detection, and mitigation of harm occur in learning environments, not in environments of blame and reprisal. Designing systems for safety requires specific, clear, and consistent efforts to develop a work culture that encourages reporting of errors and hazardous conditions, as well as communication among staff about safety concerns. Such learning also requires attention to effective knowledge transfer, including the systematic acquisition, dissemination, and incorporation of ideas, methods, and evidence that may have been developed elsewhere (Institute of Medicine, 2000). As described in detail in the committee's earlier report, *To Err Is Human* (Institute of Medicine, 2000), designing health care processes for safety involves a three-part strategy: (1) designing systems to prevent errors, (2) designing procedures to make errors visible when they do occur, and (3) designing procedures that can mitigate the harm to patients from errors that are not detected or intercepted (Nolan, 2000).

Designing systems to prevent errors includes designing jobs for safety, avoiding reliance on memory and vigilance, and simplifying and standardizing key processes (such as using checklists and protocols). Designing jobs for safety means attending to the effects of work hours, workloads, staffing ratios, appropriate training, sources of distraction and their relationship to fatigue and reduced alertness, and sleep deprivation, as well as providing appropriate training. Avoiding reliance on memory and vigilance can be accomplished in simple ways, such as instituting reminder systems and color coding, eliminating look-alike and sound-alike products, wisely using checklists and protocols, and employing more complex automated systems that may prevent many errors (though they may also introduce new sources of error). Simplification and standardization are key principles not only in delivering effective services, but also in making them safer. For example, standardization of data displays so that all are expressed in the same units, of equipment so that on–off switches are in consistent locations, of the location of supplies and equipment, of order forms, and of prescribing conventions can prevent many errors (Institute of Medicine, 2000).

Designing procedures to make errors visible can also improve safety. Although human beings will always make errors, procedures can be designed so that many errors are identified before they result in harm to patients. For example, pharmaceutical software can alert the prescriber to an incorrect dose or potential interaction with another medication (Institute of Medicine, 2000).

Designing procedures that can mitigate harm from errors is a third means of improving patient safety. Examples of this strategy are having antidotes and up-to-date information available to clinicians; having equipment that is designed to default to the least harmful mode; and ensuring that teams are trained in effective recovery from crises, such as unexpected complications during operative procedures (Institute of Medicine, 2000).

Mass Customization

Mass customization involves combining the uniqueness of customized products and services with the efficiencies of mass production. In manufacturing, this strategy has been developed as a way to give customers exactly what they want in a way that is feasible from a business standpoint—that is, quickly, at an acceptable cost, and without added complexity (Pine et al., 1995).

With reference to the three levels of predictability discussed earlier, mass customization is the design approach to Level 2 (patients with moderate levels of predictability of needs). Patients can often be grouped according to their need for a common set of services. For example, many medical conditions are defined in terms of their grade or degree of severity (e.g., cancer staging), degree of control achieved (e.g., controlled or uncontrolled hypertension), or level of risk (e.g., high- or low-risk pregnancy and the Glasgow trauma scale). With good information about the past needs and preferences of patients, it is often possible to standardize processes of care within a given stratum. It is possible to predict fairly accurately, for example, what proportion of patients will choose a variety of options, such as a group versus individual visit for management of a condition.

In a non-health care example, hotels such as the Ritz Carlton keep track of their customers' preferences so they can be offered appropriate services (Gilmore and Pine, 1997).

Yet patients thus grouped are not identical, and the health system should be responsive to differences in their preferences and special needs. Mass customization involves attempting to standardize the common set of services needed by many patients while customizing or tailoring other aspects of those services to respond to individual preferences and needs. In the computer world, Internet sites can cater to "segments of one" by efficiently providing each customer with products that match his or her preferences (Leibovich, 2000). Likewise, the use of independent modules means that computer products can be assembled into different forms quickly and inexpensively (Feitzinger and Lee, 1997). Gateway is an example of a retail computer company that uses modules (such as varying amounts of memory or hard drive capacity) in mass customizing its products for the consumer. This use of modules for mass customization can be applied to the health care arena, for example to patients with congestive heart failure who need acute care. Modules for admission to a hospital or nursing home, for family education, and for rehabilitation can be drawn on and combined for individual patients. Another example is the steps in patient care, which can be thought of as a series of modules, such as (1) prescribing a medication, (2) assessing and encouraging adherence to therapy, and (3) monitoring patient outcomes. In these examples, the 80/20 approach also applies; that is, for each module, the set of options should be appropriate for 80 percent of patients.

In applying the principle of mass customization, differentiation is the last step—in industry, an example is manufacturing all products in the same way up to the addition of the product color. A health care example is having standardized instructions for patients with a given health problem, but writing in further information for those with additional health conditions.

Continuous Flow

When a patient calls to make an appointment, our philosophy is: If your doctor is here today, you will see your doctor.—Primary care practice

We have bedside registration in the emergency department. Each room receives a portable computer rolled in on a cart. Computer orders for lab and pharmacy are entered from the bedside.—Emergency department

Each morning we make rounds on all 34 intensive care patients. The discussion includes pointed, patient-oriented reports, social as well as medical needs. All such issues can be dealt with and work begun at once.—Intensive care unit

If a patient calls in with a breast lump, she is usually seen within a day or so. First she sees her primary care provider, then she is sent to us for a mammogram—usually an ultrasound as well. We can do what we think should be done right then—a biopsy and surgery if needed. Usually everything is done within 1 or 2 days.—Breast care center

Volume has dramatically increased here. We have had to change the way we work. Although most ERs have 12-hour shifts, we shortened the shifts to 9 hours. We have a system where there is "virtual on-call." Physicians have agreed in advance that if our tracking system shows that the cycle time from the arrival of a patient to being seen by a doctor is past a specific threshold, they will stay longer, even if more help is there or on its way.—Emergency department

Continuous flow, sometimes referred to as "a batch size of one," is an important design concept in which the system is designed to match demand so there is no aggregation of persons or units during processing. It represents the theoretical optimum for any production or service delivery system. In health care, application of this principle involves examining current assumptions about patient demand and redesigning the care process to better correspond to the characteristics of the demand curve (Murray and Tantau, 1998; Nolan et al., 1996).

If clinicians and managers assume that patient demand is insatiable, health care systems and individual practitioners must find ways to manage this demand. Management of demand generally entails using barriers, such as waiting, to dissuade some people from seeking services or reducing the need to use resources that could be used elsewhere, or both. Alternatively, if the assumption is that patient demand is steady, predictable, and reasonable, then continuous flow is a more appropriate and effective solution. Some of the most advanced examples of continuous flow have been pioneered by office practices that use "open-access" scheduling (Grandinetti, 2000; Murray, 2000; Terry, 2000). Most scheduling systems rely on distinguishing between urgent and nonurgent requests for appointments; the result is often waits of 2 weeks for a nonurgent appointment and several months for a physical examination. As a result, many patients do not keep their appointments (Bowman et al., 1996; Festinger et al., 1995). In an open-access system, office staff do not triage patients who call for an appointment on the basis of whether they believe those patients need to be seen that day. Patients can schedule an appointment and be seen the same day, if they wish, by their doctor (or nurse practitioner) if that individual is in. Continuous flow does not, however, mean that patients must be fit into a lock-step process. If they prefer to wait or schedule an appointment for the future, they are always free to do so.

To implement such a program and match demand with resources requires that a practice first deal with its backlog of future appointments. Once it has implemented an open-access process, the practice will have only one scheduling system for all patients. Practices that have implemented open access report that they are able to see as many or more patients as before; that they finish the day on time and with personnel less exhausted; and that they are providing more appropriate—effective, patient-centered, timely, and probably safer—care (Institute for Healthcare Improvement, 2000).

Under a system of continuous flow, as opposed to batch flow, practitioners dictate notes, take care of other tasks after a patient's visit, and respond to telephone messages as they occur or as patients are seen, rather than "batching" such tasks to be addressed at the end of the day. In the case of telephone messages, for example, batching often results in repeated calls by patients who are not certain their message has been received, repeated calls to patients who may be on their way home from work by the time the message is returned, delays in managing medications or in providing information about laboratory tests and instructions for self-care, and sometimes greater anxiety and suffering.

Production Planning

> We reorganized into teams 2 years ago. An MD, RN, and Medical Assistant form a team. We have six or seven teams; each team sees a panel of 1200 patients. Each team sees patients for a 4 1/2-hour block of time per day. The morning starts with a 30-minute meeting to review appointments that are scheduled for the day. Then the compressed clinic day. Then time for charting each afternoon. We have practice management time that is scheduled every week. Patients are not scheduled for that time. That time is for reviewing data, collecting data. It's funny, but you can see almost the same number of patients during a compressed clinical day as during a full day. The teams are staggered throughout the day so that we can be open from 8 a.m. to 8 p.m. The number of teams is scheduled to match times when patient demand is the greatest.—Primary care practice

Production planning has been used in other industries to find the best way to allocate staff, equipment, and other resources to meet the needs of customers, as well as to reduce costs. Application of the principle depends on a detailed understanding of work processes, specifically, the identification of repetitive patterns of work.

Although the needs of patients and the work required to meet those needs will vary from day to day, all clinical practices have a natural rhythm defined by a period—for example, a week—after which the nature of the work repeats. One method of production planning involves the use of a repetitive master schedule to make the best use of resources in meeting patient needs. Creating such a schedule necessitates defining the work to be done, assembling a team suited to perform the work, understanding the time period within which the work repeats, and making work assignments based on the standard time period. If a master schedule can be built for a typical week, it can be used with minor adjustments for any week. The repetitive master schedule serves a variety of purposes. Its primary purpose is to match resources to the needs of patients, but it also provides a method for understanding complex systems and designing better production processes.

Summary

The reengineering principles described in this section—system design using the 80/20 approach, design for safety, mass customization, continuous flow, and production planning—are used by other industries, and, as indicated in the accompanying quotations, by teams across a range of health care settings that include ambulatory office practices, hospital units, emergency departments, and hospices. Such engineering principles illustrate what is meant by focusing at a system level. They enable health care teams to organize their resources effectively to better meet patient needs, and make medical practice more satisfying without driving up costs. Such deliberate crafting of systems of care results not in impersonal, one-size-fits-all care processes. Rather, it makes care safer, enables standardization where appropriate, and at the same time results in situations that meet the unique needs of each patient.

Making Effective Use of Information Technologies

Spending 1 hour each day online, I send 800–900 e-mails each month. In my former visit-based model, I would see 400–500 patients each month. Now I see 200 patients each month, in unhurried and more time intensive visits, but I communicate with over 1,000 patients each month. I feel less stressed and my patients receive better care.—Primary care practice

Chapter 7 examines in detail the potential role of information technology in improving quality. Information technology can reduce errors and harm from errors (Bates et al., 1998; Raschke et al., 1998), make up-to-date evidence and decision support systems available at the point of patient care (Berner et al., 1999; Classen, 1998; Evans et al., 1998; Hunt et al., 1998), support research (Blumenthal, 1997), help make quality measurement timely and accurate (Schneider et al., 1999), improve coordination among clinicians, and increase accountability for performance (Blumenthal, 1997; National Committee for Quality Assurance, 2000).

Increasingly, secure Internet and intranet applications are making it possible for clinicians and patients to communicate with one another more easily, for up-to-date evidence about what works to become increasingly accessible, and for clinical data to be shared in a timely fashion (Cushman and Detmer, 1998; Science Panel on Interactive Communication and Health, 1999). Some organizations have begun to implement Internet applications for their patients for such purposes as obtaining health information, communicating with one another, reading information about physicians and staff, and viewing schedules for health education classes (Kaiser Permanente Online, 2000).

Information technology can provide laboratory results and other findings, as well as tools that help clinicians apply the health literature when making diagnoses and deciding among therapeutic approaches. The validity of the information used for such decision making is obviously critical. Also important is a user interface that matches clinical workflow, cognitive style, and the time constraints of clinical practice (Kibbe and Bard, 1997b), a need that can be addressed by vendors, experts in medical informatics, and usability experts. The widespread adoption of Web-based browsers to interface with data systems has influenced medical informatics, increasing the likelihood of its acceptance and use in health care settings.

Systems that can access and combine data from many sources should be able to evolve with the uses to which they are put, the changing demands of the health care environment, and advances in technology. Such systems should be able to access all patient data wherever clinical decisions are made. They should be able to access the evidence base and decision supports, such as clinical practice guidelines. They should provide efficient means of entering orders and retrieving results. They should help practitioners coordinate activities whether they occur in the inpatient, outpatient, home, or other settings.

A handful of health care organizations have made impressive gains in automating clinical information—for example, the health systems of the Department of Veterans Affairs and Intermountain Health Care (in Salt Lake City, Utah)—but overall progress has been slow. Barriers to moving forward include the many policy (e.g., privacy concerns), technical (e.g., data standards), financial (e.g., capital requirements), and human factors (e.g., clinician acceptance) considerations discussed in Chapter 7.

Managing Clinical Knowledge and Skills

We have an intranet throughout the system that enables physicians to see the latest guidelines and recommendations about screening and to find out where each of their patients is in this care process.—Health plan–based breast care center

Our protocols for brain edema were going well. However, new literature emerged. One of the neurosurgeons recommended that we revamp the protocols to incorporate the new findings. He gathered the evidence, and the first protocol was designed by a team headed by a unit nurse. The protocol was soon standardized, and ownership was created at the physician and nurse level.—Intensive care unit

All surgeons who join the staff, regardless of seniority, start by assisting, then being assisted in 150 cases before being left on their own. If we are not completely confident they have mastered the technique, supervision is extended to another 100 cases. The secret of success is in everyone using the same technique. It decreases complications and is more cost-effective.—Small hospital specializing in two procedures

If the Respiratory Therapist notes an abnormal lab value, he or she is comfortable not just taking a blood sample and reporting it, but managing it. The technicians are caregivers. Expectations have changed. They [adjust] therapy to within physiological parameters. They are cross-trained so that they can take on nursing tasks, for example, starting IVs when needed. When fully trained and confident, they may tell an admitting doc that a patient is not ready to have a ventilator tube removed.—Intensive care unit

A key challenge for organizations, requiring a range of competencies, is translating the evidence base into practice. The competencies involved include tracking and disseminating new information, managing the clinical change that helps incorporate new information into practice, and ensuring that health care professionals have the skills they need to make use of new knowledge. All such competencies are interrelated. New information and technologies may require new skills. And new technologies, such as simulation, may enhance skills, such as those involved in performing surgical procedures or managing crises.

As described in greater detail in Chapter 6, the flood of new information that is relevant to practice can no longer be managed adequately by individual clinicians trying to keep up with the literature and attending conferences or lectures (Davis et al., 1999; Weed, 1999). One new approach to timely management of information involves including clinical librarians as a part of clinical care teams, for example, on morning rounds or on call, to note questions and search the literature for the best and most relevant information (Davidoff and Florance, 2000). Another response is to create easily accessible systematic reviews of the literature, using well-understood criteria for determining the strength of evidence and the generalizability of findings. Such systematic reviews, though important, are only the first stage, however, in disseminating the flow of new knowledge and translating it for use with individual patients. First, clinicians need evidence-based guidelines that make clear which steps are well founded and which are based on expert consensus (Institute of Medicine, 1992). These efforts may occur within practices or larger institutions, or may be developed by external entities such as specialty groups, independent organizations established for the purpose, or governmental groups. Whatever the source of such guidelines, any group that uses them needs to understand their validity and ensure that they are kept up to date.

Ensuring that new knowledge is incorporated into practice also requires a thorough understanding of how change is managed most effectively in health care, including the barriers to and facilitators of change. Knowledge about why guidelines are or are not used is accumulating, and experts now better understand the circumstances in which such strategies as education, administrative changes, incentives, penalties, feedback, and social marketing are likely to be effective (Greco and Eisenberg, 1993; Grol, 1997; Oxman et al., 1995; Solberg et al., 2000; Wensing et al., 1998) and why the translation of research findings to date has been characterized as "slow and haphazard" (Grol and Grimshaw, 1999).

One strategy for successfully managing change is to design guidelines and implementation processes so that it is easier to apply the best evidence than not to do so. This strategy begins with a systematic review of the evidence, but attends to the creation of clinical guidelines or protocols that match the logic and flow of care. Implementing this strategy also requires agreement on the part of clinicians that they will use the new guidelines and protocols, as well as the resources needed to redesign care processes (despite such resources often being scarce) so that the guidelines and protocols will become an integral and efficiently designed element of the care process.

Health care requires complex, sophisticated judgments and psychomotor skills, perhaps at a level unmatched in any other field. Other industries test judgment and psychomotor skills. In aviation, for example, simulations are used to assess competence and to help pilots improve their judgment and skills. Medicine has traditionally relied on cognitive testing of knowledge, not of judgment or skills. The field also relies on privileges granted by hospitals using various levels of rigor to assess professionals' skills, but such mechanisms do not include testing to ensure that those skills are current and have not deteriorated.

Making use of new knowledge may require that health professionals develop new skills or that their roles change. New skills might include basic technical proficiency, for example, in executing a procedure, using equipment, and interpreting data from new tests and devices. Managing new knowledge may also require the use of new psychosocial skills to elicit behavior change in patients and colleagues. Other new skills might include designing data collection efforts and managing and interpreting quality-of-care information. Finally, incorporating new knowledge requires skilled leadership to engage the participation of health professionals in collaborative teams. Leaders need to devote explicit attention to ensuring that the most appropriate individuals are trained in, maintain competence in, and are supported in their new tasks.

Developing Effective Teams

There has been a radical change since we introduced teams. You can see it even where they hang out. Before the docs were together, the nurses together, etc. But now the team hangs out with the team. At the morning meetings, you may see the medical assistants providing the leadership. The medical director calls it the "fast break"—three people on the floor and anybody can finish the play.—Primary care practice

[The doctors] are worried about managing clinical conditions. They work under pressure and stress and try to find a way to control it. They all claim that "my patients are sicker." I reply, "Give me your sickest patients—those with congestive heart failure, the ones on coumadin, patients with diabetes, hypertension, the old, sick people, anyone who seems to require more than the average resources and time." When they ask why I would say this, I reply, "Because I will enlist help, resources—clinical pathways, care managers." We provide these resources to the practice and should never charge [or penalize] the doctors for this help. Doctors have not learned yet how to enhance the team with other kinds of providers—health education, behavioral medicine, physical therapy, pharmacy.—Primary care practice

Organized work groups, or multidisciplinary teams, have become a common way to organize health care, and considerable attention has been focused on their value and functioning. Such teams are found in primary care practice, in the focused care of patients with chronic conditions, in critical acute care (the intensive care unit, trauma units, operating rooms), and in geriatrics and care at the end of life. In such settings, smooth team functioning is needed because of the increasing complexity of care, the demands of new technology, and the need to coordinate multiple patient needs (Fried et al., 2000). Nonphysician team members may increase efficiency (e.g., drawing blood, giving immunizations); substitute for physicians (e.g., care for patients with simple, well-defined problems); and complement physicians (Starfield, 1992) by filling roles that physicians may not perform well or may be reluctant to undertake, such as counseling about behavior change or performing highly technical diagnostic tests. Such distributions of roles and tasks change dramatically over time. Many tasks, such as monitoring and adjusting equipment for an ill newborn after hospital discharge, have been taken over by family members and patients themselves (Hart, 1995; Lorig et al., 1993, 1999; Von Korff et al., 1997).

An IOM study of small work teams at the front lines of patient care (Donaldson and Mohr, 2000) included asking practitioners and staff who worked together on a daily basis about that experience. Respondents cited the importance of collaborative work both for clinical care and for improvement efforts. They emphasized the need to base quality improvement work within the team and to recognize the contributions that all members of the group could make, with various individuals taking leadership roles for specific improvement activities. They also described new or expanded roles and the need for coaching and training new members of the team in their work relationships.

Effective working teams must be created and maintained. Yet members of teams are typically trained in separate disciplines and educational programs, leaving them unprepared to enter practice in complex collaborative settings. They may not appreciate each other's strengths or recognize weaknesses except in crises, and they may not have been trained together to use established or new technologies (Institute of Medicine, 2000). An enormous amount of knowledge has been accumulated about team creation and management, including effective communication among team members (Fried et al., 2000). In commercial aviation, for example, emphasis is placed on crew resource management because of its importance to airline safety, and communication among flight personnel has become a special focus of proficiency checks by certified examiners (e.g., during simulated emergencies).

Considerable research has gone into identifying the characteristics of effective teams (Fried et al., 2000). These characteristics include (1) team makeup, such as having the appropriate size and composition and the ability to reduce negative effects of status differences between, for example, physicians and nurses; (2) team processes, such as communication structures, conflict management, and leadership that emphasizes excellence and conveys clear goals and expectations; (3) the nature of the team's tasks, such as matching roles and training to the level of complexity and promoting cohesiveness when work is highly interdependent; and (4) the environmental context, such as obtaining needed resources and establishing appropriate rewards. Effective teams have a culture that fosters openness, collaboration, teamwork, and learning from mistakes. Shortell et al. (1994) have demonstrated a significant relationship between better interaction among team members in intensive care units and decreased risk-adjusted length of stay. Such interaction includes the dimensions of culture, leadership, communication, coordination, problem solving, and conflict management.

Research on team interactions has also demonstrated that teams often fall short of the expectations of their clinical leaders, members, and administrative managers (Pearson and Jones, 1994). One reason is that medical education emphasizes hierarchy and the importance of assuming individual responsibility for decision making. An emphasis on personal accountability comes at the price of losing the contribution of others who may bring added insight and relevant information, whatever their formal credentials. Acculturation to medical roles makes it difficult for members of a team to point out or admit to safety problems and thereby prevent harm. Indeed, challenges to those in positions of power and authority by nurses, physicians in training, and others is notoriously difficult and discouraged (Helmreich, 2000; Institute of Medicine, 2000). Avoiding overt hostility over a slip or lapse and acknowledging shared knowledge and proficiency when recovering from unexpected patient events (Helmreich, 2000) are examples of how strong collaborative working relationships can improve patient safety.

In health care environments characterized by uncertainty, instability, and variability (such as operating rooms and intensive care units), high levels of stress are common (Mark and Hagenmueller, 1994; Perrow, 1967). Other environments do not have the level of instability and uncertainty associated with critical care units and operating suites, yet the complexity of patients' needs still necessitates highly effective coordination of resources across a spectrum of settings, disciplines, and the community. An example is the care of frail elderly patients, in which the ability to coordinate care and assemble effectively functioning health care teams is paramount, and flexibility in role functioning may be key.

In Chapter 3, new rule 10 emphasizes the importance of collaboration for effective team functioning. What is sometimes thought to be collaboration, however, may in fact be uncoordinated or sequential action rather than collaborative work. That is, the work of each individual may be efficient from the perspective of his or her own tasks, but overall the efforts are suboptimal and do not serve the needs of patients. An example of suboptimization may occur when an elderly woman breaks her hip and comes to the emergency department. She may spend several hours receiving x-rays and being stabilized and will certainly need to be admitted. At the end of this time, someone may call to notify the nursing staff that the patient is being admitted, and several hours more may elapse while admission orders are written and the patient's room is made available. When emergency department and floor staff collaborate, notification is given immediately after the patient arrives in the emergency department so that the admission process can begin, and the patient can go from the emergency department directly to her hospital room, where she will be much more comfortable. In such cases and in many others, running parallel processes reduces delays and improves outcomes (Nugent et al., 1999).

Coordinating Care Across Patient Conditions, Services, and Settings Over Time

That is fundamental to what is important to me—that the focus be on the individual—a complex person—and you try to do the best you can for them. It seems odd to say, but that is what is fun. We did focus groups with families and learned key things that are important: (1) the organization and delivery of care, (2) shared medical decision making, (3) treating each person as an individual, and (4) attending to those who care for and love the dying person. The building blocks to accomplish this are information and education of the patient and family, coordination, and continuity.—Hospice

Another key challenge for organizations is coordination (or clinical integration) of work across services that are complementary, such as emergency response units, emergency departments, and operating suites, or across primary care practices, specialty practices, and laboratories to which patients are referred. Clinical integration can be defined as "the extent to which patient care services are coordinated across people, functions, activities, and sites over time so as to maximize the value of services delivered to patients" (Shortell et al., 2000a). In particular, coordination encompasses a set of practitioner behaviors and information systems intended to bring together health services, patient needs, and streams of information to facilitate the aims of care set forth in Chapter 2. For example, coordination may involve ensuring that treating physicians are informed about diagnostic results, therapies attempted during an earlier hospital admission, and the effectiveness of those efforts. Coordination may involve nurse case managers transmitting information to both primary and specialty care practitioners about a patient's unmet needs. Such coordination may be facilitated as well by procedures for engaging community resources (such as social and public health services) and other sites of care (such as hospice or home care) when and as appropriate.

Coordination of care across clinicians and settings has been shown to result in greater efficiency and better clinical outcomes (Aiken et al., 1997; Gittell et al., 2000; Knaus et al., 1986; Shortell et al., 1994, 2000a, 2000b). Optimizing care for a patient with a complex chronic condition is challenging enough, but optimizing care for patients with several chronic conditions and acute episodes, as well as meeting health maintenance needs, represents an extraordinary challenge for today's health care systems (MacLean et al., 2000; Shortell et al., 2000a). The challenges arise at many organizational levels and across the full range of tasks, including the design, dissemination, implementation, and modification of care processes and the payment for these tasks. What is important to patients and their families is that effective systems for transferring patient-related information be in place so that the information is accurate and available when needed. Patients and their families need to know who is responsible for decisions and can answer questions, and to be assured that gaps in responsibility will not occur.

Some problems—such as substance abuse, AIDS, and domestic violence—are so interrelated that they appear to require a comprehensive rather than problem-by-problem approach (Shortell et al., 2000a). Other problems require assembling and making the best use of an array of resources, such as the numerous federal programs that might be involved in obtaining and paying for a wheelchair for a child with special needs. In any case, if care is to move beyond single solutions crafted by individual clinicians (as in the Stage 1 delivery of care described earlier in this chapter), it will require an accurate understanding of patient needs so that standard processes can be provided and individual solutions crafted as appropriate. Newly developed infrastructures, information technologies, and well-thought-out and -implemented modes of communication can reduce the need to craft laborious, case-by-case strategies for coordinating patient care. A variety of other mechanisms can improve coordination, such as involving a combination of individuals (e.g., clinicians, members of multidisciplinary teams, care managers), along with patients and their families.

Some patients and their families become so expert in their condition that they choose to coordinate care for themselves or a family member. Those who do so are likely to need new skills in accessing information and new technologies for structuring and conveying information to others who are involved in their care. For example, patients can contribute to flow sheets, respond to questions about changes in health status, or upload data from micromonitoring devices worn on the body or from home monitoring devices. Not all patients or their families (or perhaps even most) will choose or be able to become central actors in coordinating their own care, however. In such cases, appropriate mechanisms within the delivery system must be available to meet this responsibility.

One means of improving coordination is based on what are sometimes called *clinical pathways*. These blueprints for care set forth a set of services needed for patients with a given health problem and the sequence in which they should take place. For some conditions, a set of clearly identified processes should occur. In complex adaptive systems such as health care, however, few patient care processes are linear (such as the transition from hospital to nursing home). Rather, most organizational processes are reciprocal and interdependent (Thompson, 1967), and coordination requires the design of procedures that are responsive both to variations among individual patients and to unexpected occurrences.

Incorporating Performance and Outcome Measurements for Improvement and Accountability

We have a Clinical Roadmap team for breast cancer screening. The team has formulated four criteria for success that include process and outcome measures. They are (1) the proportion of women in our population who have received care in the last 2 years; (2) the number of women who came to the screening program when invited; (3) the number of women in the program who develop a late stage disease; and (4) survey responses during the time of enrollment in the program. These criteria give us specific as well as broad measures of success.—Breast care center

We have a clinical "instrument panel." We measure cycle time, patient satisfaction, phone calls (incoming and outgoing), proportion reaching treatment goals for hypertension, operating costs per visit, proportion of patients seeing their provider of choice, available appointments, team morale, practice size, and proportion of pap smears in eligible women.—Primary care practice

The main outcome measure is risk adjusted mortality. We compare ourselves quarterly to similar institutions for observed versus predicted mortality on one axis and resource consumption on the other. Using 50 percent random sampling, we track mortality, admission and discharge rates, length of stay, number of patients readmitted to the ICU, and reintubation rates. This helps us know if changes that affect efficiency are affecting quality of care. Although our admissions are up, length of stay is down significantly, and our reintubation rate is very low.—Critical care unit

Although we generally think of individuals as learning and enhancing their capabilities, it is also possible to think of an organization as learning—increasing its competence and responsiveness and improving its work (Davies and Nutley, 2000). The committee believes moving toward the health system of the 21st century will require that health care organizations successfully address the challenge of becoming learning organizations. A decade ago, Senge and others (Argyris and Schön, 1978; Senge, 1990) described such organizations as those that can learn quickly and accurately about their environment and translate this learning to the work they do. This idea has been incorporated in the work of many companies, most outside of health care—such as 3M, Boeing, the Cadillac Division of General Motors, Fedex, Motorola, and Xerox—whose drive to reduce defects and improve quality and customer service has been recognized by the Malcolm Baldrige National Quality Award (National Institute of Standards and Technology, 2000b).

In Senge's terminology, "single-loop" learning results in incremental improvements in existing practice. In health care it might involve efforts to decrease waiting time for follow-up appointments for patients who have an abnormal laboratory test result. Another feature of learning organizations is their reexamination of mental models or assumptions on which they base their work, giving rise to "double-loop" learning. An example of double-loop learning is rethinking and reorganizing all ancillary and specialty medical services for women in a breast care center to eliminate any waiting between reporting of abnormal mammographic findings, definitive diagnosis, and therapy.

A critical feature of learning organizations is the ability to be aware of their own "behavior." In organizational terms, this means having data that allow the organization to track what has happened and what needs to happen—in other words, to assess its performance and use that information to improve. The committee is convinced that a major tool for accomplishing this critical function is the investment in and use of an effective information infrastructure to develop a balanced set of measures on, for example, clinical and financial performance, patient health outcomes, and satisfaction with care (Nelson et al., 1996). It is important that such measures be balanced—that they include a variety of measures so that when changes are made in processes, such as to increase efficiency, other outcomes, such as patient health, are not adversely affected.

Clinical practices that participated in the IOM study of exemplary practices (Donaldson and Mohr, 2000) described how routine measurement has become part of their production process. Ideally, such measures can be aggregated for external reporting, whether to support contract discussions or to help patients make choices about where and from whom to seek care. Building measurement into the production process can counter the perception on the part of many health care leaders that reporting is a burden. Such a perception results when organizations must respond to numerous demands from external groups for quality measures, especially if those measures lack specificity or relevance to the clinical teams that must generate them.

Measures need not involve expensive, large-scale, long-term evaluation projects to be useful. New methods that use sampling and small-scale rapid-cycle testing, modification, and retesting are proving useful in dynamic settings such as patient care units (Berwick, 1996; Langley et al., 1996). As other world-class businesses have learned, including American industry giants (Walton and Deming, 1986), attention to improving quality includes continuous monitoring, often based on small samples of events, that can provide organizations with timely data at the front lines to manage the processes of concern (James, 1989; Rainey et al.,

1998; Scholtes, 1988). In the IOM study of exemplary practices, several health care teams described their use of such methods to manage their care processes (Donaldson and Mohr, 2000).

> It's an incredible relief to try small changes on a small scale. It's so simple it's brilliant. We had been managing indigent diabetic patients for years and didn't think we could do any better. The providers believed that these people are so hard. But the patients responded to the changes we made. You have to craft something that is doable. You have to look for the simplicity in complex things.—Diabetic management group for underserved minorities

> We have embraced the concept of "real-time tracking." We have developed a "radar screen" that has 8 simultaneous processes continuously monitored. We get information on the census in the ER, the status of the patients, the x-ray cycle, etc. We know where in the process not only the patient is, but where the system is. Each process measured is summarized on the screen by graphs. All we have to do to obtain data is touch the screen. The graphs are equipped with goal lines that are based on customer satisfaction, for example waiting time.— Community based emergency department

> The key word to describe a micro-system is *homeostasis*. A micro-system is always changing and adapting, just like the human body. We have identified the "pathophysiology" of a micro-system. It is powerful, yet very predictable. Think about two downstream processes, x-ray cycle time and getting patients to the floor. If the downstream [processes] get out of control, there are predictable changes in the system. Occupancy in the ER goes up, the number of new patients seen in the ER goes down, the number of free beds in the ER goes down, and the cycle time between a patient's arrival to a bed goes up. Eventually, every measurement goes up. When we obtain three consecutive 15-minute intervals going the wrong way, we realize that something needs to be done.— Community based Emergency Department.

LEADERSHIP FOR MANAGING CHANGE

The role of leaders is to define and communicate the purpose of the organization clearly and establish the work of practice teams as being of highest strategic importance. Leaders must be responsible for creating and articulating the organization's vision and goals, listening to the needs and aspirations of those working on the front lines, providing direction, creating incentives for change, aligning and integrating improvement efforts, and creating a supportive environment and a culture of continuous improvement that encourage and enable success.

Learning organizations need leadership at many levels that can provide clear strategic and sustained direction and a coherent set of values and incentives to guide group and individual actions. The first criterion of performance excellence for health care organizations listed by the Baldrige National Quality Program is the provision of "a patient focus, clear and visible values, and high expectations" by the organization's senior leaders (National Institute of Standards and Technology, 2000a). Indeed, strong management leadership in hospitals is positively associated with greater clinical involvement in quality improvement (Weiner et al., 1996, 1997).

Leaders of health care organizations may need to provide an environment for innovation that allows for new and more flexible roles and responsibilities for health care workers; and supports the accomplishments of innovators despite regulatory, legal, financial, and sometimes interprofessional conflict (Donaldson and Mohr, 2000). Leaders need to provide such an environment because the learning, adaptation, and incorporation of best practices needed to effect engineering changes requires energy that is scarce in a demanding and rapidly changing environment.

At the level of front-line teams, leaders should encourage the members of the team to engage in deliberate inquiry—using their own observations and ideas to improve safety and quality. The individual who serves as leader may not be constant over time or across innovative efforts, or be associated with a particular discipline, such as medicine. What is important is for the leader to understand how units relate to each other—a form of systems thinking—and to facilitate the transfer of learning across units and practices.

Leaders of health care organizations must fill a number of specific roles. First, they must identify and prioritize community health needs and support the organization's ability to meet these needs. Addressing community needs might involve collaboration with other community or health care organizations and the creation of new services. Examples include providing CPR training for a major employer and identifying and alerting the community to patterns of injury, such as the number of children with head injuries from bicycle accidents, or a newly appearing occupational illness. Other examples include addressing the more complex needs for coordinated local social and health services presented by low-income ill elderly individuals or the need for more accessible substance abuse treatment facilities. Leaders of organizations can support accountability to individual patients while also assuming responsibility for accountability to public bodies and the community at large for the populations they serve.

Second, leaders can help obtain resources and respond to changes in the health care environment, which have been rapid and unrelenting. Leaders must ensure that their organization has the ability to change. Yet many leaders now view their role as shielding and protecting the organization from environmental pressures that may require them to change. Leadership should support innovation and provide a forum so that individuals can continuously learn from each other. Organizations must invest in innovation and redesign.

Third, and perhaps the most difficult leadership role, is to optimize the performance of teams that provide various services in pursuit of a shared set of aims. In any complex organization, there is danger in supporting some clinical services (perhaps those that are most profitable) to the detriment of the whole system. Leaders must strive to align the strategic priorities of their organization, its resources (financial and human), and support mechanisms (e.g., information systems). Balancing these elements can be extremely difficult and requires leaders to have a performance measurement capability that includes measures of safety, effectiveness, patient-centeredness, timeliness, efficiency, and equity.

Fourth, leaders can support reward and recognition systems that are consistent with and supportive of the new rules set forth in Chapter 3 and that facilitate coordination of work across sets of services as necessary. Organizations should support an environment in which incentives to provide effective care are not distorted before they reach caregivers. An example of distortion is a payment system based solely on the numbers of home care visits made by a visiting nurse per day. This sort of productivity measure prevents nurses from focusing on patient needs. A system based on effectively caring for a given number of patients recognizes that a predictable mix of needs will occur over a period of time, and can encourage small teams to organize themselves to meet those needs. Such decision making can be very difficult, especially in the current economic environment and payment system (see Chapter 8).

Fifth, leaders need to invest in their workforce to help them achieve their full potential, both individually and as a team, in serving their patients. The resulting interpersonal and technical competence can produce the synergies and improved outcomes that emerge from collaborative work.

Although the leadership roles described are not novel, the orientation toward facilitating the work of health care teams represents a fundamental shift in perspective. The new rules set forth in Chapter 3 and the engineering principles described in this chapter will require strong and visible leadership with corresponding reward structures. All organizations must overcome their inherent resistance to change. It is role of leaders to surmount these barriers by visibly promoting the need for improvement, becoming role models for the required new behaviors, providing the necessary resources, and aligning recognition and reward systems in support of improvement goals. Leadership's role in promoting innovation, gathering feedback, and recognizing progress is essential to successful and sustained improvement.

Finally, leaders must recognize the interdependence of changes at all levels of the organization—individual, group or team, organizational, and interorganizational—in addressing the six challenges discussed in this chapter. For example, providing additional training in error correction or technical skill development to individuals without recognizing that they work as part of a team will have little impact. Similarly, working to develop more effective teams without recognizing that they are part of a complex organization with frequently misaligned incentives will have little effect on improving quality. Likewise, trying to redesign organizational structures and incentives and revise organizational cultures without taking into account the specific needs of teams and individuals is likely to be an exercise in frustration. And attempting to make changes at any of these levels without recognizing the larger interorganizational networks that include other providers, payers, and legal and regulatory bodies (as discussed in subsequent chapters) is likely to result in the waste of well-intended plans and energy.

REFERENCES

Aiken, L. H., J. Sochalski, and E. T. Lake. Studying Outcomes of Organizational Change in Health Services. *Medical Care* 35(11 Suppl):NS6–18, 1997.

Anderson, John C., Manus Rungtusanatham, and Roger G. Schroeder. A Theory of Quality Management Underlying the Deming Management Method. *Academy of Management Review* 19(3): 472–509, 1994.

Argyris, Chris and Donald A. Schön. *Organizational Learning.* Reading, Mass.: Addison-Wesley Pub. Co., 1978.

Bates, David W., Lucian L. Leape, David J. Cullen, et al. Effect of Computerized Physician Order Entry and a Team Intervention on Prevention of Serious Medication Errors. *JAMA* 280(15): 1311–6, 1998.

Bennis, Warren and Michael Mische. *The 21st Century Organization: Reinventing Through Reengineering.* San Diego, CA: Pfeiffer & Company, 1995.

Berner, Eta S., Richard S. Maisiak, C. Glenn Cobbs, and O. D. Taunton. Effects of a Decision Support System on Physicians' Diagnostic Performance. *J Am Med Inform Assoc* 6(5):420–7, 1999.

Berwick, Donald M. A Primer on Leading the Improvement of Systems. *BMJ* 312:619–22, 1996.

Blumenthal, David. The Future of Quality Measurement and Management in a Transforming Health Care System. *JAMA* 278(19):1622–5, 1997.

Blumenthal, David and Charles M. Kilo. A Report Card on Continuous Quality Improvement. *Milbank Quarterly* 76(4):625–48, 1998.

Bowman, R. J. C., H. J. B. Bennet, C. A. Houston, et al. Waiting Times For and Attendance at Paediatric Ophthalmology Outpatient Appointments. *BMJ* 313:1244, 1996.

Carey, J. C. Health Supervision and Anticipatory Guidance for Children with Genetic Disorders (including specific recommendations for trisomy 21, trisomy 18, and neurofibromatosis I). *Pediatr Clin North Am* 39(1):25–53, 1992.

Christensen, Clayton M., Richard Bohmer, and John Kenagy. Will Disruptive Innovations Cure Health Care? *Harvard Business Review* September/October:102–12, 2000.

Classen, David C. Clinical Decision Support Systems to Improve Clinical Practice and Quality of Care. *JAMA* 280(15):1360–1, 1998.

Collins, James C. and Jerry I. Porras. *Built to Last: Successful Habits of Visionary Companies.* New York, NY: Harperbusiness, 1997.

COR Health LLC. Collaboratives Are the Hot Ticket to Success with Performance Improvement Initiatives. *COR Clinical Excellence* 1:1–3, 2000.

COR Healthcare Resources. It Takes a Network to Manage the Full Continuum of Stroke Care. *Medical Management Network* 8(3):1–7, 2000.

Cushman, F. Reid and Don E. Detmer. 1998. "Information Policy for the U.S. Health Sector: Engineering, Political Economy, and Ethics." Online. Available at http://www.milbank.org/art/ intro.html [accessed Dec. 1, 2000].

Davidoff, Frank and Valerie Florance. The Informationist: A New Health Profession? *Ann Int Med* 132(12):996–8, 2000.

Davies, Huw T. O. and Sandra M. Nutley. Developing Learning Organisations in the New NHS. *BMJ* 320:998–1001, 2000.

Davis, David A., Mary Ann Thomson, Nick Freemantle, et al. Impact of Formal Continuing Medical Education. Do Conferences, Workshops, Rounds, and Other Traditional Continuing Education Activities Change Physician Behavior or Health Care Outcomes? *JAMA* 282(9):867–74, 1999.

Desai, J., P. J. O'Connor, D. B. Bishop, et al. Variation in Process and Outcomes of Diabetes Care in HMO Owned and Controlled Clinics. *Proceedings, CDC Diabetes Trans. Conference.* Atlanta, GA: 1997.

Donaldson, Molla S. and Julie J. Mohr. *Exploring Innovation and Quality Improvement in Health Care Micro-Systems: A Cross-Case Analysis.* Washington, D.C.: Institute of Medicine, National Academy Press, 2000.

Evans, R. Scott, Stanley L. Pestotnik, David C. Classen, et al. A Computer-Assisted Management Program for Antibiotics and Other Antiinfective Agents. *N Engl J Med* 338(4):232–8, 1998.

Feitzinger, Edward and Hau L. Lee. Mass Customization at Hewlett-Packard: The Power of Postponement. *Harvard Business Review* Jan/Feb:116–21, 1997.

Festinger, D. S., R. J. Lamb, M. R. Kountz, et al. Pretreatment Dropout as a Function of Treatment Delay and Client Variables. *Addictive Behaviors* 20(1):111–5, 1995.

Fried, Bruce J., Sharon Topping, and Thomas G. Rundall. Groups and Teams in Health Services Organizations (Chapter 6). *Health Care Management. Organization and Design and Behavior.* 4th edition S. M. Shortell and A. D. Kaluzny, eds. Albany, NY: Delmar, 2000.

Galvin, Robert W., personal communication. Washington, D.C.: Meeting of the National Roundtable on Health Care Quality, 1998.

Gilmore, James H. and B. Joseph Pine, II. The Four Faces of Mass Customization. *Harvard Business Review* Jan/Feb:91–101, 1997.

Gittell, J. H., K. M. Fairfield, B. Bierbaum, et al. Impact of Relational Coordination on Quality of Care, Postoperative Pain and Functioning, and Length of Stay: A Nine-Hospital Study of Surgical Patients. *Medical Care* 38(8):807–19, 2000.

Glymph, Minnie. 2000. "Keeping Our Patients Safe . . . in the Pediatric Emergency Department." Online. Available at http://www2.md.duke.edu/news/inside/000710/4.html [accessed Nov. 30, 2000].

Goldsmith, Jeff C. Integration Reconsidered: Five Strategies for Improved Performance. *Healthcare Strateg* 2(11):1–8, 1998.

Grandinetti, Deborah A. You mean I can see the doctor today? *Medical Economics* 77(6):102–14, 2000.

Greco, Peter J. and John M. Eisenberg. Changing Physicians' Practice. *N Engl J Med* 329(17):1271–3, 1993.

Griffin, S. and A. L. Kinmouth. *Diabetes Care: The Effectiveness of Systems for Routine Surveillance for People with Diabetes (Cochrane Review).* The Cochrane Library, Oxford: Update Software, 1998.

Grol, Richard. Personal paper: Beliefs and Evidence in Changing Clinical Practice. *BMJ* 315:418–21, 1997.

Grol, Richard and Jeremy Grimshaw. Evidence-Based Implementation of Evidence-Based Medicine. *Joint Commission Journal on Quality Improvement* 25(10):503–13, 1999.

Hart, Julian Tudor. Clinical and Economic Consequences of Patients as Producers. *Journal of Public Health Medicine* 17(4):383–6, 1995.

Helmreich, Robert L. On Error Management: Lessons from Aviation. *BMJ* 320:781–5, 2000.

Hodgetts, Richard M. *Measures of Quality and High Performance: Simple Tools and Lessons Learned from America's Most Successful Corporations.* New York, NY: American Management Association, 1998.

Hunt, Dereck L., R. Brian Haynes, Steven E. Hanna, and Kristina Smith. Effects of Computer-Based Clinical Decision Support Systems on Physician Performance and Patient Outcomes: A Systematic Review. *JAMA* 280(15):1339–46, 1998.

Institute for Healthcare Improvement. 2000. "Idealized Design of Clinical Office Practices." Online. Available at http://www.ihi.org/idealized [accessed Aug. 23, 2000].

Institute of Medicine. *Guidelines for Clinical Practice: From Development to Use.* Marilyn J. Field and Kathleen N. Lohr, eds. Washington, D.C.: National Academy Press, 1992.

———. *To Err Is Human: Building a Safer Health System.* Linda T. Kohn, Janet M. Corrigan, and Molla S. Donaldson, eds. Washington, D.C: National Academy Press, 2000.

James, Brent C. *Quality Management for Health Care Delivery.* Chicago, IL: Hospital Research and Educational Trust, American Hospital Association, 1989.

Juran, J. M. *Juran on Leadership for Quality: An Executive Handbook.* New York, NY: The Free Press, 1989.

Kaiser Permanente Online. 2000. "Sample Version of Kaiser Permanente's Members Only Web Site." Online. Available at http://www.kaiserpermanente.org/membersonly/overview.htm [accessed Oct. 31, 2000].

Kegan, Robert. *In Over Our Heads: The Mental Demand of Modern Life.* Cambridge, Massachusetts: Harvard University Press, 1994.

Kibbe, David C. and Mark Bard. Applying Clinical Informatics to Health Care Improvement: Making Progress is More Difficult Than We Thought It Would Be. *Joint Commission Journal on Quality Improvement* 23(12):619–22, 1997a.

Kibbe, David and Mark Bard. A Roundtable Discussion: Have Computerized Patient Records Kept Their Promise of Improving Patient Care? *Joint Commission Journal on Quality Improvement* 23(12):695–702, 1997b.

Knaus, William A. Draper Elizabeth A. Wagner Douglas, et al. An Evaluation of Outcome from Intensive Care in Major Medical Centers. *Ann Int Med* 104(3):410–8, 1986.

Langley, Gerald J., Kevin M. Nolan, Thomas W. Nolan, et al. *The Improvement Guide. A Practical Approach to Enhancing Organizational Performance.* San Francisco, CA: Jossey-Bass, 1996.

Leibovich, Mark. Child Prodigy, Online Pioneer. *Washington Post.* A-23, Sept. 3, 2000.

Lorig, Kate R., Peter D. Mazonson, and Halsted R. Holman. Evidence Suggesting that Health Education for Self Management in Chronic Arthritis has Sustained Health Benefits While Reducing Health Care Costs. *Arthritis Rheumatism* 36(4):439–46, 1993.

Lorig, Kate R., David S. Sobel, Anita L. Steward, et al. Evidence Suggesting that a Chronic Disease Self-Management Program Can Improve Health Status While Reducing Hospitalization: A Randomized Trial. *Medical Care* 37(1):5–14, 1999.

MacLean, Catherine H., Rachel Louie, Barbara Leake, et al. Quality of Care for Patients With Rheumatoid Arthritis. *JAMA* 284(8):984–92, 2000.

Mark, Barbara and Alice C. Hagenmueller. Technological and Environmental Characteristics of Intensive Care Units. Implications for Job Redesign. *J Nurs Adm* 24(4 Suppl):65–71, 1994.

Mundinger, Mary O., Robert L. Kane, Elizabeth R. Lenz, et al. Primary Care Outcomes in Patients Treated by Nurse Practitioners or Physicians: A Randomized Trial. *JAMA* 283(1):59–68, 2000.

Murray, Mark. Modernising the NHS. Patient Care: Access. *BMJ* 320:1594–6, 2000.

Murray, Mark and Catherine Tantau. Must Patients Wait? *Joint Commission Journal on Quality Improvement* 24(8):423–5, 1998.

National Committee for Quality Assurance. *The State of Managed Care Quality 2000.* Washington, D.C.: National Committee for Quality Assurance, 2000.

National Committee for Quality Health Care. *Innovative Quality Health Care Strategies. Best Practices of NCQHC National Quality Health Care Award Winners, 1994–1999.* Ashburn, VA: The Severyn Group, 1999.

National Institute of Standards and Technology. 2000a. "Health Care Criteria for Performance Excellence. Baldrige National Quality Program, 2000." Online. Available at http://www. quality.nist.gov/bcpg.pdf.htm#HEALTH CARE [accessed Nov. 21, 2000].

———. 2000b. "National Quality Program: Home of the Malcolm Baldrige National Quality Award." Online. Available at http://www.quality.nist.gov [accessed Dec. 4, 2000].

Nelson, Eugene C., Julie J. Mohr, Paul B. Batalden, and Stephen K. Plume. Improving Health Care, Part 1: The Clinical Value Compass. *Joint Commission Journal on Quality Improvement* 22(4):243–58, 1996.

Nolan, Thomas W. System Changes to Improve Patient Safety. *BMJ* 320:771–3, 2000.

Nolan, Thomas W., Marie W. Schall, Donald M. Berwick, et al. *Reducing Delays and Waiting Times Throughout the Healthcare System.* Boston, MA: Institute for Healthcare Improvement, 1996.

Norman, Donald A. *The Design of Everyday Things.* New York, NY: Doubleday/Currency, 1988.

Nugent, William C., Charles M. Kilo, Cathy S. Ross, et al. *Improving Outcomes and Reducing Costs in Adult Cardiac Surgery.* Boston, MA: Institute for Healthcare Improvement, 1999.

Oxman, A., M. Thomason, D. Davis, et al. No Magic Bullets: A Systematic Review of 102 Trials of Interventions to Improve Professional Practice. *CMAJ* 153(10):1423–31, 1995.

Pearson, Pauline and Kevin Jones. The Primary Health Care Non-team? *BMJ* 309:1387–8, 1994.

Perrow, Charles. A Framework for the Comparative Analysis of Organizations. *American Sociological Review* 32:194–208, 1967.

Peters, Thomas J. and Robert H. Waterman, Jr. *In Search of Excellence: Lessons from America's Best-Run Companies.* New York, NY: Warner Books, Inc., 1982.

Pine, B. Joseph, II, Don Peppers, and Martha Rogers. Do You Want to Keep Customers Forever? *Harvard Business Review* Mar/Apr, 1995.

Rainey, Thomas G., Andrea Kabcenell, Donald M. Berwick, and Jane Roessner. *Reducing Costs and Improving Outcomes in Adult Intensive Care.* Boston, MA: Institute for Healthcare Improvement, 1998.

Raschke, Robert A., Bea Bollihare, Thomas A. Wunderlich, et al. A Computer Alert System to Prevent Injury From Adverse Drug Events: Development and Evaluation in a Community Teaching Hospital. *JAMA* 280(15):1317–20, 1998.

Robinson, James C. and Lawrence P. Casalino. Vertical Integration and Organizational Networks in Health Care. *Health Affairs* 15(1):7–22, 1996.

Rosenstein, Alan H. Using Information Management to Implement a Clinical Resource Management Program. *Joint Commission Journal on Quality Improvement* 23(12):653–66, 1997.

Schneider, Eric C., Virginia Riehl, Sonja Courte-Wienecke, et al. Enhancing Performance Measurement. NCQA's Road Map for a Health Information Framework. *JAMA* 282(12):1184–90, 1999.

Scholtes, Peter R. *The Team Handbook: How to Use Teams to Improve Quality.* Madison, WI: Joiner Associates, 1988.

Science Panel on Interactive Communication and Health. *Wired for Health and Well-Being. The Emergence of Interactive Health Communication.* T. R. Eng and D. H. Gustafson, eds. Washington, D.C.: U.S. Department of Health and Human Services, U.S. Government Printing Office, 1999.

Senge, Peter M. *The Fifth Discipline: The Art and Practice of the Learning Organization.* New York, NY: Doubleday/Currency, 1990.

Shortell, Stephen M., Charles L. Bennett, and Gayle R. Byck. Assessing the Impact of Continuous Quality Improvement on Clinical Practice: What It Will Take to Accelerate Progress. *Milbank Quarterly* 76(4):593–624, 1998.

Shortell, Stephen M., Robin R. Gillies, and David A. Anderson. *Remaking Health Care in America, Second Edition.* San Francisco, CA: Jossey-Bass, 2000a.

Shortell, Stephen M., Robert H. Jones, Alfred W. Rademaker, et al. Assessing the Impact of Total Quality Management and Organizational Culture on Multiple Outcomes of Care for Coronary Artery Bypass Graft Surgery Patients. *Medical Care* 38(2):207–17, 2000b.

Shortell, Stephen M., Jack E. Zimmerman, Denise M. Rousseau, et al. The Performance of Intensive Care Units: Does Good Management Make a Difference? *Medical Care* 32(5):508–25, 1994.

Shum, Chau, Ann Humphreys, David Wheeler, et al. Nurse Management of Patients with Minor Illnesses in General Practice: Multicentre, Randomised Controlled Trial. *BMJ* 320:1038–43, 2000.

Solberg, Leif I., Milo L. Brekke, Charles J. Fazio, et al. Lessons from Experienced Guideline Implementers: Attend to Many Factors and Use Multiple Strategies. *Joint Commission Journal on Quality Improvement* 26(4):171–88, 2000.

Starfield, Barbara. *Primary Care: Concept, Evaluation, and Policy*. New York, NY: Oxford University, 1992.

Terry, Ken. Re-engineer Your Practice—Starting Today. *Medical Economics* 77(2):174, 2000.

Thompson, James D. *Organizations in Action; Social Science Bases of Administrative Theory*. New York, NY: McGraw-Hill, 1967.

Transit Cooperative Research Program. *Report 8. The Quality Journey: A TQM Roadmap for Public Transportation*. National Research Council - Transportation Research Board. Washington, D.C.: National Academy Press, 1995.

Von Korff, Michael, Jessie Gruman, Judith Schaefer, Susan J. Curry, and Edward H. Wagner. Collaborative Management of Chronic Illness. *Ann Int Med* 127(12):1097–102, 1997.

Walton, Mary and W. Edwards Deming. *Deming Management Method*. New York, NY: Dodd, Mead, and Company, 1986.

Washington Business Group on Health. *Managing Care, Operations and Performance: Innovations in Organized Systems of Care*. Sally Coberly, Principal Investigator. Washington, D.C.: Washington Business Group on Health, 1998.

Weed, Lawrence L. Opening the Black Box of Clinical Judgment—An Overview. *BMJ* 319:1–4, 1999. Online. Available at http://www.bmj.com/cgi/reprint/319/7220/1279.pdf [accessed Jan. 24, 2001].

Weiner, Bryan J., Jeffrey A. Alexander, and Stephen M. Shortell. Leadership for Quality Improvement in Health Care: Empirical Evidence on Hospital Boards, Managers, and Physicians. *Medical Care Research and Review* 53(4):397–416, 1996.

Weiner, Bryan J., Stephen M. Shortell, and Jeffrey Alexander. Promoting Clinical Involvement in Hospital Quality Improvement Efforts: The Effects of Top Management, Board, and Physician Leadership. *Health Services Research* 32(4):491–510, 1997.

Wensing, M., T. van der Weijden, and R. Grol. Implementing Guidelines and Innovations in General Practice: Which Interventions are Effective? *British Journal of General Practioner* 48(427): 991–7, 1998.

6

Applying Evidence to Health Care Delivery

Substantial investments have been made in clinical research and development over the last 30 years, resulting in an enormous increase in the medical knowledge base and the availability of many more drugs and devices. Unfortunately, Americans are not reaping the full benefit of these investments. The lag between the discovery of more efficacious forms of treatment and their incorporation into routine patient care is unnecessarily long, in the range of about 15 to 20 years (Balas and Boren, 2000). Even then, adherence of clinical practice to the evidence is highly uneven.

A far more effective infrastructure is needed to apply evidence to health care delivery. Greater emphasis should be placed on systematic approaches to analyzing and synthesizing medical evidence for both clinicians and patients. Many promising private- and public-sector efforts now under way, including the Cochrane Collaboration, the *ACP Journal Club*, and the Evidence-Based Practice Centers supported by the Agency for Healthcare Research and Quality, represent excellent models and building blocks for a more comprehensive effort. Yet synthesizing the evidence is only the first step in making knowledge more usable by both clinicians and patients. Many efforts to develop clinical practice guidelines, defined as "systematically developed statements to assist practitioner and patient decisions about appropriate health care for specific clinical circumstances," flourished during the 1980s and early 1990s (Institute of Medicine, 1992). Although the translation of evidence into clinical practice guidelines is an important first step, however, the dissemination of guidelines alone has not been a very effective method of improving clinical practice (Cabana et al., 1999).

Far more sophisticated clinical decision support systems will be needed to assist clinicians and patients in selecting the best treatment options and delivering safe and effective care. Certain types of clinical decision support applications, most notably preventive service reminder systems and drug dosing systems, have been demonstrated to improve clinical decisions and should be adopted on a widespread basis (Balas et al., 2000; Bates et al., 1999). More complex applications, such as computer-aided diagnosis, are in earlier stages of development (Kassirer, 1994), but the potential for these systems to contribute to evidence-based practice and consumer-oriented care is great.

The spread of the Internet has opened up many new opportunities to make medical evidence more accessible to clinicians and consumers. The efforts of the National Library of Medicine to facilitate access to the medical literature by both consumers and health care professionals and to design Web sites that organize large amounts of information on particular health needs are particularly promising (Lindberg and Humphreys, 1999).

The development of a more effective infrastructure to synthesize and organize evidence around priority conditions and to improve clinician and consumer access to the evidence base through the Internet offers new opportunities to enhance quality measurement and reporting. A stronger and more organized evidence base should facilitate the development of valid and reliable quality measures for priority conditions that can be used for both internal quality improvement and external accountability. Broad-based involvement of private- and public-sector groups and strong leadership from within the medical and other health professions are critical to ensuring the success of this effort.

Recommendation 8: The Secretary of the Department of Health and Human Services should be given the responsibility and necessary resources to establish and maintain a comprehensive program aimed at making scientific evidence more useful and accessible to clinicians and patients. In developing this program, the Secretary should work with federal agencies and in collaboration with professional and health care associations, the academic and research communities, and the National Quality Forum and other organizations involved in quality measurement and accountability.

The infrastructure developed through this public- and private-sector partnership should focus initially on priority conditions (see Chapter 4, Recommendation 5). Its activities should include the following:

- Ongoing analysis and synthesis of the medical evidence
- Delineation of specific practice guidelines
- Enhanced dissemination efforts to communicate evidence and guidelines to the general public and professional communities

- Development of decision support tools to assist clinicians and patients in applying the evidence
  - Identification of best practices in the design of care processes
  - Development of quality measures for priority conditions

It is critical that leadership from the private sector, both professional and other health care leaders and consumer representatives, be involved in all aspects of this effort to ensure its applicability and acceptability to clinicians and patients.

BACKGROUND

Early definitions of evidence-based medicine or practice emphasized the "conscientious, explicit and judicious use of current best evidence in making decisions about the care of individual patients" (Sackett et al., 1996). In response to concerns that this definition failed to recognize the importance of other factors in making clinical decisions, more recent definitions explicitly incorporate clinical expertise and patient values into the decision-making process (Lohr et al., 1998). Contemporary definitions also clarify that "evidence" is intended to refer not only to randomized controlled trials, the "gold standard," but also to other types of systematically acquired information.

For purposes of this report, the following definition of evidence-based practice, adapted from Sackett et al. (2000), is used:

> Evidence-based practice is the integration of best research evidence with clinical expertise and patient values. *Best research evidence* refers to clinically relevant research, often from the basic health and medical sciences, but especially from patient-centered clinical research into the accuracy and precision of diagnostic tests (including the clinical examination); the power of prognostic markers; and the efficacy and safety of therapeutic, rehabilitative, and preventive regimens. *Clinical expertise* means the ability to use clinical skills and past experience to rapidly identify each patient's unique health state and diagnosis, individual risks and benefits of potential interventions, and personal values and expectations. *Patient values* refers to the unique preferences, concerns, and expectations that each patient brings to a clinical encounter and that must be integrated into clinical decisions if they are to serve the patient.

Evidence-based practice is not a new concept. One of its earliest proponents was Archie Cochrane, a British epidemiologist who wrote extensively in the 1950s and 1960s about the importance of conducting randomized controlled trials to upgrade the quality of medical evidence (Mechanic, 1998).

Evidence has always contributed to clinical decision making, but the standards for evidence have become more stringent, and the tools for its assembly and analysis have become more powerful and widely available (Davidoff, 1999). Prior to 1950, clinical evidence consisted of case reports, whereas during the latter half of the 20th century, results of about 131,000 randomized controlled trials of medical interventions were published. Study designs and methods of analysis have also become more sophisticated, and now include decision analysis, systematic review of the literature, meta-analysis, and cost-effectiveness analysis.

Prior to 1990, efforts to incorporate evidence-based decision making into practice encouraged clinicians to follow four steps. According to this approach, when a patient presents a problem for which the decision is not apparent, the clinician should (1) formulate a clear clinical question from that problem, (2) search for the relevant information from the best possible published or unpublished sources, (3) evaluate that evidence for its validity and usefulness, and (4) implement the appropriate findings (Davidoff, 1999).

During the last decade, it has become apparent that this strategy of training and encouraging clinicians to independently find, appraise, and apply the best evidence will not alone lead to major improvements in practice (Guyatt et al., 2000; McColl et al., 1998). The relevant information is widely scattered across the medical literature and of varying quality in terms of methodological rigor (Davidoff, 1999). Advanced study is required to master and apply state-of-the-art approaches to analysis of the literature. The demands and rigors of clinical practice do not allow clinicians the time required to undertake this process on a regular basis. Some have proposed a greater role for specially trained clinical librarians to assist clinicians in framing clinical questions and identifying the relevant literature (Davidoff and Florance, 2000). Many efforts are also under way to make it easier for clinicians and patients to access and interpret the findings of the literature.

SYNTHESIZING CLINICAL EVIDENCE

The most common approaches to synthesizing and integrating the results of primary studies are the conduct of systematic reviews and the development of evidence-based practice guidelines. Interest in applying both techniques has increased dramatically in the last 15 years (Chalmers and Haynes, 1994; Chalmers and Lau, 1993).

Systematic Reviews

Systematic reviews are scientific investigations that synthesize the results of multiple primary investigations. Conduct of a systematic review to answer a specific clinical question generally involves four steps (Cook et al., 1997):

• Conduct of a comprehensive search of potentially relevant articles using explicit, reproducible criteria in the selection of articles for review
• Critical appraisal of the scientific soundness of the research designs of the primary studies, including the selection of patients, sample size, and methods of accounting for confounding variables (Cook et al., 1997; Lohr and Carey, 1999)

- Synthesis of data
- Interpretation of results

There are two types of systematic reviews—qualitative and quantitative (Cook et al., 1997). In a qualitative review, the results of primary studies are summarized but not statistically combined. Quantitative reviews, sometimes called meta-analyses, use statistical methods to combine the data and results of two or more studies.

When applied properly, meta-analysis can be a powerful tool for reaching a decision about the efficacy of alternative treatments in a more timely fashion than is possible through the qualitative review of individual studies. A classic example is the case of the efficacy of thrombolysis in treating myocardial infarction (Davidoff, 1999). In a review of 33 randomized controlled trials published between 1959 and 1988 that examined the efficacy of thrombolysis in reducing acute mortality, it was found that most studies "suggested" some benefit of therapy; however, the outcomes varied considerably from one study to another, and for the most part, the studies did not achieve statistical significance (Lau et al., 1992). But through the use of meta-analysis techniques to combine the results of multiple studies (thus increasing the statistical power), it was possible to demonstrate by 1973 that the therapeutic efficacy of thrombolysis was statistically significant at the 0.05 level. Unfortunately, some medical textbooks in the early 1990s still contained statements that thrombolysis was an unproven therapy (Davidoff, 1999).

Systematic reviews are highly variable in their methodological rigor. In a critical evaluation of 50 articles describing a systematic review or meta-analysis of the treatment of asthma, for example, Jadad et al. (2000b) concluded that 40 publications had serious or extensive flaws. Reviews conducted by the Cochrane Collaboration, discussed below, were found to be far more rigorous than those published in peer-reviewed journals.

Two organized efforts are directed at conducting systematic reviews or meta-analyses. The first, the Cochrane Collaboration, was started in 1992 in Oxford, England. The second, the Agency for Healthcare Research and Quality's Evidence-Based Practice Centers program, started in 1997 and has resulted in the establishment of 12 centers, located mainly in universities, medical centers, and private research centers, that produce evidence-based reports on specific topics (Agency for Healthcare Research and Quality, 2000b).

The Cochrane Collaboration is an international network of health care professionals, researchers, and consumers that develops and maintains regularly updated reviews of evidence from randomized controlled trials and other research studies (Cochrane Collaboration, 1999). It currently comprises about 50 Collaborative Review Groups, which produce systematic reviews of various prevention and health care issues. The Collaboration maintains the Cochrane Library, a collection of several databases that is updated quarterly and distributed annually to subscribers on disk, on CD-ROM, and via the Internet. One of the databases, *The Cochrane Database of Systematic Reviews*, contains Cochrane reviews, and another, *The Cochrane Controlled Trials Register*, is a bibliographic database of controlled trials. *The Database of Abstracts of Reviews of Effectiveness* includes structured abstracts of systematic reviews that have been critically appraised by the National Health Services Centre for Reviews and Dissemination in York, England; the *American College of Physicians' Journal Club;* and the journal *Evidence-Based Medicine*. The library also includes a registry of bibliographic information on nearly 160,000 controlled trials that provide high-quality evidence on health care outcomes.

The Agency for Healthcare Research and Quality's 12 Evidence-Based Practice Centers conduct systematic, comprehensive analyses and syntheses of the scientific literature on clinical conditions/problems that are common, account for a sizable proportion of resources, and are significant for the Medicare or Medicaid populations (Agency for Healthcare Research and Quality, 2000b). The centers include universities (Duke University, The Johns Hopkins University, McMaster University, Oregon Health Sciences University, the University of California at San Francisco, and Stanford University); research organizations (Meta-Works, the Research Triangle Institute, and the RAND Corporation); and health care organizations and associations (New England Medical Center, and Blue Cross and Blue Shield Association). Since December 1998, evidence reports have been released on the following topics: sleep apnea, traumatic brain injury, alcohol dependence, cervical cytology, urinary tract infection, depression, dysphagia, sinusitis, testosterone suppression, attention deficit/hyperactivity disorder, and atrial fibrillation (Eisenberg, 2000a).

In response to the rapid increase in the volume of and interest in systematic reviews generated by the Cochrane Collaboration, the Evidence-Based Practice Centers, and many other smaller-scale efforts, numerous journals specializing in evidence-based publications have emerged. The first journal devoted exclusively to systematic reviews and meta-analyses was the *ACP Journal Club*, first published in 1991. There are now a number of evidence-based journals, including *Evidence-Based Medicine, Journal of Evidence-Based Health Care, Evidence-Based Cardiovascular Medicine, Evidence-Based Mental Health*, and *Evidence-Based Nursing*, as well as numerous "best-evidence" departments in other journals (Sackett et al., 2000).

One of the most recent evidence-based resources is *Clinical Evidence*, an "evidence formulary" resulting from a collaborative effort of the *British Medical Journal* and the American College of Physicians (Godlee et al., 1999). *Clinical Evidence* is noteworthy because of its focus and organization around common conditions. First published in June 1999, it includes summaries on the prevention and treatment of about 70 such conditions. The summaries are based on systematic reviews and, when these are lacking, individual randomized controlled trials.

Clinical Evidence will be updated periodically, and eventually will lead to a family of products available in electronic and print form.

Practice Guidelines

Clinical practice guidelines can be defined as "systematically developed statements to assist practitioner and patient decisions about appropriate health care for specific clinical circumstances" (Institute of Medicine, 1992). Guidelines build on syntheses of the evidence, but go one step further to provide formal conclusions or recommendations about appropriate and necessary care for specific types of patients (Lohr et al., 1998). As a practical tool to influence practice, guidelines have been used in continuing medical education and clinical practice, as well as to make decisions about benefits coverage and medical necessity.

Guidelines have proliferated at a rapid pace during the last decade. During the early 1990s, the Agency for Health Care Policy and Research (now the Agency for Healthcare Research and Quality) sponsored an ambitious program for guideline development, which led to the specification of about 20 guidelines across a wide variety of clinical areas (Agency for Healthcare Research and Quality, 2000a; Perfetto and Stockwell Morris, 1996). The efforts in this area were eventually curtailed in favor of establishing the Evidence-Based Practice Centers in partnership with private-sector organizations (Lohr et al., 1998). Specialty societies, professional groups, health plans, medical centers, utilization review organizations, and others have also developed many practice guidelines.

Guidelines vary greatly in the degree to which they are derived from and consistent with the evidence base, for several reasons. First, as noted above, there is much variability in the quality of systematic reviews, which are the foundation for guidelines. Second, guideline development generally relies on expert panels to arrive at specific clinical conclusions. Judgment must be exercised in this process because the evidence base is sometimes weak or conflicting, or lacking in the specificity needed to develop recommendations useful for making decisions about individual patients in particular settings (Lohr et al., 1998).

In an effort to organize information on practice guidelines and to identify those having an adequate evidence base, the Agency for Healthcare Research and Quality, in partnership with the American Medical Association and the American Association of Health Plans, has developed a National Guideline Clearinghouse, which became fully operational in 1999 (Eisenberg, 2000a). The Clearinghouse provides online access to a large and growing repository of evidence-based practice guidelines.

Developing and disseminating practice guidelines alone has minimal effect on clinical practice (Cabana et al., 1999; Hayward, 1997; Lomas et al., 1989; Woolf, 1993). But a growing body of evidence indicates that guidelines implemented with patient-specific feedback and/or computer-generated reminders lead to significant improvements (Dowie, 1998; Grimshaw and Russell, 1993). More recent literature in this area also recognizes the importance of breaking down cultural, financial, organizational, and other barriers, both internal and external to health care organizations, to achieve widespread compliance with evidence-based guidelines (Solberg et al., 2000). To this end, up-front involvement of leaders from the health professions and representatives of patients in the guideline development process would likely help to ensure widespread adoption of the guidelines developed.

USING COMPUTER-BASED CLINICAL DECISION SUPPORT SYSTEMS

Until now, we have believed that the best way to transmit knowledge from its source to its use in patient care is to first load the knowledge into human minds . . . and then expect those minds, at great expense, to apply the knowledge to those who need it. However, there are enormous 'voltage drops' along this transmission line for medical knowledge.—Lawrence Weed, 1997

A clinical decision support system (CDSS) is defined as software that integrates information on the characteristics of individual patients with a computerized knowledge base for the purpose of generating patient-specific assessments or recommendations designed to aid clinicians and/or patients in making clinical decisions.[1] Work on such systems has been under way for decades with minimal impact on health care delivery. Interest in CDSSs has grown dramatically during the last decade, however, in part because of the promise such systems hold for assisting clinicians and patients in applying science to practice.

Publications reporting the results of clinical trials evaluating the effectiveness of CDSSs have also increased in number and quality in recent years. In a systematic review of controlled clinical trials assessing the effects of CDSSs on physician performance and patient outcomes, Hunt and colleagues identified 68 publications during the period 1974 through 1998, with 40 of these having been published in the most recent 6-year period (Hunt et al., 1998; Johnston et al., 1994).

CDSS applications assist clinicians and patients with three types of clinical decisions: preventive and monitoring tasks, prescribing of drugs, and diagnosis and management. Applications in the first category and most applications to date in the second category deal with less complex and frequently occurring clinical decisions. The software required to assist clinicians and patients with these types of decisions can be constructed using relatively simple rule-based logic, often based on practice guidelines (Delaney et al., 1999; Shea et al., 1996). Applications in the third category are far more complex and require more comprehensive

---

[1]This definition is adapted from a physician-oriented definition developed by Hunt et al., 1998.

patient-specific data, access to a much larger repository of up-to-date clinical knowledge, and more sophisticated probabilistic mathematical models.

Use of a CDSS for prevention and monitoring purposes has been shown to improve compliance with guidelines in many clinical areas. In a meta-analysis of 16 randomized controlled trials, computer reminders were found to improve preventive practices for vaccinations, breast cancer screening, colorectal cancer screening, and cardiovascular risk reduction, but not for cervical cancer screening or other preventive services (e.g., glaucoma screening, TB skin test) (Shea et al., 1996). In another meta-analysis of 33 studies of the effect of prompting clinicians, 25 of which used computer-generated prompts, the technique was found to enhance performance significantly in all 16 preventive care procedures studied (Balas et al., 2000). Computer-generated reminder systems targeting patients have also been shown to be effective (Balas et al., 2000; McDowell et al., 1986, 1989).

Computerized prescribing of drugs offers great potential benefit in such areas as dosing calculations and scheduling, drug selection, screening for interactions, and monitoring and documentation of adverse side effects (Schiff and Rucker, 1998). Many studies have been conducted on the use of CDSSs to improve drug dosing, and most (9 out of 15) show some positive effect (Hunt et al., 1998). The use of CDSSs for drug selection, screening for interactions, and monitoring and documentation of adverse side effects is far more limited because these applications generally require the linkage of more comprehensive patient-specific clinical information with the medication knowledge base. Although comprehensive medication order entry systems have been implemented in only a limited number of health care settings, the results of several recent studies have demonstrated that these systems reduce medical errors and costs (Bates et al., 1997, 1998, 1999). Computer-assisted disease management programs in areas in which decision making about medications is complex, such as the use of antibiotic and anti-infective agents, also have been shown to have a positive impact on quality and cost reduction (Classen et al., 1992; Evans et al., 1998).

The third category, computer-assisted diagnostic and management aids, is by far the most challenging. These systems require (1) an expansive knowledge base covering the full range of diseases and conditions, (2) detailed patient-specific clinical information (e.g., history, physical examination, laboratory data), and (3) a powerful computational engine that employs some form of probabilistic decision analysis.

Interest in computer-assisted diagnosis goes back more than four decades, and yet there have been only a few evaluations of its performance (Kassirer, 1994). In a systematic review of 68 CDSS controlled trials between 1974 and 1998, Hunt and colleagues found only 5 studies (4 of the 5 published before 1990) that assessed the role of CDSSs in diagnosis, only one of which found a benefit from their use (Chase et al., 1983; Hunt et al., 1998; Pozen et al., 1984; Wellwood et al., 1992; Wexler et al., 1975; Wyatt, 1989).

These early studies generally evaluated how well a computer performed in making or generating plausible diagnoses as compared with the decisions of experts, not the ability of a computer in partnership with a practicing clinician to perform better than the clinician alone (Kassirer, 1994). One recent study compared the performance of practicing clinicians with and without the aid of a diagnostic CDSS, and found among the former a significant improvement in the generation of correct diagnoses in hypothesis lists (Friedman et al., 1999). The study included faculty, residents, and fourth-year medical students; while all three groups performed better with the help of the computer, the magnitude of the improvement was greatest for students and smallest for faculty.

Studies conducted to date do not provide a convincing case in support of CDSS diagnostic tools. Yet it is important to recognize that changes under way in health care and computing will likely result in the development of far superior tools in the near future, for three reasons. First, CDSS diagnostic programs have been limited to date in terms of their clinical knowledge base. The cost of maintaining updated syntheses of the evidence for most conditions and translating these syntheses into decision rules has been prohibitively high for commercial developers of these systems. As discussed above, however, interest in evidence-based practice has led to a logarithmic increase in systematic reviews of the clinical evidence on particular clinical questions, which are available in the public domain.

Second, advances in computer technology, accompanied by dramatic decreases in the cost of hardware and software, have greatly reduced concerns about the computing requirements of CDSS diagnostic systems. Furthermore, there are early signs of CDSS diagnostic systems becoming available on the Internet, thus further reducing the capital investment and operational costs incurred at the level of a clinical practice (McDonald et al., 1998).

Third, the Internet has opened up new opportunities to address issues related to patient data. As noted, to be effective, CDSS diagnostic systems require detailed, patient-specific clinical information (history, physical results, medications, laboratory test results), which in most health care settings resides in a variety of paper and automated datasets that cannot easily be integrated. Past efforts to develop automated medical record systems have not been very successful because of the lack of common standards for coding data, the absence of a data network connecting the many health care organizations and clinicians involved in patient care, and a number of other factors. The Internet has the potential to overcome many of these barriers to automated patient data. The World Wide Web offers much of the standardization technology needed to combine independent sources of clinical data (McDonald et al., 1998). The willingness of patients and clinicians to use these systems will depend to a great extent on finding ways to adequately address concerns about the confidentiality of personally identifiable clinical information and a host of technical, legal, policy, and organizational issues that currently impede many health applications on the

Internet. But numerous efforts are under way to address these issues as they apply to both the current and the next-generation Internet (Elhanan et al., 1996; National Research Council, 2000).

Fourth, the extraordinary advances achieved in molecular medicine in recent years will further increase the complexity of both the evidence base and the clinical decision-making process, making it imperative that clinicians use computer-aided decision supports. Molecular medicine introduces a huge new body of knowledge that will affect virtually every area of practice, and also opens up the possibility of developing individualized treatments linked to a patient's genetic definition (Rienhoff, 2000). CDSS programs offer the prospect of applying more sophisticated forms of decision analysis to the evaluation of various treatment options, taking into account both the patient's genetic definition and preferences (Lilford et al., 1998).

Given the potential of CDSSs to enhance evidence-based practice and provide greater opportunity for patients to participate in clinical decision making, the committee believes greater public investment in research and development on such systems is warranted. In fiscal year 1999, the Agency for Healthcare Research and Quality began a new initiative, Translating Research into Practice, aimed at implementing evidence-based tools and information in health care settings (Eisenberg, 2000a). The focus of the initiative is on cultivating partnerships between researchers and health care organizations for the conduct of practice-based, patient outcome research in applied settings. In fiscal year 1999, 3-year grants were awarded in support of projects to identify effective approaches to smoking cessation, chlamydia screening of adolescents, diabetes care in medically underserved areas, and treatment of respiratory distress syndrome in preterm infants. The resources for this program should be expanded to support an applied research and development agenda specific to CDSSs.

MAKING INFORMATION AVAILABLE ON THE INTERNET

The Internet is rapidly becoming the principal vehicle for communication of health information to both consumers and clinicians. It is predicted that 90 percent of households will have Internet access by 2005–2010 (Rosenberg, 1999). The number of Americans who use the Internet to retrieve health-related information is estimated to be about 70 million (Cain et al., 2000). The connectivity of health care organizations has also increased. For example, between 1993 and 1997, the percentage of academic medical libraries with Internet connections increased from 72 to 96 percent, and that of community hospital libraries rose from 24 to 72 percent (Lyon et al., 1998).

The volume of health care information available on the Internet is enormous. Estimates of the number of health-related Web sites vary from 10,000 to 100,000 (Benton Foundation, 1999; Eysenbach et al., 1999). A survey conducted by *USA Today* found that consumers access health-related Web sites to research an illness or disease (62 percent), seek nutrition and fitness information (20 percent), research drugs and their interactions (12 percent), find a doctor or hospital (4 percent), and look for online medical support groups (2 percent) (*USA Today*, 1998).

It is easy for a user to be overwhelmed by the volume of information available on the Web. For example, there are some 61,000 Web sites that contain information on breast cancer (Boodman, 1999), and a simple search for "diabetes mellitus" returns more than 40,000 sites (National Research Council, 2000). Information available on the Internet is also of varying quality: some is incorrect, and some is misleading (Achenbach, 1996; Biermann et al., 1999). Several options have been proposed to assist users in distinguishing the good information from the bad. Silberg et al. (1997) have encouraged Web site sponsors to adhere voluntarily to a set of rules including (1) inclusion of information on authors, along with their affiliations and credentials; (2) attribution, including references and sources for all content; (3) disclosure of Web site ownership, sponsorship, advertising, underwriting, commercial funding, and potential conflicts of interest; and (4) dates on which content was posted and updated.

To identify valuable information, users can rely on a number of rating services that review and rate Web sites, but there are problems with many of these rating services as well. In a recent review, Jadad and Gagliardi (1998) identified 47 rating services, of which only 14 provided a description of the criteria used to produce the ratings, and none gave information on interobserver reliability or construct validity.

One of the richest sources of clinical information on the Internet is the National Library of Medicine's (NLM) MEDLINE. MEDLINE contains more than 9 million citations and abstracts of articles drawn mainly from professional journals (Miller et al., 2000). In June 1997, NLM made MEDLINE available free of charge on the Web, and usage jumped about 10-fold to 75 million searches annually (Lindberg and Humphreys, 1998).

When MEDLINE was established, it was assumed that its primary audience would be health care professionals, but it is now recognized that the lay public has a keen interest in accessing the clinical knowledge base as well. It is estimated that about 30 percent of MEDLINE searches are by members of the general public and students, 34 percent by health care professionals, and 36 percent by researchers (Lindberg, 1998). In 1998, NLM added 12 consumer health journals to MEDLINE to increase its coverage of information written for the general public, and also launched MEDLINE*plus*, a Web site specifically for consumers (Lindberg and Humphreys, 1999). MEDLINE*plus* is divided into eight sections (e.g., health topics, databases, organizations, clearinghouses), each of which provides links to reputable Web sites maintained by the National Institutes of Health, the Centers for Disease Control and Prevention, the Food and Drug Administration, and professional organizations and associations.

The MEDLINE*plus* section HealthTopics provides users with access to pre-formulated MEDLINE searches on common topics, most of which are diseases or conditions. The topics included were identified through an analysis of the most common search terms used on the NLM home page, which revealed that 90 percent or more were for specific diseases, conditions, or other common medical terms (e.g., Viagra, St. John's Wort) (Miller et al., 2000). The HealthTopics list numbers more than 300, with some of the most frequently searched topics being diabetes, shingles, prostate, hypertension, asthma, lupus, fibromyalgia, multiple sclerosis, and cancer.

There are many other sources of filtered evidence-based information as well, including the Cochrane Library discussed above. Access to evidence-based guidelines is provided in the United States by the National Guideline Clearinghouse (sponsored by the Agency for Healthcare Research and Quality), the American Medical Association, and the American Association of Health Plans (Agency for Healthcare Research and Quality et al., 2000), and in Canada by the CPG Infobase (sponsored by the Canadian Medical Association) (Canadian Medical Association, 2000). NOAH (New York Online Access to Health) is a library collaboration for bilingual consumer health information on the Internet (Voge, 1998).

Thus many efforts are under way to assist users in accessing useful health care information on the Web. Some believe, however, that much more could be done to achieve a more "powerful and efficient synergy" between the Internet and evidence-based decision making (Jadad et al., 2000a).

DEFINING QUALITY MEASURES

The enhanced interest in and infrastructure to support evidence-based practice have implications for quality measurement, improvement, and accountability (Eisenberg, 2000b). The use of priority conditions as a framework for organizing the evidence base, as discussed in Chapter 4, may also have implications for external accountability programs.

Systematic reviews and practice guidelines provide a strong foundation for the development of a richer set of quality measures focused on medical care processes and outcomes. To date, a good deal of quality measurement for purposes of external accountability has focused on a limited number of "rate-based" indicators—rates of occurrence of desired or undesired events. The National Committee for Quality Assurance, through its Health Plan Employer Data and Information Set, makes comparative quality data available on participating health plans and includes such measures as childhood immunization rates, mammography rates, and the percentage of diabetics who had an annual eye exam (National Committee for Quality Assurance, 1999). The Joint Commission on the Accreditation of Healthcare Organizations sponsors the ORYX system for hospitals, which includes measures such as infection rates and postsurgical complication rates. Syntheses of the evidence base and the development of practice guidelines should contribute to more valid and meaningful quality measurement and reporting.

As systematic reviews, development of practice guidelines, and efforts to disseminate evidence focus increasingly on priority conditions—a unit of analysis that is meaningful to patients and clinicians—so, too, must accountability processes. To date, efforts to make comparative quality data available in the public domain have focused on types of health care organizations, for the most part health plans and hospitals, and, as noted above, measurement of a limited number of discrete quality indicators for these organizations. Numerous efforts are under way, however, to develop comprehensive measurement sets for various conditions and quality reporting mechanisms. These include the efforts of the Foundation for Accountability, the Health Care Financing Administration's peer review organizations, and a variety of collaborations involving leading medical associations and accrediting bodies.

The Foundation for Accountability (2000b) has developed condition-specific measurement guides related to a number of common conditions: adult asthma, alcohol misuse, breast cancer, diabetes, health status under age 65, and major depressive disorders. The Foundation continues to work on child and adolescent health, coronary heart disease, end of life, and HIV/AIDS. In addition, it has created FACCT | ONE, a survey tool designed to gather information directly from patients about important aspects of their health care (Foundation for Accountability, 2000a). The first phase of the survey addresses quality of care for people living with the chronic illnesses of asthma, diabetes, and coronary artery disease. It assesses performance related to patient education and knowledge, obtaining of essential treatments, access, involvement in care decisions, communication with providers, patient self-management behaviors, coping, symptom control, maintenance of regular activities, and functional status.

Since 1992, the Health Care Financing Administration, through its Peer Review Organizations, has been developing core sets of performance measures for a number of common conditions, including acute myocardial infarction, heart failure, stroke, pneumonia, breast cancer, and diabetes (Health Care Financing Administration, 2000). Comparative performance data for Medicare fee-for-service beneficiaries by state were recently released for each of these conditions (Jencks et al., 2000). Quality-of-care measures for beneficiaries experiencing acute myocardial infarction have been piloted in four states as part of the Cooperative Cardiovascular Project (Ellerbeck et al., 1995; Marciniak et al., 1998).

The Diabetes Quality Improvement Project, a collaborative quality measurement effort involving the American Diabetes Association, the Foundation for Accountability, the Health Care Financing Administration, the National Committee for Quality Assurance, the American Academy of Physicians, the American College of Physicians, and the Veterans Administration, has been under way for several years. The project has identified seven accountability measures (i.e., hemoglobin A1c tested, poor hemoglobin A1c control, eye exam performed, lipid profile performed, lipids controlled, monitoring for kidney disease, and blood pressure controlled), six of which will be included in the National Committee for Quality Assurance's Year 2000 Health Plan Employer Data and Information Set (Health Care Financing Administration, 1999).

The American Medical Association, working with experts from national medical specialty societies and the quality measurement community, has developed measure sets for physician clinical performance in the areas of adult diabetes, prenatal testing, and chronic stable coronary artery disease. The core measure set for adult diabetes, developed with input from the Iowa Foundation for Medical Care, was approved by the American Medical Association in July 2000, while the other two measure sets are undergoing public review and comment (American Medical Association, 2000).

It will be important for the National Quality Forum, a recently created public–private partnership developed to foster collaboration across public and private oversight organizations, to consider carefully how best to align comparative quality reporting with the developing infrastructure in support of evidence-based practice and consumer-centered health care. The National Quality Forum, a not-for-profit organization established in 1999 with the participation of both public and private purchasers, is currently developing a strategic measurement framework to guide the future development of external quality reporting for purposes of accountability and consumer choice (Kizer, 2000). This activity, now under way, presents a unique opportunity to influence the direction of quality measurement.

REFERENCES

Achenbach, Joel. Reality Check. You Can't Believe Everything You Read. But You'd Better Believe This. *Washington Post.* E–C01, Dec. 4, 1996.

Agency for Healthcare Research and Quality. 2000a. "Clinical Practice Guidelines Online." Online. Available at http://www.ahcpr.gov/clinic/cpgonline.htm [accessed Jan. 2, 2001].

———. 2000b. "Evidence-based Practice Centers. Synthesizing Scientific Evidence to Improve Quality and Effectiveness in Clinical Care. AHRQ Publication No. 00–P013." Online. Available at http://www.ahcpr.gov/clinic/epc/ [accessed Oct. 11, 2000].

Agency for Healthcare Research and Quality, American Medical Association, and American Association of Health Plans. 2000. "National Guideline Clearinghouse." Online. Available at http://www.guideline.gov [accessed Jan. 2, 2001].

American Medical Association. *Adult Diabetes Core Physician Performance Measurement Set.* Chicago, IL: American Medical Association, 2000.

Balas, E. Andrew and Suzanne A. Boren. Managing Clinical Knowledge for Health Care Improvement. *Yearbook of Medical Informatics.* National Library of Medicine, Bethesda, MD:65–70, 2000.

Balas, E. Andrew, Scott Weingarten, Candace T. Garb, et al. Improving Preventive Care by Prompting Physicians. *Arch Int Med* 160(3):301–8, 2000.

Bates, David W., Lucian L. Leape, David J. Cullen, et al. Effect of Computerized Physician Order Entry and a Team Intervention on Prevention of Serious Medication Errors. *JAMA* 280(15): 1311–6, 1998.

Bates, David W., Nathan Spell, David J. Cullen, et al. The Costs of Adverse Drug Events in Hospitalized Patients. *JAMA* 277(4):307–11, 1997.

Bates, David W., Jonathan M. Teich, Joshua Lee, et al. The Impact of Computerized Physician Order Entry on Medication Error Prevention. *J Am Med Inform Assoc* 6(4):313–21, 1999.

Benton Foundation. 1999. "Networking for Better Care: Health Care in the Information Age." Online. Available at http://www.benton.org/Library/health/ [accessed Sept. 18, 2000].

Biermann, J. Sybil, Gregory J. Golladay, Mary Lou V. H. Greenfield, and Laurence H. Baker. Evaluation of Cancer Information on the Internet. *Cancer* 86(3):381–90, 1999.

Boodman, Sandra G. Medical Web Sites Can Steer You Wrong. Study Finds Erroneous and Misleading Information on Many Pages Dedicated to a Rare Cancer. *Washington Post.* Health–Z07, Aug. 10, 1999.

Cabana, Michael D., Cynthia S. Rand, Neil R. Powe, et al. Why Don't Physicians Follow Clinical Practice Guidelines? A Framework for Improvement. *JAMA* 282(15):1458–65, 1999.

Cain, Mary M., Robert Mittman, Jane Sarasohn-Kahn, and Jennifer C. Wayne. *Health e-People: The Online Consumer Experience.* Oakland, CA: Institute for the Future, California Health Care Foundation, 2000.

Canadian Medical Association. 2000. "CMA Infobase - Clinical Practice Guidelines." Online. Available at http://www.cma.ca/cpgs/index.asp [accessed Jan. 2, 2001].

Chalmers, Iain and Brian Haynes. Systematic Reviews: Reporting, Updating, and Correcting Systematic Reviews of the Effects of Health Care. *BMJ* 309:862–5, 1994.

Chalmers, T. C. and J. Lau. Meta-Analytic Stimulus for Changes in Clinical Trials. *Statistical Methods in Medical Research* 2:161–72, 1993.

Chase, Christopher R., Pamela M. Vacek, Tamotsu Shinozaki, et al. Medical Information Management: Improving the Transfer of Research Results to Presurgical Evaluation. *Medical Care* 21(3):410–24, 1983.

Classen, David C., R. Scott Evans, Stanley L. Pestotnik, et al. The Timing of Prophylactic Administration of Antibiotics and the Risk of Surgical-Wound Infection. *N Engl J Med* 326(5):281–6, 1992.

Cochrane Collaboration. 1999. "Cochrane Brochure." Online. Available at http://hiru.mcmaster.ca/cochrane/cochrane/cc-broch.htm [accessed Jan. 2, 2001].

Cook, Deborah J., Cynthia D. Mulrow, and R. Brian Haynes. Systematic Reviews: Synthesis of Best Evidence for Clinical Decisions. *Ann Int Med* 126(5):376–80, 1997.

Davidoff, Frank. In the Teeth of the Evidence. The Curious Case of Evidence-Based Medicine. *The Mount Sinai Journal of Medicine* 66(2):75–83, 1999.

Davidoff, Frank and Valerie Florance. The Informationist: A New Health Profession? *Ann Int Med* 132(12):996–8, 2000.

Delaney, Brendan C., David A. Fitzmaurice, Amjid Riaz, and F. D. Richard Hobbs. Changing the Doctor–Patient Relationship: Can Computerised Decision Support Systems Deliver Improved Quality in Primary Care? *BMJ* 319:1281, 1999.

Dowie, Robin. A Review of Research in the United Kingdom to Evaluate the Implementation of Clinical Guidelines in General Practice. *Family Practice* 15(5):462–70, 1998.

Eisenberg, John M. Quality Research for Quality Healthcare: The Data Connection. *Health Services Research* 35:xii–xvii, 2000a.

———. A Research Agenda for Quality. Washington, D.C.: Presentation at the Institute of Medicine Thirtieth Annual Meeting, The National Academies, 2000b.

Elhanan, G., S. A. Socratous, and J. J. Cimino. Integrating DXplain into a Clinical Information System Using the World Wide Web. *Proc AMIA Annual Fall Symp*:348–52, 1996.

Ellerbeck, Edward F., Stephen F. Jencks, Martha J. Radford, et al. Quality of Care for Medicare Patients With Acute Myocardial Infarction: A Four-State Pilot Study from the Cooperative Cardiovascular Project. *JAMA* 273(19):1509–14, 1995.

Evans, R. Scott, Stanley L. Pestotnik, David C. Classen, et al. A Computer-Assisted Management Program for Antibiotics and Other Antiinfective Agents. *N Engl J Med* 338(4):232–8, 1998.

Eysenbach, Gunther, Eun Ryoung Sa, and Thomas L. Diepgen. Shopping Around the Internet Today and Tomorrow: Towards the Millennium of Cybermedicine. *BMJ* 319:1294, 1999.

Foundation for Accountability. 2000a. "FACCT│ONE: A Tool for Evaluating the Performance of Health Care Organizations." Online. Available at http://www.facct.org/measures/Develop/FACCTONE.htm [accessed Jan. 2, 2001].

———. 2000b. "Supporting Quality-Based Decisions. The FACCT Consumer Information Network, Comparative Information for Better Health Care Decisions." Online. Available at http://www.facct.org/information.html [accessed Jan. 2, 2001].

Friedman, Charles P., Arthur S. Elstein, Fredric M. Wolf, et al. Enhancement of Clinicians' Diagnostic Reasoning by Computer-Based Consultation. *JAMA* 282(19):1851–6, 1999.

Godlee, Fiona, Richard Smith, and David Goldmann. Clinical Evidence: This month sees the publication of a new resource for clinicians. *BMJ* 318:1570–1, 1999.

Grimshaw, Jeremy M. and Ian T. Russell. Effect of Clinical Guidelines on Medical Practice: A Systematic Review of Rigorous Evaluations. *The Lancet* 342:1317–22, 1993.

Guyatt, Gordon H., Maureen O. Meade, Roman Z. Jaeschke, et al. Practitioners of Evidence Based Care: Not All Clinicians Need to Appraise Evidence from Scratch but All Need Some Skills. *BMJ* 320:954–5, 2000.

Hayward, Robert S. A. Clinical Practice Guidelines on Trial. *Can Med Assoc J* 156:1725–7, 1997.

Health Care Financing Administration. 1999. "Quality of Care—National Projects. Diabetes Quality Improvement Project (DQIP)." Online. Available at http://www.hcfa.gov/quality/3l.htm [accessed Jan. 2, 2001].

———. 2000. "Quality of Care - PRO Priorities. National Clinical Topics (Task 1)." Online. Available at http://www.hcfa.gov/quality/11a.htm [accessed Jan. 2, 2001].

Hunt, Dereck L., R. Brian Haynes, Steven E. Hanna, and Kristina Smith. Effects of Computer-Based Clinical Decision Support Systems on Physician Performance and Patient Outcomes: A Systematic Review. *JAMA* 280(15):1339–46, 1998.

Institute of Medicine. *Guidelines for Clinical Practice: From Development to Use.* Marilyn J. Field and Kathleen N. Lohr, eds. Washington, D.C.: National Academy Press, 1992.

Jadad, Alejandro R. and Anna Gagliardi. Rating Health Information on the Internet: Navigating to Knowledge or to Babel? *JAMA* 279(8):611–4, 1998.

Jadad, Alejandro R., R. Brian Haynes, Dereck Hunt, and George P. Browman. The Internet and Evidence-Based Decision-Making: A Needed Synergy for Efficient Knowledge Management in Health Care. *Journal of the Canadian Medical Association* 162(3):362–5, 2000a.

Jadad, Alejandro R., Michael Moher, George P. Browman, et al. Systematic Reviews and Meta-Analysis on Treatment of Asthma: Critical Evaluation. *BMJ* 320(7234):537, 2000b.

Jencks, Stephen F., Timothy Cuerdon, Dale R. Burwen, et al. Quality of Medical Care Delivered to Medicare Beneficiaries: A Profile at State and National Levels. *JAMA* 284(13):1670–6, 2000.

Johnston, Mary E., Karl B. Langton, R. Brian Haynes, and Alix Mathieu. Effects of Computer-Based Clinical Decision Support Systems on Clinician Performance and Patient Outcome: A Critical Appraisal of Research. *Ann Int Med* 120:135–42, 1994.

Kassirer, Jerome P. A Report Card on Computer-Assisted Diagnosis—The Grade: C. *N Engl J Med* 330(25):1824–5, 1994.

Kizer, Kenneth W. The National Quality Forum Enters the Game. *International Journal for Quality in Health Care* 12(2):85–7, 2000.

Lau, Joseph, Elliott M. Antman, Jeanette Jimenez-Silva, et al. Cumulative Meta-Analysis of the Therapeutic Trials for Myocardial Infarction. *N Engl J Med* 327(4):248–54, 1992.

Lilford, R. J., S. G. Pauker, D. A. Draunholtz, and Jiri Chard. Getting Research Findings into Practice: Decision Analysis and the Implementation of Research Findings. *BMJ* 317:405–9, 1998.

Lindberg, Donald A. B. 1998. "Fiscal Year 1999 President's Budget Request for the National Library of Medicine." Online. Available at http://www.nlm.nih.gov/pubs/staffpubs/od/budget99. html [accessed Sept. 18, 2000].

Lindberg, Donald A. B. and Betsy L. Humphreys. Updates Linking Evidence and Experience. Medicine and Health on the Internet: The Good, the Bad, and the Ugly. *JAMA* 280(15):1303–4, 1998.

———. A Time of Change for Medical Informatics in the USA. *Yearbook of Medical Informatics* National Library of Medicine, Bethesda, MD:53–7, 1999.

Lohr, Kathleen N. and Tomothy S. Carey. Asessing "Best Evidence:" Issues in Grading the Quality of Studies for Systematic Reviews. *Journal on Quality Improvement* 25(9):470–9, 1999.

Lohr, Kathleen N., Kristen Eleazer, and Josephine Mauskopf. Health Policy Issues and Applications for Evidence-Based Medicine and Clinical Practice Guidelines. *Health Policy* 46:1–19, 1998.

Lomas, Jonathan Anderson Geoffrey M., Karin Domnick-Pierre, et al. Do Practice Guidelines Guide Practice? The Effect of a Consensus Statement on the Practice of Physicians. *N Engl J Med* 321(19):1306–11, 1989.

Lyon, Becky J., P. Zoë Stavri, D. Colette Hochstein, and Holly Grossetta Nardini. Internet Access in the Libraries of the National Network of Libraries of Medicine. *Bull Med Libr Assoc* 86(4):486–90, 1998.

Marciniak, Thomas A., Edward F. Ellerbeck, Martha J. Radford, et al. Improving the Quality of Care for Medicare Patients With Acute Myocardial Infarction: Results from the Cooperative Cardiovascular Project. *JAMA* 279(17):1351–7, 1998.

McColl, Alastair, Helen Smith, Peter White, and Jenny Field. General Practitioners' Perceptions of the Route to Evidence Based Medicine: A Questionnaire Survey. *BMJ* 316:361–5, 1998.

McDonald, Clement J., J. Marc Overhage, Paul R. Dexter, et al. Canopy Computing: Using the Web in Clinical Practice. *JAMA* 280(15):1325–9, 1998.

McDowell, Ian, Claire Newell, and Walter Rosser. Comparison of Three Methods of Recalling Patients for Influenza Vaccination. *Can Med Assoc J* 135:991–7, 1986.

———. A Randomized Trial of Computerized Reminders for Blood Pressure Screening in Primary Care. *Medical Care* 27(3):297–305, 1989.

Mechanic, David. Bringing Science to Medicine: The Origins of Evidence-Based Practice. *Health Affairs* 17(6):250–1, 1998.

Miller, Naomi, Eve-Marie Lacroix, and Joyce E. B. Backus. MEDLINEplus: Building and Maintaining the National Library of Medicine's Consumer Health Web Service. *Bull Med Libr Assoc* 88(1):11–7, 2000.

National Committee for Quality Assurance. *Health Plan Employer Data and Information Set, Version 3.0*. Washington, D.C.: National Committee for Quality Assurance, 1999.

National Research Council. *Networking Health: Prescriptions for the Internet*. Washington D.C.: National Academy Press, 2000.

Perfetto, Eleanor M. and Lisa Stockwell Morris. Agency for Health Care Policy and Research Clinical Practice Guidelines. *The Annals of Pharmacotherapy* 30:1117–21, 1996.

Pozen, Michael W., Ralph B. D'Agostino, Harry P. Selker, et al. A Predictive Instrument to Improve Coronary-Care-Unit Admission Practices in Acute Ischemic Heart Disease. *N Engl J Med* 310(20):1273–8, 1984.

Rienhoff, Otto. Retooling Practitioners in the Information Age. *Information Technology Strategies from the United States and the European Union: Transferring Research to Practice for Health Care Improvement.* E. Andrew Balas, ed. Washington, D.C.:IOS Press, 2000.

Rosenberg, Matt. Popularity of Internet Won't Peak for Years: Not Until Today's Middle-Schoolers Reach Adulthood Will the Technology Really Take Off. *Puget Sound Business Journal.* May 24, 1999. Online. Available at http://www.bizjournals.com/seattle/stories/1999/05/24/focus9.html [accessed Jan. 22. 2001].

Sackett, David L., William M. C. Rosenberg, J. A. Muir Gray, et al. Evidence Based Medicine: What It Is and What It Isn't. *BMJ* 312:71–2, 1996.

Sackett, David L., Sharon E. Straus, W. Scott Richardson, et al. *Evidence-Based Medicine: How to Practice & Teach EBM.* 2nd edition. London, England: Churchill Livingstone, 2000.

Schiff, Gordon D. and T. Donald Rucker. Computerized Prescribing: Building the Electronic Infrastructure for Better Medication Usage. *JAMA* 279(13):1024–9, 1998.

Shea, Steven, William DuMouchel, and Lisa Bahamonde. A Meta-Analysis of 16 Randomized Controlled Trials to Evaluate Computer-Based Clinical Reminder Systems for Preventive Care in the Ambulatory Setting. *J Am Med Inform Assoc* 3(6):399–409, 1996.

Silberg, William M., George D. Lundberg, and Robert A. Musacchio. Assessing, Controlling, and Assuring the Quality of Medical Information on the Internet. *JAMA* 277(15):1244–5, 1997.

Solberg, Leif I., Milo L. Brekke, Charles J. Fazio, et al. Lessons from Experienced Guideline Implementers: Attend to Many Factors and Use Multiple Strategies. *Joint Commission Journal on Quality Improvement* 26(4):171–88, 2000.

USA Today. Health-Related Activities Conducted Online. Health, July 10, 1998.

Voge, Susan. NOAH-New York Online Access to Health: Library Collaboration for Bilingual Consumer Health Information on the Internet. *Bull Med Libr Assoc* 86(3):326–34, 1998.

Wellwood, J., S. Johannessen, and D. J. Spiegelhalter. How Does Computer-Aided Diagnosis Improve the Management of Acute Abdominal Pain? *Annals of the Royal College of Surgeons of England* 74:40–6, 1992.

Wexler, Jerry R., Phillip T. Swender, Walter W. Tunnessen, and Frank A. Oski. Impact of a System of Computer-Assisted Diagnosis: Initial Evaluation of the Hospitalized Patient. *Am J Dis Child* 129:203–5, 1975.

Woolf, Steven H. Practice Guidelines: A New Reality in Medicine. III. Impact on Patient Care. *Arch Int Med* 153:2646–55, 1993.

Wyatt, J. R. Lessons Learnt from the Field Trial of ACORN, An Expert System to Advise on Chest Pain. *Proceedings of the Sixth World Conference on Medical Informatics, Singapore.* 111–5, 1989.

7

Using Information Technology

Throughout this report, the committee has emphasized that health care should be supported by systems that are carefully and consciously designed to produce care that is safe, effective, patient-centered, timely, efficient, and equitable. This chapter examines the critical role of information technology (IT) in the design of those systems.

IT has enormous potential to improve the quality of health care with regard to all six of the aims set forth in Chapter 2. In the area of *safety,* there is growing evidence that automated order entry systems can reduce errors in drug prescribing and dosing (Bates et al., 1997, 1998a, 1999). In the area of *effectiveness,* there is considerable evidence that automated reminder systems improve compliance with clinical practice guidelines (Balas et al., 2000; Shea et al., 1996), and some promising studies, although few in number, indicate that computer-assisted diagnosis and management can improve quality (Durieux et al., 2000; Evans et al., 1998). There are many opportunities to use IT to make care more *patient-centered,* for example, by facilitating access to clinical knowledge through understandable and reliable Web sites and online support groups (Cain et al., 2000); customized health education and disease management messages (Goldsmith, 2000); and the use of clinical decision support systems to tailor information according to an individual patient's characteristics, genetic makeup, and specific conditions (Garibaldi, 1998) (see Chapter 6 for additional discussion). Both patients and clinicians can benefit from improvements in *timeliness* through the use of Internet-based communication (i.e., e-visits, telemedicine) and immediate access to automated clinical information, diagnostic tests, and treatment results. Clinical decision support systems have been shown to improve *efficiency* by reducing redundant laboratory tests (Bates et al., 1998b). Finally, Internet-based health communication can enhance *equity* by providing a broader array of options for interacting with clinicians, although this can only happen if all people, regardless of race, ethnicity, socioeconomic status, geographic location, and other factors, have access to the technology infrastructure (Science Panel on Interactive Communication and Health, 1999).

The committee believes IT must play a central role in the redesign of the health care system if a substantial improvement in health care quality is to be achieved during the coming decade. This is a theme underlying many of the topics addressed in this report. Chapter 5 emphasizes the importance of a strong information infrastructure in supporting efforts to reengineer care processes, manage the burgeoning clinical knowledge base, coordinate patient care across clinicians and settings and over time, support multidisciplinary team functioning, and facilitate performance and outcome measurements for improvement and accountability. Chapter 6 stresses the importance of building such an infrastructure to support evidence-based practice, including the provision of more organized and reliable information sources on the Internet for both consumers and clinicians, and the development and application of clinical decision support tools. And Chapter 9 considers the need to build information-rich environments for undergraduate and graduate health education, as well as the potential to enhance continuing education through Internet-based programs.

Central to many IT applications is the automation of patient-specific clinical information. Efforts to automate clinical data date back several decades, and have tended to focus on creation of an automated medical record. For example, in 1991 the IOM set forth a vision and issued a strong call for nationwide implementation of computer-based patient records (Institute of Medicine, 1991). But progress has been slow. It is important to recognize that a fully electronic medical record, including all types of patient information, is not necessary to achieve many if not most of the benefits of automated clinical data. For example, use of medication order entry systems using data on patient diagnoses, current medications, and history of drug interactions or allergies can result in sizable reductions in prescribing errors (Bates et al., 1998a; Leapfrog Group, 2000). The automation and linking of data on services provided to patients in ambulatory and institutional settings (e.g., encounters, procedures, ancillary tests) would provide a rich source of information for quality measurement and improvement purposes.

The challenges of applying IT to health care should not be underestimated. Consumers and policy makers share concerns about the privacy and confidentiality of these data (Cain et al., 2000). The United States still lacks national standards for the protection of health data and the capture, storage, communication, processing, and presentation of health information (Work Group on Computerization of Patient Records, 2000). Sizable capital investments will also be required. Moreover, widespread adoption of many IT applications will require behavioral adaptations on the part of large numbers of patients, clinicians, and organizations.

The committee believes solutions to these barriers can and must be found given the critical importance of the judicious application of IT to addressing the nation's health care quality concerns. The time has come to establish a national health information infrastructure that will encourage public- and private-sector investments in IT while providing adequate safeguards for consumers. As discussed in Chapter 4, a sizable portion of the resources of the recommended Health Care Quality Innovation Fund (see Recommendation 6) should be invested in projects that implement and evaluate IT applications and are likely to contribute to quality improvements.

> **Recommendation 9: Congress, the executive branch, leaders of health care organizations, public and private purchasers, and health informatics associations and vendors should make a renewed national commitment to building an information infrastructure to support health care delivery, consumer health, quality measurement and improvement, public accountability, clinical and health services research, and clinical education. This commitment should lead to the elimination of most handwritten clinical data by the end of the decade.**

POTENTIAL BENEFITS OF INFORMATION TECHNOLOGY

In less than 5 years, the IT landscape has changed dramatically. The share of households with Internet access grew from 26.2 percent in December 1998 to 41.5 percent in August 2000, an increase of 58 percent in 20 months (U.S. Department of Commerce, 2000). The explosive growth of the Internet has opened up many new promising applications that have implications for the roles of consumers, clinicians, and organizations in the delivery of health care services. A recent report by the National Research Council of The National Academies identified six major health-related application domains: consumer health, clinical care, administrative and financial transactions, public health, professional education, and research (see Table 7-1) (National Research Council, 2000). Many of the applications in these domains, such as online searching for health information by patients and providers, are commonplace. Others, such as remote and virtual surgery and simulations of surgical procedures, are in the early stages of development.

• *Consumer Health.* A September 1999 poll conducted by Harris Interactive found that 70 million of the 97 million American adults who were online had searched for health information in the last year (Cain et al., 2000). Consumers are using the Internet to search for health information, to obtain information useful in selecting a health plan or provider, and to participate in formal and informal support groups. Comparative performance data are available on the Internet for many health plans (National Committee for Quality Assurance, 2000), and depending on the geographic area of interest, there may be relevant information on hospitals and providers. The Internet can also be used to post customized health education messages according to a person's profile and needs (Kendall and Levine, 1997).

• *Clinical Care.* The Internet has the potential to make health care delivery more timely and responsive to consumer preferences. As discussed in Chapter 6, the Internet is playing an increasingly critical role in making scientific publications, syntheses of the evidence, practice guidelines, and other tools required to support evidence-based practice available to both patients and clinicians. Examples of information technologies that are of growing importance in the health care arena are reminder systems (Alemi et al., 1996); telemedicine applications, such as teleradiology and e-mail; and online prescribing (National Health Policy Forum, 2000; Schiff and Rucker, 1998).

• *Administrative and Financial Transactions.* To date, the area in which information systems have been used most extensively in health care has been to improve the service and efficiency of various administrative and financial transactions (Starr, 1997; Turban et al., 1996). In 1999, almost 65 percent of the 4.6 billion medical claims processed by private and public health insurance plans were transmitted electronically (Goldsmith, 2000).

• *Public Health.* IT can be used to improve the quality of health care at the population level. Applications include incident reporting, videoconferencing among public health officials during emergency situations, disease surveillance, transfer of epidemiology maps and other image files for monitoring of the spread of disease, delivery of alerts and other information to clinicians and health workers, and maintenance of registries.

• *Professional Education.* The Internet can be a powerful tool for undergraduate, graduate, and continuing medical education for all types of health professionals. A variety of Internet-based educational programs have made their curricula and training materials available on the Web. There are also educational videos, lectures, virtual classrooms, and simulation programs to teach surgical skills.

• *Research.* The Internet opens up many options for improving researchers' access to databases and literature, enhancing collegial interaction, and shortening the time required to conduct certain types of research and disseminate results to the field. These applications are already gaining widespread acceptance.

Of course, not all computer health applications are Internet-based. There are computerized order entry systems, reminder systems, and other applications that run on legacy systems (older IT systems, often built around mainframes, owned

TABLE 7-1 Health-Related Applications for the Internet

Application Domain	Types of Applications
Consumer health	• Online searching for health information • Searches of medical literature • Downloading of educational videos • Search for a clinician or health plan • Participation in chat and support groups • Online access to personal health records • Completion of patient surveys
Clinical care	• Searches of medical literature • Routine care delivery (e.g., e-visits) and chronic disease management (e.g., periodic reports on health conditions to clinicians) • Reminders and alerts; decision support systems • Consultations among clinicians (perhaps involving manipulation of digital images) • Remote monitoring of patients in home and long-term care settings • Transfer of medical records and images • Remote and virtual surgery
Administrative and financial transactions	• Videoconferencing with real-time sharing of documents • Enrollment of patients • Scheduling of appointments • Billing for services, payment of providers • Certain aspects of clinician credentialing • Consumer access to information about health plans, participating providers, eligibility for procedures, covered drugs in formulary, etc.

Public health	• Videoconferencing among public health officials during emergency situations
	• Incident reporting
	• Collection of information from local public health departments
	• Surveillance for emerging diseases or epidemics
	• Transfer of epidemiology maps or other image files for monitoring the spread of a disease
	• Delivery of alerts and other information to providers and health workers
Professional education	• Accessing reference material
	• Distance education with real-time transmission of lectures or prerecorded videos
	• Real-time consultations with experts about difficult cases
	• Virtual classrooms, distributed collaborative projects and discussions
	• Simulation of surgical procedures
	• Virtual exploration of three-dimensional environments
Health services, biomedical, and clinical outcomes research	• Health services research using administrative and clinical data
	• Searching of remote databases and professional literature
	• Collaboration among researchers, peer review, interactive virtual conferences
	• Control of experimental equipment, such as electron microscopes, visual feedback from remote instrumentation
	• Real-time monitoring of compliance with protocols
	• Transfer of large datasets between computers for high-speed computation and comparisons
	• Enrolling of populations in clinical trials

SOURCE: Adapted from National Research Council, 2000.

by some hospitals, medical centers, and group practices) (Turban et al., 1996). In the future, however, the Internet will likely be the platform of choice for many if not most health applications because of the ready access it provides to both consumers and clinicians, as well as other financial and technical considerations.

It must be acknowledged that although the potential benefits of IT are compelling, the evidence in support of these benefits varies greatly by type of application. As discussed in Chapter 6, there is strong evidence to support the effectiveness of computerized reminder systems in improving compliance with practice guidelines. For computerized medication order entry systems, recent studies substantiate reductions in errors and unnecessary services, but such studies are few in number (Bates et al., 1998a). A recent review of 80 controlled trials carried out between 1966 and 1996 concluded that telephone-based distance medicine or telemedicine technologies are beneficial in the areas of preventive care and the management of osteoarthritis, cardiac rehabilitation, and diabetes care (Balas et al., 1997). In a review of 15 controlled trials in which diabetic patients received computer-generated information, it was found that 12 of the 15 trials documented positive clinical outcomes, such as improved hemoglobin and blood glucose levels (Balas et al., 1998).

In summary, the strength of the evidence on the effects of various IT applications is highly varied. Many applications, such as simulation of surgical procedures for educational purposes and remote and virtual surgery, are in the early developmental stages. Others may be highly promising, but their adoption and testing are hampered by the lack of computerized patient information (e.g., computer-aided diagnosis), regulatory or legal impediments (e.g., e-mail communications across state lines), and payment issues (e.g., for e-visits). Still other applications, such as telemedicine, have not been rigorously evaluated (Grigsby and Sanders, 1998; Institute of Medicine, 1996).

AUTOMATED CLINICAL INFORMATION

Much of the potential of IT to improve quality is predicated on the automation of at least some types of clinical data. Automated clinical data are required by many of the most promising IT applications, including computer-aided decision support systems that couple medical evidence with patient-specific clinical data to assist clinicians and patients in making diagnoses and evaluating treatment options (see Chapter 6) (Burger, 1997; Weed and Weed, 1999). Automated clinical data also open up the potential to glean medical knowledge from patient care (Institute of Medicine, 2000). An example is the extraordinary gains in cancer survival for children as compared with adults, attributable in part to the participation of virtually all pediatric cancer patients in clinical trials that systematically collect, pool, and analyze data and disseminate results to all participants (Simone and Lyons, 2000). Automated clinical and administrative data also enable many types of health service research applications, such as assessment of

clinical outcomes associated with alternative treatment options and care processes; identification of best practices; and evaluation of the effects of different
methods of financing, organizing, and delivering services.

Both private- and public-sector groups have identified the need to move
forward expeditiously with the automation of clinical information. In 1991, the
IOM issued a report concluding that computer-based patient records are an "essential technology" for health care and that electronic records should be the
standard for medical and all other records related to health care. In that same
year, the U.S. General Accounting Office issued a report stating that automated
medical records offer great potential to improve patient care, increase efficiency,
and reduce costs, and calling for the development of standards to ensure uniform
electronic recording and transmission of medical information. A 1993 report of
the U.S. General Accounting Office called for leadership and the acceleration of
efforts to develop standards. In 1997, a revised edition of the 1991 IOM report
noted the strides that had been made in the power and capacity of personal
computers and other computer-based technologies, the remarkable growth of the
Internet for research and some health applications, the increasing level of computer literacy among health professionals and the public, and the linkage of
organizations and individuals in local and regional networks that were beginning
to tackle the development of population databases.

Some health care organizations have made important advances, but overall
progress has been slow. In a few large systems—most notably the health systems
of the Department of Veterans Health Affairs—integrated electronic records systems have been implemented. There are also examples of robust, well-integrated
hospital-based information systems (National Research Council, 2000), such as
Intermountain Health Care (in Salt Lake City, Utah), but they are few and notable
for their rarity. Many other organizations have automated major portions of
clinical information systems—laboratory data, order entry, and the like—and
others are on their way to becoming paperless in the next few years (McDonald et
al., 1997; Warden and Lawrence, 2000).

There are numerous barriers to the automation of clinical information. The
remainder of this section addresses four of these barriers: privacy concerns, the
need for standards, financial requirements, and human factors issues.

Privacy Concerns and the Need for Standards

Two of the greatest impediments to the widespread automation of clinical
information are the absence of national policies pertaining to privacy, security,
and confidentiality and the lack of standards for the coding and exchange of
clinical information (e.g., definitions and nomenclature, patient identifiers, and
electronic transfer) (Dwyer, 1999; Kleinke, 1998; McDonald, 1998; U.S. Department of Commerce, 1994). Indeed, the issues of protecting privacy and data
standardization are closely interrelated. In 1998, for example, plans of the De-

partment of Health and Human Services to issue recommendations for establishing unique patient identifiers were put on hold in response to public outcry over potential violations of medical privacy (Goldman, 1998).

There is general agreement that privacy protections are needed for consumers, but there is also recognition that unless carefully balanced, such protections may limit the future prospects of IT (Detmer, 2000a). Public opinion polls conducted during the last decade document high and increasing levels of concern about privacy, raising questions about whether people's fear of violations of their privacy may lead some to forego seeking necessary health services or to withhold personal information from clinicians (Goldman, 1998). Others point out that, if too stringent, privacy protections will impede the adoption of many IT applications critical to addressing health care quality concerns (Detmer, 2000a).

The demands of health care with regard to security and availability are both more stringent and more varied than those of other industries (Institute of Medicine, 1994). Automated records can make it much easier for hackers to assemble lists or to find (or alter) information about individuals. At the same time, there are many different sources and types of health data, and clinical information must be available to all clinicians and others involved in care delivery whenever needed. Well-crafted policies can be implemented to ensure timely access for those with a valid need to access the data, including treating clinicians and patients, while denying access to unauthorized users. Information security technologies, such as encryption, authentication of both the sender and receiver of data, and audit trails to detect unauthorized users, are available to support such policies (Detmer, 2000a; National Research Council, 1998; U.S. General Accounting Office, 1999). Legal enforcement of privacy and confidentiality rights with strong remedies can serve as both a deterrent to unauthorized users and a method of redress for individuals whose privacy rights have been violated.

The lack of commonly accepted definitions and nomenclature for the collection and coding of data and standards for the exchange of information has also been recognized as an obstacle to broad adoption of clinical information technologies (Dwyer, 1999; Kleinke, 1998; McDonald, 1998; U.S. Department of Commerce, 1994). Data standards are needed to facilitate sharing and communication of the data across different health care information systems, and to ensure that the data are complete, accurate, and comparable (National Committee on Vital and Health Statistics, 2000). Numerous groups, including the American National Standards Institute's Healthcare Informatics Standards Board, High Level 7, the American Sociey for Testing and Material, the American Standards Committee, the Institute of Electrical and Electronics Engineers, international organizations, and numerous governmental groups, have developed standards for claims forms, datasets, diagnostic and procedure classifications, vocabularies, and messaging formats (Agency for Healthcare Research and Quality, 1999; Cushman and Detmer, 1998). The Library of Medicine has made extensive efforts to standardize vocabulary (including the construction and maintenance of a metathesaurus as part of the unified medical language system). But these efforts, as important as they are, amount to a patchwork of standards that address some areas and not others, and are not adhered to by all users.

To begin addressing the need for comprehensive national standards, Congress passed the Health Insurance Portability and Accountability Act in 1996, creating a federal mandate to develop standards for all electronic health transmissions (Health Care Financing Administration, 2000). The law directed the Secretary of Health and Human Services to make recommendations to Congress regarding the privacy of individually identifiable health information by August 1997, and if Congress failed to pass privacy legislation by August 1999, the Secretary of DHHS was directed to issue health privacy regulations by January 2000. The law also provided that the National Committee on Vital and Health Statistics was to report to the Secretary of DHHS by August 21, 2000, on recommendations and legislative proposals pertaining to data standards for patient medical record information (National Committee on Vital and Health Statistics, 2000).

Congress failed to enact legislation implementing a comprehensive package of privacy protections by the August 1999 deadline. Therefore, DHHS worked to develop these regulations, based on the Secretary's recommendations to Congress in 1997 (U.S. Department of Health and Human Services, 1997). These regulations were extremely controversial and generated over 50,000 comments when published in proposed rulemaking form. However, DHHS was able to finalize and announce them in December 2000 (U.S. Department of Health and Human Services, 2000).

DHHS also has efforts under way to develop national standards for the definition, collection, coding, and exchange of patient medical record information, but progress has been slow. In July 2000, the National Committee on Vital Health Statistics forwarded a report to the Secretary of Health and Human Services addressing a variety of process, technical, organizational, financing, and other issues related to the development of national standards (National Committee on Vital and Health Statistics, 2000). Some progress has been made toward developing coding standards for data elements; however, none has emerged as a comprehensive standard (Institute of Medicine, 1997), and, as noted above, the adoption of a standardized health identifier has been suspended. Chief information officers and other health care executives have reported they do not believe that health records can be restructured to comply with electronic formats in the time frame required by the law (Shinkman and Jonathan, 2000).

In the absence of strong national leadership in establishing standards and defining appropriate legal and regulatory structures for an IT-driven health care delivery system, states and various branches of the federal government have responded to issues and concerns primarily on an ad hoc basis. For example, more than two-thirds of states have made legislative efforts to affect various types of health information practices, resulting in an increasingly complex array of laws (Cushman and Detmer, 1998). In other instances, existing legal and regulatory structures are being applied to IT issues, creating confusion and probably ineffective oversight. For example, online pharmacies, whereby the physician enters orders into pharmacy computers often using a handheld wireless electronic prescription pad, have given rise to a set of jurisdictional issues. These issues relate both to federal and state responsibilities and, at the federal level, to questions about the responsibilities of different agencies (i.e., Federal Trade Commission, Food and Drug Administration, Drug Enforcement Administration, Department of Justice, U.S. Customs Service, and U.S. Postal Service) for consumer protection, rooting out of fraud and misinformation, drug quality, advertising of prescription drugs, and importation and domestic mailing of pharmaceutical products (National Health Policy Forum, 2000).

Financial Requirements

The 21st-century health care system will require a significant financial investment in information technology—far greater than current investments by most health care organizations. Capital will be needed to purchase and install new technology, while installation of the new systems is likely to produce temporary disruptions in the delivery of patient care and result in sizable short-term costs to manage the transition. Some specialized training and education will also be needed to help the workforce adapt to the new environment.

In addition, some health care organizations have invested heavily in legacy systems—older computer systems built around mainframes (Turban et al., 1996). There is no easy way to shift from such systems to state-of-the-art information systems based on an open client–server architecture, personal computer networks, and more flexible, nonproprietary protocols. These are important considerations for all health care organizations when making decisions about investing in IT. Recent reductions in Medicare payments under the 1997 Balanced Budget Act have likely contributed to an even more cautious approach to long-term investment in technology on the part of many health care institutions.

Access to capital may be particularly limited for certain types of health care organizations. Not-for-profit hospitals and health plans must obtain capital from bond rather than equity markets. Many small physician group practices have a limited ability to obtain capital. Large for-profit health plans may have ready capital to invest in IT, but absent strong, long-term partnerships with provider groups, lack the leverage and incentive to implement such systems.

These capital decisions are also being made in an environment in which benefits are difficult to quantify. Unlike billing or pharmaceutical transactions, clinical transactions have only an indirect effect on profitability, and demonstrating the value of clinical information systems in improving the quality of care has been difficult although, as discussed above, evidence has begun to accumulate about their usefulness in specific settings and applications. Moreover, as discussed in Chapter 8, current payment policies do not adequately reward improvements in quality.

There are some indications that the use of IT is slowly becoming more widespread. In 1997, the health information technology industry sold $15 billion worth of products to health care organizations (Kleinke, 1998). The development of Web-based applications for use on the Internet may also open the door to new forms of financing the expenses of IT. For example, if IT shifts from an equipment purchase to a service expense, it can be bought on a monthly basis and upgraded easily in response to both technological advances and changes in medical practice. Maintaining up-to-date applications that reflect the evolution of technology and the knowledge base and making them available by subscription at a Web site rather than requiring users in individual organizations to purchase and maintain them is likely to provide great impetus for the development and use of these systems.

Human Factors Issues

One of the most challenging, and least understood, barriers to the application of useful information technologies in health care relates to human factors. These barriers include both workforce and patient issues.

The health care sector is labor-intensive, with about 700,000 physicians, over 2 million nurses, and many other health care workers being involved in the delivery of patient care to varying degrees (Health Resources and Services Administration, 2000). The workforce is highly variable in terms of IT-related knowledge and experience, and probably also in terms of receptivity to learning or acquiring these skills. Some clinicians may also be wary of embracing new IT applications because of frustrating experience with earlier IT applications that failed to prove useful in solving diagnostic and therapeutic problems (Kassirer, 2000). Moreover, the development of new data infrastructures and the incorporation of new IT applications into clinical practice generally entails disruptions in patient care, resulting in lost revenues for many clinicians.

Many IT applications require the forging of new relationships between clinicians and institutional providers, which may be slow to develop. For example, some have observed that the deeply ingrained economic distrust and cultural conflict between physicians and hospitals has impeded the adoption of IT applications that require Web-based integration (Kleinke, 2000).

IT will undoubtedly alter the clinician and patient relationship, and in some cases, these changes may be threatening to clinicians. The standardization and automation of various types of clinical data opens up many new opportunities to make comparative quality data available to consumers who must chose among clinicians, sites of care, and treatment options, and to bolster oversight and accountability programs (Kleinke, 2000). The availability of clinical knowledge on the Internet will lead to more informed patients who will be increasingly likely to question clinician recommendations.

Not all patients will embrace these new roles of IT. Although consumers are migrating to the Internet at a rapid pace, there will likely be some proportion of individuals who do not have access either by personal choice or because of economic or other constraints (Conte, 1999). Consequently, there will be a need for the health system to operate in the old and the new, automated ways in parallel for the foreseeable future (Ferguson, 1999).

NEED FOR A NATIONAL HEALTH INFORMATION INFRASTRUCTURE

Many developments now under way augur well for the future adoption of IT by the health care sector. A growing body of evidence supports the conclusion that various types of IT applications lead to improvements in safety, effectiveness, patient-centeredness, timeliness, efficiency, and equity. Some progress is being made on the specification of standards for protecting privacy, and various private- and public-sector standardization efforts are being undertaken to provide the foundation for a more expansive effort focused on achieving national consensus. The extraordinary growth of the Internet has opened up a plethora of new applications; provided a highly accessible platform for tapping the clinical knowledge base, running applications, and sharing data; and lowered capital requirements.

Nonetheless, IT has barely touched patient care. The vast majority of clinical information is still stored in paper form. Only a fraction of clinicians offer e-mail as a communication option to patients (Hoffman, 1997). Few patients benefit even from very simple decision aids, such as reminder systems, which have been shown repeatedly to improve compliance with practice guidelines. Many medical errors, ubiquitous throughout the health care system, could be prevented if only clinical data were accessible and readable, and prescriptions were entered into automated order entry systems with built-in logic to check for errors and oversights in drug selection and dosing. The pace of change is unacceptably slow. Much more can and should be done.

To achieve a substantial improvement in quality, the United States, like other industrialized countries, will need to begin developing a comprehensive national health information infrastructure (Detmer, 2000b). As defined by the National Committee on Vital and Health Statistics, such a structure is "a set of technologies, standards, applications, systems, values, and laws that support all facets of individual health, health care, and public health (Work Group on Computerization of Patient Records, 2000). A national health information infrastructure is not a centralized government database, but rather "rules for the road" that offer a way to connect distributed health data in the framework of a secure network.

As discussed above, some elements of such a structure are in various stages of development, but at the current pace, many more years will be required for its completion. To further the development process, the country must move forward expeditiously with the promulgation of national standards to protect data privacy. Moreover, these standards should be reevaluated and fine-tuned periodically to strike the right balance between protecting consumer privacy and providing access to clinical data for legitimate purposes, such as care delivery, quality evaluation, research, and public health (Detmer, 2000a). A high priority for the coming 2 years should be to achieve national consensus on comprehensive standards for the definition, collection, coding, and exchange of clinical data.

As technological barriers are overcome, much greater attention should be focused on legal, societal, organizational, and cultural issues (Work Group on Computerization of Patient Records, 2000). Legal and regulatory structures that have the unintended consequence of impeding the adoption of useful IT applications must be identified and modified (Moran, 1998). Health care organizations and the health professions will need strong leadership and a clear direction as they move forward with what will be a dramatic transformation of care delivery (Shortliffe, 2000).

Finally, efforts should also be made to better inform the American public about IT issues, and to ensure that all individuals have the opportunity to benefit from the extraordinary innovations now under way. The American public should be fully informed of both the benefits and risks of automated clinical data and electronic communication, as well as the various options available for protecting privacy. Steps must also be taken to ensure that all Americans have ready access to the Internet, should they so desire, and that the benefits of IT reach practice settings that serve a disproportionate share of the most vulnerable populations.

REFERENCES

Agency for Healthcare Research and Quality. 1999. "Health Care Informatics Standards: Activities of Selected Federal Agencies." Online. Available at http://www.ahcpr.gov/data/infostd1.htm [accessed Dec. 15, 2000].

Alemi, Farrokh, Sonia A. Allemango, Jeffrey Goldhagen, et al. Comptuer Reminders Improve On-time Immunization Rates. *Medical Care* 34(10[Supplement]):OS45–51, 1996.

Balas, E. Andrew, Suzanne A. Boren, and G. Griffing. Computerized Management of Diabetes: A Synthesis of Controlled Trials. *A Paradigm Shift in Health Care Information Systems: Clinical Infrastuctures for the 21st Century: Proceedings of the 1998 AMIA Annual Symposium.* Christopher G. Chute, ed., 295–9, 1998.

Balas, E. Andrew, Farah Jaffrey, Gilad J. Kuperman, et al. Electronic Communication With Patients: Evaluation of Distance Medicine Technology. *JAMA* 278(2):152–9, 1997.

Balas, E. Andrew, Scott Weingarten, Candace T. Garb, et al. Improving Preventive Care by Prompting Physicians. *Arch Int Med* 160(3):301–8, 2000.

Bates, David W., Lucian L. Leape, David J. Cullen, et al. Effect of Computerized Physician Order Entry and a Team Intervention on Prevention of Serious Medication Errors. *JAMA* 280(15): 1311–6, 1998a.

Bates, David W., Elizabeth M. Pappius, Gilad J. Kupperman, et al. Measuring and Improving Quality Using Information Systems. *MedInfo 1998: Proceedings of the Ninth World Congress on Medical Informatics.* B. Cesnik, A. T. McCray, and J. R. Scherrer, eds., 814–8 in Part 2. Amsterdam: IOS Press, 1998b.

Bates, David W., Nathan Spell, David J. Cullen, et al. The Costs of Adverse Drug Events in Hospitalized Patients. *JAMA* 277(4):307–11, 1997.

Bates, David W., Jonathan M. Teich, Joshua Lee, et al. The Impact of Computerized Physician Order Entry on Medication Error Prevention. *J Am Med Inform Assoc* 6(4):313–21, 1999.

Burger, C. S. The Use of Problem Knowledge Couplers in a Primary Care Practice. *Healthcare Information Management* Winter;11(4):13–26, 1997.

Cain, Mary M., Robert Mittman, Jane Sarasohn-Kahn, and Jennifer C. Wayne. *Health e-People: The Online Consumer Experience.* Oakland, CA: Institute for the Future, California Health Care Foundation, 2000.

Conte, Christopher *Networking for Better Care: Health Care in the Information Age.* Jean Smith and Rachel Anderson, eds.Benton Foundation, 1999.

Cushman, F. Reid and Don E. Detmer. 1998. "Information Policy for the U.S. Health Sector: Engineering, Political Economy, and Ethics." Online. Available at http://www.milbank.org/art/intro.html [accessed Dec. 1, 2000].

Detmer, Don E. Your Privacy or Your Health: Will Medical Privacy Legislation Stop Quality Health Care? *International Journal for Quality in Health Care* 12:1–3, 2000a.

———. *Information Technology for Quality Healthcare: A Summary of United Kingdom and United States Experiences.* Background Paper for the Ditchley Park Conference: Co-sponsored by The Commonwealth Fund and the Nuffield Trust, Oxfordshire, England, 2000b.

Durieux, Pierre, Remy Nizard, Philippe Ravaud, et al. A Clinical Decision Support System for Prevention of Venous Thromboembolism. *JAMA* 283(21):2816–21, 2000.

Dwyer, Chris. Ideas and Trends: Medical Informatics and Health Care Computing. *Ann Int Med* 130(2):170–2, 1999.

Evans, R. Scott, Stanley L. Pestotnik, David C. Classen, et al. A Computer-Assisted Management Program for Antibiotics and Other Antiinfective Agents. *N Engl J Med* 338(4):232–8, 1998.

Ferguson, Roger, Vice Chairman of the Federal Reserve Board, Boston, MA. Presentation at the IOM Workshop on Information Technology and Quality. Sept. 29, 1999.

Garibaldi, Richard A. Computers and the Quality of Care — A Clinician's Perspective. *N Engl J Med* 338(4):259–60, 1998.

Goldman, Janlori. Protecting Privacy To Improve Health Care. *Health Affairs* 17(6):47–60, 1998.

Goldsmith, Jeff. The Internet and Managed Care: A New Wave of Information. *Health Affairs* 19(6):42–56, 2000.

Grigsby, Jim and Jay H. Sanders. Telemedicine: Where It Is and Where It's Going. *Ann Int Med* 129:123–7, 1998.

Health Care Financing Administration. 2000. "Medicare EDI (Electronic Data Exchange)." Online. Available at http://www.hcfa.gov/medicare/edi/edi.htm [accessed Jan. 3, 2001].

Health Resources and Services Administration. *United States Health Workforce Personnel Factbook.* Washington, D.C.: Bureau of Health Professions, 2000.

Hoffman, A. Take 2 and E-mail Me in the Morning: Doctors Consult Patients Electronically. *New York Times*, June 3, 1997.

Institute of Medicine. *The Computer-Based Patient Record: An Essential Technology for Health Care.* Richard S. Dick and Elaine B. Steen, eds. Washington, D.C.: National Academy Press, 1991.

———. *Health Data in the Information Age: Use, Disclosure, and Privacy.* M. S. Donaldson and K. N. Lohr, eds. Washington, D.C.: National Academy Press, 1994.

———. *Telemedicine: A Guide to Assessing Telecommunications for Health Care.* Marilyn J. Field, ed. Washington, D.C.: National Academy Press, 1996.

———. *The Computer-Based Patient Record: An Essential Technology for Health Care.* Revised edition. Richard S. Dick, Elaine B. Steen, and Don E. Detmer, eds. Washington, D.C.: National Academy Press, 1997.

———. *Enhancing Data Systems to Improve the Quality of Cancer Care.* Maria Hewitt and Joseph V. Simone, eds. Washington, D.C.: National Academy Press, 2000.

Kassirer, Jerome P. Patients, Physicians, And The Internet. *Health Affairs* 19(6):115–23, 2000.

Kendall, David B. and S. Robert Levine *Creating a Health Information Network. Stage Two of the Health Care Revolution.* Washington, D.C.: Progressive Policy Institute, Policy Report, 1997. Online. Available at http://www.ppionline.org/ppi_ci.cfm?contentid=1941&knlgAreaID=111&subsecid=138 [accessed Jan. 31, 2001].

Kleinke, J. D. Release 0.0: Clinical Information Technology In The Real World. *Health Affairs* 17(6):23–38, 1998.

———. Vaporware.com: The Failed Promise of the Health Care Internet. *Health Affairs* 19(6):57–71, 2000.

Leapfrog Group. 2000. "Leapfrog Patient Safety Standards: The Potential Benefit of Universal Adoption." Online. Available at http://www.leapfroggroup.org [accessed Jan. 3, 2001].

McDonald, Clement J., et al. The Three Legged Stool: Regenstrief Institute for Health Care. *Third Annual Nicholas E. Davies Award Proceedings of the CPR Recognition Symposium.* Computer-Based Patient Record Institute. Burr Ridge, IL: McGraw-Hill Healthcare Education Group, 1997.

McDonald, Clement J. Need For Standards In Health Information. *Health Affairs* 17(6):44–6, 1998.

Moran, Donald W. Health Information Policy: On Preparing For The Next War. *Health Affairs* 17(6):9–22, 1998.

National Committee for Quality Assurance. *The State of Managed Care Quality 2000.* Washington, D.C.: National Committee for Quality Assurance, 2000.

National Committee on Vital and Health Statistics. *Uniform Data Standards for Patient Medical Record Information: Report to the Secretary of the U.S. Department of Health and Human Services.* Washington, D.C.: U.S. Department of Health and Human Services, 2000.

National Health Policy Forum. Physician Connectivity: Electronic Prescribing. Issue Brief, No. 752. Washington, D.C.: The George Washington University, 2000.

National Research Council. *Privacy Issues in Biomedical and Clinical Research.* Washington, D.C.: National Academy Press, 1998.

———. *Networking Health: Prescriptions for the Internet.* Washington, D.C.: National Academy Press, 2000.

Schiff, Gordon D. and T. Donald Rucker. Computerized Prescribing: Building the Electronic Infrastructure for Better Medication Usage. *JAMA* 279(13):1024–9, 1998.

Science Panel on Interactive Communication and Health *Wired for Health and Well-Being. The Emergence of Interactive Health Communication.* T. R. Eng and D. H. Gustafson, eds. Washington, D.C.: U.S. Department of Health and Human Services, U.S. Government Printing Office, 1999.

Shea, Steven, William DuMouchel, and Lisa Bahamonde. A Meta-Analysis of 16 Randomized Controlled Trials to Evaluate Computer-Based Clinical Reminder Systems for Preventive Care in the Ambulatory Setting. *J Am Med Inform Assoc* 3(6):399–409, 1996.

Shinkman, Ron and Gardner Jonathan. The HIPAA Lurks. Just when CIOs thought it was safe for business as usual. . . . *Modern Healthcare* 30(5):24–9, 2000.

Shortliffe, Edward H. Networking Health: Learning From Others, Taking The Lead. *Health Affairs* 19(6):9–22, 2000.

Simone, Joseph V. and Jane Lyons. *Superior Cancer Survival in Children Compared to Adults: A Superior System of Cancer Care.* National Cancer Policy Board Background Paper. Washington, D.C.: Institute of Medicine, 2000. Online. Available at http://www.iom.edu/IOM/IOMHome.nsf/WFiles/Manuscript/$file/Manuscript.PDF [accessed Jan. 26, 2001].

Starr, Paul. Smart Technology, Stunted Policy: Developing Health Information Networks. *Health Affairs* 16(3):91–105, 1997.

Turban, Efraim, Ephraim McLean, and James Wetherbe. *Information Technology for Management: Improving Quality and Productivity.* New York, NY: John Wiley & Sons, 1996.

U.S. Department of Commerce. *Putting the Information Infrastructure to Work. Report of the information infrastructure task force committee on applications and technology.* Washington, D.C.: National Institute of Standards and Technology, 1994. PB94–163383.

———. *Falling Through the Net: Toward Digital Inclusion. A Report on American's Access to Technology Tools.* Washington, D.C.: Economics and Statistics Administration; National Telecommunications and Information Administration, 2000. Online. Available at: http://www.ntia.doc.gov/ntiahome/digitaldivide/ [accessed Sept. 19, 2000].

U.S. Department of Health and Human Services. *Confidentiality of Individually Identifiable Health Information: Recommendations Submitted by the Secretary of Health and Human Services to Congress for Federal Health Record Confidentiality Legislation.* Washington, D.C.: U.S. Department of Health and Human Services, 1997. Submitted on September 11, 1997. Online. Available at http://www.hhs.gov/news/press/1997pres/970911c.html [accessed Jan. 28, 2001].

———. *Press Briefing on Final Privacy Regulation.* Washington, D.C.: U.S. Department of Health and Human Services, 2000. Released on December 20, 2000. Online. Available at http://www.hhs.gov/ocr/briefs.html [accessed Jan. 30, 2001].

U.S. General Accounting Office. Automated Medical Records: Leadership Needed to Expedite Standards Development. GAO/IMTEC-93-17. Washington, D.C.: U.S. General Accounting Office, 1993.

———. Medical Records Privacy: Access Needed for Health Research, But Oversight of Privacy Protection is Limited. Report B-280657. Washington, D.C.: U.S. General Accounting Office, 1999.

Warden, Gail, The Henry Ford Health System and David Lawrence, Kaiser Permanente. Personal communication: telephone conversation. September, 2000.

Weed, Lawrence L. and Lincoln Weed. Opening the Black Box of Clinical Judgment. Part III: Medical Science and Education. *EBMJ.* November 13, 1999. Online. Available at http://www.bmj.com/cgi/content/full/319/7220/1279/DC2 [accessed Jan. 24, 2001].

Work Group on Computerization of Patient Records. *Toward a National Health Information Infrastructure: Report of the Work Group on Computerization of Patient Records.* Washington, D.C.: U.S. Department of Health and Human Services, 2000.

8

Aligning Payment Policies with Quality Improvement

Many factors influence how health care organizations and professionals deliver care to patients. For example, information can be used to compare performance with that of peers and motivate improvement. Similarly, tools such as practice guidelines, clinical pathways, or protocols aim to change clinical practice to make it more consistent around a definition of best practice. Health care professionals and organizations are also motivated by public acknowledgment and honorary recognition. Recognition of professional accomplishment and innovation is a strong motivator of improvement.

Payment policies are another strong influence on how health care organizations and professionals deliver care and how patients select and use that care (Hillman, 1991). Thus, to achieve the aims of the 21st-century health care system set forth in Chapter 2, it is critical that payment policies be aligned to encourage and support quality improvement. Yet financial barriers embodied in current payment methods can create significant obstacles to higher-quality health care. Even among health professionals motivated to provide the best care possible, the structure of payment incentives may not facilitate the actions needed to systematically improve the quality of care, and may even prevent such actions. For example, redesigning care processes to improve follow-up for chronically ill patients through electronic communication may reduce office visits and decrease revenues for a medical group under some payment methods. Current payment policies are complex and contradictory, and although incremental improvements are possible, more fundamental reform will be needed over the long run.

The goals of any payment method should be to reward high-quality care and to permit the development of more effective ways of delivering care to improve the value obtained for the resources expended. These goals are relevant regardless of whether care is delivered in a predominantly competitive or regulated environment, and whether the ultimate purchaser is an employer or the patient/consumer. Payment policies should not create barriers to improving the quality of care.

> **Recommendation 10: Private and public purchasers should examine their current payment methods to remove barriers that currently impede quality improvement, and to build in stronger incentives for quality enhancement.**

Although some purchasers are pursuing payment approaches that include rewards for quality, all existing payment methods could be modified to create stronger incentives for quality improvement. Purchasers should identify ways to (1) recognize quality, (2) reward quality, and (3) support quality improvement. For example, quality could be recognized by developing better quality measures and making their results more broadly available to covered populations, whether through new forms of information or improvements in the ways existing information is shared. Quality could be rewarded by using direct payment mechanisms or by redirecting volume to health plans and providers recognized for providing high-quality care by offering stronger incentives for people to seek out better quality care (e.g., adjustments to out-of-pocket costs). Quality improvement could be supported by exploring the potential for shared-risk arrangements that could encourage making significant changes in care processes to improve quality. Although more fundamental change may be required in the long run, immediate improvements can and should be pursued.

> **Recommendation 11: The Health Care Financing Administration and the Agency for Healthcare Research and Quality, with input from private payers, health care organizations, and clinicians, should develop a research agenda to identify, pilot test, and evaluate various options for better aligning current payment methods with quality improvement goals.**

Although most payment methods have an objective of cost containment or reflect consideration of issues of access (e.g., in determining levels of copayments), they do not have the explicit goal of ensuring quality care or facilitating quality improvement. Approaches to incorporating such an explicit goal into payment policy should be explored. This research agenda should include work in the following areas: blended or bundled methods of payment for providers, multiyear contracts, payment modifications to encourage use of electronic interactions between providers and patients, risk adjustment, and alternative approaches for addressing the capital requirements necessary to improve quality. Blended or bundled payments may offer providers greater flexibility in incorporating quality. Multiyear contracts can encourage longer-term relationships among providers, purchasers, and payers to permit investment in improved quality of care. Payment methods that support electronic or other forms of communication between providers and patients can improve contacts with the health system. Payment methods that are appropriately adjusted for the risk of the patients served can support the provision of needed care and improved sources. Capital will be needed for the redesigning and reengineering of health care that will be required to improve quality. A better understanding is needed of how these, as well as other mechanisms, can enhance the effects of payment policy on the provision of high-quality health care.

The potential to link payment methods to priority conditions should also be explored. As noted in Chapter 4, priority conditions can provide a framework for aligning payment methods with patient needs and the ways care is organized and measured. If payment methods were designed to encompass the scope of services received by patients, providers could allocate resources according to patient needs, across provider types and settings of care. Pilot testing should include an evaluation of the use of bundled payments for priority conditions to provide incentives for redesigning care processes and to permit resources to be allocated according to the scope and types of services needed by patients.

The committee believes certain principles should guide the development of payment policies to reward quality, regardless of the specific payment method used for any given transaction. The aim of these principles is to guide payment policy reforms that can support care that is more patient-centered, evidence-based, and systems-based. Payment arrangements should facilitate alignment of the units of patient care delivered (including consistency with best practice) with the needs of consumers and patients, the unit of payment, and the level at which information is collected and shared. To achieve alignment that can reward quality care, payment methods should:

- Provide fair payment for good clinical management of the types of patients seen. Clinicians should be adequately compensated for taking good care of all types of patients, neither gaining nor losing financially for caring for sicker patients or those with more complicated conditions. The risk of random incidence of disease in the population should reside with a larger risk pool, whether that be large groups of providers, health plans, or insurance companies.
- Provide an opportunity for providers to share in the benefits of quality improvement. Rewards should be located close to the level at which the re-engineering and process redesign needed to improve quality are likely to take place.
- Provide the opportunity for consumers and purchasers to recognize quality differences in health care and direct their decisions accordingly. In particular, consumers need to have good information on quality and the ability to use that information as they see fit to meet their needs.

- Align financial incentives with the implementation of care processes based on best practices and the achievement of better patient outcomes. Substantial improvements in quality are most likely to be obtained when providers are highly motivated and rewarded for carefully designing and fine-tuning care processes to achieve increasingly higher levels of safety, effectiveness, patient-centeredness, timeliness, efficiency, and equity.
- Reduce fragmentation of care. Payment methods should not pose a barrier to providers' ability to coordinate care for patients across settings and over time.

The remainder of this chapter examines in greater detail the relationship between payment methods and the ability of health care organizations and professionals to undertake quality improvement activities. In the first section, the theoretical incentives of current payment methods are briefly reviewed. The second section focuses on barriers in the payment system that inhibit the achievement of significant improvements in quality. The third section describes how existing payment methods could be adapted to support quality improvement. Although difficult to accomplish in today's environment, examples are provided to illustrate how some health care organizations are attempting to incorporate greater attention to quality in their payment arrangements. Any payment method can be improved to support quality. However, fundamental misalignments will remain; thus fixing current payment methods may be important, but not sufficient. The final section therefore explores the need for a new approach to payment policy that can better align the needs of patients with the unit and type of payment method.

INCENTIVES OF CURRENT PAYMENT METHODS

Payment processes link together many different actors in health care. Purchasers, consumers and patients, health plans and insurers, and health care providers are all connected through various financial transactions (see Figure 8-1). Purchasers or funders of health care include public and private purchasers, such as employers and the Health Care Financing Administration; individual consumers and families; and federal, state, and local governments that may offer direct subsidies to certain providers (e.g., public hospitals) or for certain services (e.g., immunizations). Many purchasers buy coverage for their employees or covered populations through contractual arrangements with health plans or insurers. These health plans and insurers, in turn, contract with individual providers and/or provider groups to deliver health care services. In some cases, purchasers and providers may also be directly linked through contracting approaches under which employers contract directly with a provider group to deliver care.

Payment linkages also exist within the boxes shown in Figure 8-1. Purchasers and individuals are linked when purchasers provide a choice of coverage to

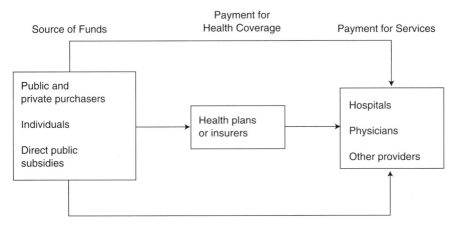

FIGURE 8-1 Linkages through payment arrangements.

their workers or covered populations and when individuals contribute to the cost of that coverage. Similarly, different types of providers can be linked through payment, such as when individual physicians receive payment through a larger medical group or when hospitals and physicians are linked financially in shared-risk arrangements. Because of these complex and diverse linkages, any given approach to payment policy can exert a powerful influence on the way services are provided to consumers and patients, and can produce unintended consequences.

Although this chapter focuses primarily on payments involving a payer and a provider, the committee recognizes the need to have a better understanding of how consumer decision making influences payment relationships. Consumers pay for health coverage both when they contribute to the cost of premiums and when they pay directly for health services through copayments, deductibles and payment for noncovered services. Although a great deal of research has been done recently on how consumers use information in selecting a health plan, less attention has been focused on how their decision making affects the payment relationship.

The committee believes consumers and patients should have a direct role in rewarding quality care. To have this role, consumers should have choices, receive information about their choices, and have the power to act on those choices. Not all consumers have a choice of health plans (Trude, 2000), but all have a choice of providers (and some services) within even a single health plan.[1] Yet

---

[1]Increasing interest in defined contribution plans suggests the potential for consumers to entertain more choices.

little information is made available to consumers at the level of providers or specific services, particularly relative to quality differences. As a consequence, consumers rarely switch health plans or providers for quality reasons (Cunningham and Kohn, 2000). Additional research is needed to understand how consumer decision making might affect the way payment flows may be altered in the future. A better understanding is also needed of how to communicate effectively with patients about best practices and evidence-based practice so that quantity is not automatically equated with quality.

The remainder of this section focuses on the right side of Figure 8-1— payment to providers for the direct delivery of services, especially the relationship between a health plan or insurer and providers. Other issues of financing health care, such as the source of funds or insurance coverage, are beyond the scope of this report, although the committee believes they are important issues and merit analysis. The following subsections provide a brief overview of common payment methods and the theoretical incentives offered by each. Four types of payment methods are reviewed: methods that pay by prospectively determined budgets regardless of whether services are used, per case payment methods that pay for a bundle of services used in a case, methods that pay by a unit of care as the units are used, and blended methods that combine approaches (Aas, 1995).

Budget Approaches

Under budgeted payment approaches, a budget is set for some defined set of services over a specified period of time and becomes a spending ceiling. A total budget can be set on a per capita basis or be based on historical costs (Aas, 1995). Capitation is a form of budgeting in which the budget is based on a fixed fee for each enrolled person to cover a specified level of health care, regardless of the amount of service actually provided (Aas, 1995; Anderson and Weller, 1999).

The advantages of a budgetary approach are that it provides an incentive to control costs and produce care efficiently, and can encourage innovation in cost-reducing technologies, use of lower-cost settings of care, and investment in health promotion and disease prevention. The approach also can make costs more predictable for the funder. Additionally, it can provide flexibility to providers in deciding how to spend the budgeted amount and coordinate care with other providers encompassed by the budget. Disadvantages include the potential for risk selection to avoid patients who might be high-cost users of care, and the potential to provide insufficient or reduced quality of services to minimize costs and stay within budget (Aas, 1995; Barnum et al., 1995; Lee, 1997). There is also the potential for conflicting incentives if physicians and hospitals are paid under separate risk pools, which could encourage a physician to admit a patient to the hospital (or refer the patient to a specialist) to reduce his or her own costs (Aas, 1995; Barnum et al., 1995).

A variant of the budget approach applied specifically to physician payment is salary. The advantage of the salary approach is good control over total costs and the dissociation of treatment decisions from a physician's financial gain or loss. The main disadvantage is the potential for reduced productivity if sufficient rewards are not built in (Aas, 1995).

Per Case Payment

Per case payment methods were introduced in 1983 by Medicare for short-term hospitals providing acute care services to Medicare beneficiaries (Cleverley, 1992). A prospectively set payment amount is determined on the basis of the diagnosis that resulted in the patient's hospital admission. From the hospital's perspective, the incentive is to reduce the costs of caring for patients within each diagnosis related group (DRG) in order to benefit from the savings achieved. From the purchaser's perspective, spending can be controlled directly through payment rates and updates (Medicare Payment Advisory Commission, 2000a). Medicare prospective payment for hospitals is generally believed to have reduced spending growth and increased efforts by hospitals to control costs, as evidenced by shorter lengths of stay and increased margins (Medicare Payment Advisory Commission, 2000a). On August 1, 2000, Medicare instituted a per case payment method for hospital outpatient care using ambulatory payment classification (APC) groups (Hallam, 2000; Medicare Payment Advisory Commission, 2000b).

Per case payment methods could be applied to the concept of priority conditions. For example, the mix of services covered under a payment method could be extended to include a comprehensive bundle of services that could be provided across different settings of care and over a defined period of time, similar to an episode of care. The advantage of this approach is that it would permit providers to design care and allocate resources for a population of patients (e.g., diabetics). Such an approach could also support the formation of multidisciplinary teams that would span settings of care to improve coordination among providers and foster the use of alternative modalities for treatment, such as e-mail for monitoring patients over time. Additional research would be needed to determine how to define an episode of care, particularly as applied to a chronic condition (Aas, 1995).

Payment by Unit of Care

Payment methods may be based on some unit of care. For example, under fee-for-service payment for physicians, the unit of payment is a visit or procedure. For hospitals, the unit of payment might be a patient day (per diem payment). These are retrospective payment methods in that care is paid for after it is used, although the rate to be paid may be set in advance.

In general, payment by unit of care offers little incentive to contain total costs since the incentive is to produce more of the unit of care that is being reimbursed. Under fee-for-service specifically, there is a potential for overuse of services by increasing the intensity of care and treating more patients. Also, since the method is based on individual units of care or service, it can be difficult to coordinate payment across the many members of a care team. The main advantages of payment by some unit of care are that it reduces the incentive for risk selection (i.e., avoiding people who are likely to be high users of care), and that physicians may specialize in difficult-to-treat medical problems. For per diem payment methods, there can also be an incentive to produce care efficiently to maximize profits per day (Aas, 1995; Barnum et al., 1995; Dudley et al., 1998).

Blended Methods

Approaches for bundling payments to providers have received increasing attention in recent years as a mechanism to align more closely the incentives faced by different providers involved in the care of a single patient. The central characteristic of bundled payment is that it covers multiple providers. The advantage of bundled payment methods is the opportunity to use resources more efficiently if some services across the continuum of care are substitutes for each other. For example, monitored home care could substitute for some office visits. Even if there is no substitution, a payer can make one entity responsible for a bundle of services and provide that entity with an incentive to deliver an efficient combination of services (Welch, 1998). Any possible gains associated with shifting patients among services is diminished.

Concerns with bundled payment approaches include questions about which entity should receive the payment and be held responsible for care (Welch, 1998). Possible responsible entities include health plans, hospitals, and physician groups. Another concern is feasibility in rural areas, where providers may face special difficulties in managing a continuum of services. Concerns have also been raised regarding the technical issues involved in building billing systems that can combine services offered by multiple providers (Schmitz, 1999). Additionally, legislative changes may be required to bundle payments for some combination of services, such as acute and postacute care (Welch, 1998).

One evaluated program that illustrates the potential of bundled payment is found in the Medicare Participating Heart Bypass Center demonstration, begun in 1991 by the Health Care Financing Administration (Cromwell et al., 1997). Four hospitals were paid a single fee for all inpatient institutional and physician care for heart bypass patients. Hospitals and physicians could split the fee in whatever manner they chose; however, no additional inpatient billing was permitted. The average total costs fell in three of four hospitals, and length of stay for patients in the program declined in all four hospitals. The savings were achieved because of changes in physician practice patterns that occurred when hospital and physician incentives were aligned. Surgeons took a more active role in discharge planning, review of drug protocols, and elimination of unnecessary standard orders for routine testing.

Payment methods could be combined along several dimensions (Aas, 1995; Barnum et al., 1995). First, a payment approach could blend methods for a specific type of provider. For example, physicians could be paid using a combination of fee for service and a target rate of growth in overall spending for physician services. Medicare applied this approach when it combined a fee schedule with a sustainable growth rate system for updating physician payment rates (Medicare Payment Advisory Commission, 2000c). Second, methods could be blended by the type of service provided. For example, a provider could be paid under capitation, with certain services designated for separate payment (Maguire et al., 1998). Third, methods could be blended by category of provider. For example, in an integrated delivery system, physicians could be paid under capitation and hospitals paid on a per diem basis. Finally, methods could be blended by time horizon. For example, providers could be paid under a prospectively determined budget, with a retrospective adjustment for the mix of patients actually seen.

Summary

In general, payment methods based on budget for a range of care are better at controlling the total costs of that care, but can create concerns regarding underuse. They may also require greater institutional investment in information and management systems so the provider organization can monitor care and costs. Payment on a per unit basis has the opposite effect: it is often easier for providers to manage, but is usually less amenable to controlling total costs.

The payment methods used most commonly today are based on payment for some unit of care as it is used (see Table 8-1). Physicians are typically paid through fee-for-service methods and hospitals through billed (discounted) charges, per diem or per case. Some surveys suggest that capitation may be increasing for physicians (Kane et al., 1998; Simon and Emmons, 1997); however, other sources suggest its use may be flat or declining (Lesser and Ginsburg, 2000). The use of capitation for hospitals may also be declining in favor of per diem, perhaps influenced by reductions in length of stay so that health plans prefer to "rent beds" on as as-needed basis (Rauber, 1999). Information is not available on the frequency of use of budget approaches. It is important to note, however, that most providers receive payment from a variety of payers that may rely on different methods. Therefore, any given provider faces a mix of incentives and rewards, rather than a consistent set of expectations. This mix has a significant influence on how payment methods can inhibit quality improvement, as discussed in the following section.

TABLE 8-1 Current Payment Methods for Physicians and Hospitals Based on Privately Insured Patients

Payment Methods For Physicians			Payment Methods For Hospitals			
Fee for Service/ Discounted Fee for Service	Salaried	Capitation	Billed Charges or Discounted Charges	Per Diem	Per Case	Capitation
Primary care: 72% Specialty care: 82%	Primary care: 3% Specialty care: 3%	Primary care: 25% Specialty care: 15%	30%	43%	18%	8%

NOTE: Data are based on Community Tracking Study (CTS), Insurance Followback Survey, 1996-1997, conducted by the Center for Studying Health System Change. The CTS Insurance Followback Survey is a supplement to the CTS Household Survey, a large, nationally representative longitudinal survey. Information on the privately insured obtained from the Household Survey was used to contact insurers/health plans and obtain information on characteristics of the health insurance products they offer. Insurers and health plans were asked to report the typical method of payment used for each type of service for each product. These responses were then matched to Household Survey respondents to describe their insurance coverage. Estimates are enrollee-weighted, representing all people under age 65 with private insurance. Totals may not sum to 100 because of rounding error.

Medicare pays physicians predominantly by fee-for-service using a fee schedule and hospitals on a per-case basis using diagnosis related groups (DRG). For beneficiaries enrolled in Medicare+Choice, health plans are paid on a capitated basis. According to a June 2000 Fact Sheet, about 16 percent of Medicare beneficiaries had selected Medicare HMOs ("The Medicare+Choice Payment Methodology," Fact Sheet, June 2000; www.hcfa.gov/facts/fs0006a.htm). In Medicaid, 55.6 percent are enrolled in managed care; the remainder are in fee for service (*National Summary of Medicaid Managed Care Programs and Enrollment*, June 30, 1999, Health Care Financing Administration, U.S. Department of Health and Human Services; http://www.hcfa.gov/medicaid/trends99.htm).

Finally, as was noted at the beginning of the chapter, different payment methods are designed to meet different objectives, but none automatically has quality improvement as an objective. Such an objective must therefore be explicitly designed into any payment method.

BARRIERS TO QUALITY IMPROVEMENT
IN CURRENT PAYMENT METHODS[2]

There is a growing body of evidence that quality improvement can translate into dollar savings (Classen et al., 1997; Clemmer et al., 1999; Conrad et al., 1996; Jarlier and Charvet-Protat, 2000). Poor quality is costly in several ways. First, quality-related problems can result in waste, such as when a step in the care process fails so that treatment must be repeated (e.g., the CT scan has to be redone), or extra resources are required to fix the failed process (e.g., treat an avoidable complication). Second, quality-related problems can lead to inefficiencies, as when two processes can produce the same outcome, but the more costly alternative is selected. An additional issue is that some processes may produce superior outcomes but utilize more resources, therefore resulting in cost increases. There is no advantage to this kind of quality improvement. In an environment that evaluates costs but not results, Anderson and Daigh (1991) suggest that quality waste accounts for 25–40 percent of all hospital costs.

Despite the evidence that poor quality costs money, however, health care organizations and professionals have not adopted quality-based process management to compete in today's marketplace. In fact, there are cases in which significant financial losses have resulted in the elimination of quality projects rather than the intensification of such efforts (Shulkin, 2000). Indeed, a variety of barriers embodied in current payment methods prevent health care organizations from pursuing quality improvement. The following subsections describe examples of four such payment barriers: perverse payment methods, adverse risk selection, annual contracting arrangements, and up-front investments required by provider groups.

Perverse Payment Mechanisms

Two examples of how payment mechanisms can inhibit quality improvement were provided at the IOM workshop held on April 24, 2000, by Dr. Brent James of the Intermountain Health System, Salt Lake City, Utah:

---

[2]Much of the discussion in this section draws on a paper prepared by Brent James, M.D. presented at an IOM-sponsored workshop on the relationship between payment and quality improvement held on April 24, 2000.

Example 1

A physician group paid primarily on a fee-for-service basis instituted a new program to improve blood sugar control for diabetic patients. Specifically, pilot studies suggested that tighter diabetic management could decrease hemoglobin A1c levels by 2 percentage points for about 40 percent of all diabetic patients managed by the physician group. Data from two randomized controlled trials demonstrated that better sugar controls should translate into lower rates of retinopathy, nephropathy, peripheral neurological damage, and heart disease (The Diabetes Control and Complications Trial Research Group, 1993). The savings in direct health care costs (i.e., reduced visits and hospital episodes) from avoided complications have been estimated to generate a net savings of about $2,000 per patient per year, on average, over 15 years (Demers et al., 1997). Across the more than 13,000 diabetic patients managed by the physician group, the project had the potential to generate over $10 million in net savings each year. The project was costly to the medical group in two ways. First, expenses to conduct the project, including extra clinical time for tighter management, fell to the physician group. Second, over time, as diabetic complication rates fell, the project would reduce patient visits and, thus revenues as well. The savings from avoided complications would fall to the insurer or a self-funded purchaser.

Example 2

A delivery system refined and implemented the American Thoracic Society's practice guideline on community-acquired pneumonia in ten rural Utah hospitals, focusing on indications for hospitalization and choice of initial antibiotics. In a prospective nonrandomized controlled trial using other Utah hospitals as controls, compliance with the guideline in the intervention hospitals increased from 22 to 40 percent ($p < 0.001$); the proportion of patients suffering significant complications fell from 15.3 to 11.6 percent ($p < 0.001$); inpatient mortality rates fell from 7.2 to 5.3 percent ($p = 0.015$); and costs fell by 12.3 percent ($p < 0.001$), primarily as a result of expenses avoided through the lower complication rate. The cost savings in those ten small rural hospitals totaled more than $500,000 per year, but an analysis of net operating income showed a loss to the facilities of over $200,000 per year. The reason was that as the complication rate fell, patients shifted from diagnosis related groups (DRGs) associated with complications (such as DRG 475, respiratory system diagnosis with ventilator support, carrying a per case payment of about $16,500 and providing a small excess of payment beyond treatment costs) to classifications such as DRG 89 (simple pneumonia and pleurisy, age > 17, with complications or comorbidities, carrying a per case payment of about $4,730, which failed to cover the full costs of care).

Quality problems can be grouped in three categories (Chassin et al., 1998). *Overuse* is the provision of a health care service under circumstances in which its potential for harm exceeds the possible benefit. *Underuse* is the failure to provide a health care service when it would have produced a favorable outcome for a patient. With *misuse* an appropriate service is provided, but a preventable complication occurs, and the patient does not receive the full potential benefit of the service. Efforts to correct each of these kinds of problems are affected differently by alternative payment methods, given the theoretical incentives described in the previous section. An example is provided below of what happens at the delivery level in trying to correct each type of quality problem, along with the effects of different payment methods.

Correcting Problems of Overuse. An example of correcting problems of overuse is a reduction in unnecessary surgical procedures. If a physician (or medical group) were paid under fee-for-service methods, the physician would lose revenues because fewer procedures would be performed. However, physicians paid under a budgeted approach (such as capitation or a shared risk arrangement) could benefit financially because fewer resources would be used in caring for affected patients. Hospitals would lose revenues under most payment methods (billed charges, per case, or per diem) because of the reduced volume of care, but, like physicians, would potentially gain financially under a capitation or shared-risk arrangement.

Correcting Problems of Underuse. An example of correcting problems of underuse is the provision of needed services to those who were previously untreated. Physicians paid under fee-for-service methods would potentially gain financially by seeing more patients who need care, but could lose under capitation or risk-sharing arrangements if patients in their current panel received more services. Similarly, hospitals would gain under most payment methods (billed charges, per diem, per case) because they would be serving more patients, but could suffer financial losses under capitation or shared-risk methods for the same reasons as physicians.

Correcting Problems of Misuse. An example of correcting problems of misuse is a reduction in infections acquired by patients while receiving needed health care services. Under fee-for-service payment, physicians would potentially lose revenues if fewer services were needed by patients because there were fewer infections. Under capitation or risk-sharing arrangements, physicians could benefit by expending fewer resources to manage the avoided infections. Hospitals would face a potentially mixed set of effects. Under billed charges, the hospital could lose revenues if reduced infections meant fewer services provided. Hospitals could gain under per diem methods if the length of stay remained the same for patients, but they used fewer resources each day because of the avoided infections. However, hospitals could also potentially lose under per diem payment if the avoided infections reduced patients' length of stay. A mixed effect is possible as well under per case payment. A hospital could gain financially if fewer resources were required per case, but could potentially lose financially if patients fell into a lower-paying DRG because of avoided infections (as in example 2). Generally, hospitals would gain financially under capitation or risk-sharing arrangements because patients would require fewer resources.

In sum, efforts to improve quality by correcting overuse, underuse, or misuse all have an impact on provider revenues; no payment method is neutral. Under the most common payment methods, correcting problems of underuse and those of overuse would have opposite effects: providers would gain financially by correcting the former problems, but they would lose by correcting the latter. Correcting problems of misuse would produce mixed effects for both physicians and hospitals, especially since physicians get most of their revenues from fee-for-service payment, and hospitals get a substantial portion of their revenues from per case payment. Thus the most common payment methods have insufficient incentives to fix problems of overuse and present great difficulties in fixing problems of misuse (because of the mixed effects, which can also make it difficult for hospitals and physicians to work together). There is a greater likelihood of financial gain from fixing problems of underuse. This reinforces the perception that improving quality costs money.

Even when care delivery groups want to improve the quality of the clinical processes and outcomes they routinely deliver to their patients, they can be severely limited in their ability to pursue such strategies if providers lose revenues from many quality improvement activities because of the expenses of implementing the improvements and the revenues lost as a result of reduced care delivery. Many health care professionals and organizations conduct activities that are harmful to their bottom line (e.g., provision of uncompensated care). However, it is not possible to sustain broad-based efforts to achieve a substantial improvement in quality if such efforts are financially harmful to those undertaking them. Furthermore, as earlier improvement efforts worsen their financial position, provider groups will not have the resources necessary to pursue additional clinical improvement projects. Therefore, although a payer may reap the initial benefits from quality improvement through reduced intensity or volume of care, the inability of providers to sustain such strategies on a long-term basis will hinder the ability to achieve continuous and lasting improvement.

Two broad options are possible to address problems associated with perverse payment mechanisms. One possible approach is to provide mechanisms to facilitate more shared-risk arrangements that include not only hospitals and physicians aligning purpose, but also payer involvement. Shared-risk arrangements could include capitation, but could also include negotiated arrangements around an agreed-upon budget amount, which might or might not result in per capita payment. Payers gain from reduced care delivery, but hospitals and physicians are responsible for changing the way care is delivered. Shared-risk arrangements could provide mechanisms for all parties involved to gain from changes in care. Alternatively, since fee-for-service payments (or billed charges for hospitals) remain in common use, mechanisms could be developed to compensate providers for the expenses associated with developing and implementing quality improvement programs. This compensation could take the form of making a direct payment or directing increased volume to those providers with recognized and measurable quality improvement initiatives. Both of those options reflect the need for resources to shift if broad-based and lasting quality improvement is to be achieved.

Adverse Risk Selection

Adverse risk selection occurs when an organization that bears financial risk (whether a health plan or provider group) attempts to avoid enrolling or caring for sick patients who have conditions that result in high and/or continuing costs. Both insurers and providers are concerned that undertaking quality improvement and publicizing quality outcomes will attract patients more likely to have conditions that make them high users of care and high-cost (Dudley et al., 1998). For example, if a health plan has a good program for identifying and managing those with diabetes, it is likely to enroll more diabetic patients. Since few purchasers adjust payment for this type of risk, the health plan bears the burden. Such health plans in turn, are unlikely to give their providers incentives to design programs that will attract a disproportionate share of people with diabetes. If financial risk is delegated to the provider group, the providers bear the financial burden of care for this population. The concern is related mainly to chronic conditions rather than acute care needs since the former represent ongoing expenses.

Risk-adjustment methods are an attempt to provide payment to health plans and providers that is commensurate with the health risks of the population served so that the organizations compete on efficiency, service, and quality instead of risk selection (Bowen, 1995). In the context of payment policy, risk is defined as how precisely future medical costs of an enrollee or group can be predicted (Gauthier et al., 1995). Risk adjustment is important because the distribution of medical expenditures is highly skewed, with a small fraction of individuals accounting for a substantial proportion of expenditures in any given year (Luft, 1995; Maguire et al., 1998). It has been estimated that the top 1 percent of spenders account for 30 percent of health care expenditures, whereas the bottom 50 percent account for only 3 percent (Berk and Monheit, 1992). Although some expenditures are unpredictable (such as trauma related to an auto accident), some are predictable (such as people with a chronic illness who are recognized as incurring continuing costs). Since some expenditures are predictable, organizations that assume financial risk for the care of a group can potentially avoid recognized high users of care and their costs.

There are a number of different approaches to adjust for risk, such as use of specific adjustment methods, withholds and risk pools, carve-outs, and reinsurance (Newhouse et al., 1997). Prospective risk-adjustment methods, several of which have been developed in recent years, have gained attention (particularly by the Health Care Financing Administration). Two leading models are adjusted clinical groups (ACGs, formerly referred to as ambulatory care groups) and diagnostic cost groups (DCGs) (Newhouse et al., 1997). Both methods use diagnostic information to improve predictability as compared with the demographic adjustments used by Medicare to pay health plans.

ACGs were developed at The Johns Hopkins University to classify risks by using diagnoses reported in ambulatory visits (Starfield et al., 1991). The system assigns diagnoses to a risk group based on five clinical dimensions, such as a condition's duration, severity, and diagnostic certainty. Both inpatient and ambulatory versions are available.

Initial development on DCGs was conducted through a consortium of researchers at Boston University, Health Economics Research, and the Harvard University School of Medicine, and is based on inpatient diagnoses for prior hospitalizations. The DCG model has been expanded to include both inpatient and ambulatory information and to account for multiple medical conditions patients may experience (Ellis et al., 1996).

Another method is clinical risk groups (CRGs), developed by 3M Health Information Systems (Averill et al., 1999). This clinical classification system assigns each patient to a risk group that relates past clinical information to the amount and type of health services the individual will consume in the future. Additionally, a survey-based approach has been developed at Kaiser-Permanente Health Plan for the working-age population. This method uses a chronic disease checklist and self-reported health status and functional status (using the RAND SF-36) to assess health risk (Hornbrook and Goodman, 1996).

The challenges involved in developing a fair and adequate risk-adjustment system cannot be underestimated. All current methods are limited in their ability to predict variation in expenditures. The Health Care Financing Administration implemented a transitional risk-adjustment system in January 2000 using a form of the DCG model, and is moving forward with an expanded model that will include inpatient, hospital outpatient, and physician encounter data. A number of models for this more comprehensive approach are being considered. It should be noted that improving risk-adjustment methods will likely necessitate more clinical information (rather than just claims information), which in turn will require significantly improved information systems (Dudley et al., 2000).

The goals for risk adjustment need to be balanced with the goals of quality improvement. In risk adjustment, the objective is to identify the subpopulation at risk of high utilization and high cost, whereas in quality improvement, the objective is to identify all patients with a particular condition who could benefit from treatment (Dudley et al., 2000). On the one hand, if there is a potential for higher payment, health care organizations are likely to identify as many at-risk patients as possible and collect whatever information is necessary. On the other hand, doing so could bias quality measures through possible upcoding and might not provide incentives to design efficient and effective systems of care. The potential for payment methods to be based on similar patients with common conditions, including definitions of best practice, may help mediate some of the possible adverse effects.

Annual Contracting Arrangements

In theory, capitation and shared-risk arrangements provide incentives to pursue quality improvement strategies that minimize costs over the long term by keeping people healthy. To the extent that turnover in health plan membership and contracting arrangements occurs, however, suboptimization may result if the organization that undertakes the quality improvement does not see the benefits from those efforts.

Annual contracting arrangements can produce turnover in three ways. First, health plans and purchasers can alter annually the plans offered to consumers and force a change in health plan enrollment. Second, health plans and providers can alter annually the composition of provider networks, forcing patients to switch providers. Third, annual enrollment by individuals in health plans can produce turnover for the plans even if there is no change in the two former arrangements.

Annual contracting cycles may hinder a health care organization's ability to pursue quality improvement initiatives if the organization believes the benefits will accrue to a competitor. If a health plan has even modest enrollee turnover, and a quality improvement project requires an up-front investment while the financial savings span years, patients may very well have shifted to another plan by the time the health benefits and related savings accrue. The same is true for a provider group that may develop a good program for difficult-to-manage diabetics and is able to improve compliance with treatment, but is dropped from the health plan's provider panel, so that those now well-controlled patients go to a competitor's diabetic program. Such turnover can eliminate the benefit for many proposed clinical improvement projects.

Longer-term arrangements among provider groups, health plans, and purchasers may be advisable to facilitate the investments needed to achieve quality improvement and ensure gains to the partners from the benefits that are generated over time (whether in the form of savings or improved outcomes). However, patients and consumers should be able to shift coverage or source of care for quality-related reasons. The ability of consumers and patients to do so can be a strong motivator for clinicians and health plans to offer such good care that people will not want to leave.

Up-Front Investments Required by Provider Groups

Provider groups face two specific managerial issues that are affected by payment arrangements and can hamper efforts by health care organizations to pursue quality improvement: (1) the difficulty of measuring the impact of quality improvement on the organization's bottom line and (2) infrastructure challenges encountered by those organizations seeking to implement broad-based quality improvement programs. Up-front investments are likely to be required to address both of these issues.

Difficulty of Measuring the Impact of Quality Improvement on the Bottom Line

When evaluating the potential for a quality improvement project to improve a health care organization's bottom line, the expense of the proposed improvement is compared with the potential savings in variable costs. Variable costs are expenses that fluctuate directly with patient volumes, such as medications, disposable equipment, other supplies, and staffing levels, and are achieved relatively quickly. The impact of the proposed clinical quality improvement initiative is rarely evaluated in terms of savings in fixed costs, since those costs accrue over a longer time period. Fixed costs are expenses that a physician, clinic, hospital, or delivery system must pay regardless of patient volumes, such as payments for buildings, diagnostic and other equipment, licensing and regulatory fees, malpractice insurance, and minimum required staffing.

Most health care costs are considered fixed, although there is likely variation in how individual health care organizations define their fixed or variable costs. For example, many consider labor costs to be fixed in the short term, but variable over the long term. However, it has been estimated that 60 to 75 percent of all expenses fall into the fixed cost category (Lave and Lave, 1984; Williams, 1996), leaving only about 25 to 40 percent of the savings generated by quality-based elimination of clinical waste (the proportion accounted as variable expenses) to appear quickly on an organization's balance sheet. The remaining 60 to 75 percent of the potential savings, representing the fixed cost portion, appears as unused capacity within the organization. If a care delivery group can recruit additional patients to reduce excess capacity, an immediate benefit will be realized. The organization's fixed costs will be spread across a larger patient population (all of the old patients, plus a number of new ones) so that the effective fixed cost per patient will fall, creating a larger financial margin for each patient treated. However, if the organization cannot increase patient volume, several years can be required to affect the fixed costs. Thus, the proportion of fixed costs in health care affects the ability to measure the impact of quality improvement efforts on an organization's bottom line.

Infrastructure Investments

An organization that wants to use clinical quality as a business strategy must make a substantial investment in skill building and culture change. Clinical process management, a health care delivery organization's core business function, has traditionally been seen as a secondary responsibility of the voluntary medical staff. Practicing physicians are asked to contribute time without compensation and to serve on clinical oversight committees, taking time away from their primary patient care role. An organization must make a substantial investment in medical and other clinical leadership, as well as build an effective management and information infrastructure to use for tracking outcomes, assessing performance, and setting clinical improvement goals. This investment should include tools and training in quality methods, but also adequate information systems that can be applied to clinical quality improvement (see Chapter 7).

ADAPTING EXISTING PAYMENT METHODS TO SUPPORT QUALITY IMPROVEMENT

As noted earlier, the IOM held a workshop on April 24, 2000, to discuss the relationship between payment and quality improvement. At the workshop, several examples were provided to illustrate how various existing payment methods—including fee for service, capitation, a blended method, and a shared-risk (budget) method—could be adapted to support quality improvement. This section describes the examples presented at the workshop.

Adapting Fee-for-Service Payment

Dr. Glenn Littenberg described how fee-for-service payment could be adapted to provide incentives for quality improvement by encouraging cooperation and providing reimbursement for care outside of the traditional office visit, which is not always optimal for meeting patients' needs. The approach involves developing relative values for the elements of work performed over time by physicians and other health professionals. For example, physicians provide care between visits, including coordination of complex cases, phone consults with patients and other professionals, and follow-up on tests performed. These activities do not require face-to-face contact, but can occupy a significant amount of professional time. A Current Procedural Technology (CPT) code could be developed for use of electronic media with the patient not present for specific communications, for research, for clinical updates, and for coordination of care with other health professionals within a 30-day period. Codes could also be developed and relative values assigned for other organizational innovations designed to improve quality (e.g., anticoagulation clinics, which would include the clinical groups that have key roles, such as physicians, pharmacists, nurses, and dietary staff).

Despite the growth of alternative payment methods, fee-for-service payment remains important. Even in capitated systems, many individual physicians are paid using a fee-for-service method. Additionally, fee-for-service payment levels often serve as the benchmark for other payment methods. As a result, financial support for activities that would improve quality care and rely on fee-for-service payment remains one avenue for building in rewards for quality care.

Adapting Capitation Payment

Dr. Sam Ho described how PacifiCare Health System has developed a payment structure that rewards quality care provided by the 700 medical groups with which the plan contracts. PacifiCare pays the majority of medical groups by capitation for all professional services. Hospitals are also paid predominantly through capitation. The health plan retains risk for certain hospital, pharmacy, and ancillary services (e.g., durable medical equipment). The core of the system is a report card program that provides quality performance information to both physicians and consumers. The provider profile contains about 80 measures enabling medical groups to compare their own performance over time, as well as with regional and national benchmarks. The consumer-focused performance report currently contains 32 indicators, with more being added each year. Preliminary analysis conducted by PacifiCare indicates that the medical groups with higher scores on "best practice" are seeing statistically significant increases in membership and high member retention rates.

Two specific elements of the PacifiCare approach are worth noting. First, the approach focuses on the availability of data, relying on depth and breadth of data. Second, much of the information is directed toward consumers as decision makers. Rather than being directed at selection of a health plan, the information is at the medical group level, where consumers can evaluate their own trade-offs among cost, quality, access, and any other dimensions of importance to them.

Adapting Blended Payment Methods

Ann Robinow of the Buyers Health Care Action Group, Minneapolis, Minnesota, described what some have termed a direct contracting approach. The group contracts with "care systems," defined as groups of primary care physicians and affiliated specialists and facilities that could assume responsibility for the provision of a full continuum of care (Christianson et al., 1999). Payment is blended in that a budget target is set prospectively and adjusted retrospectively. Each year, care systems set a financial target for all care to enrollees (including pharmacy) that becomes the price to consumers and the benchmark for financial performance. The prices are risk adjusted every quarter using ACGs by comparing the care system's performance for the most recent 12-month period with the target (Christianson et al., 1999), which is adjusted each quarter to reflect the relative illness burden of patients during the same time period for which financial information is being collected. Because it is a claims-based system in which each employer pays its own fees, fee levels are increased or decreased over time so that the fees approximate the target submitted (fees increase if the organization is below target and decrease if the target is exceeded). Consumers receive comparative information at the care system level. Ms. Robinow indicated that the group's own analysis indicates people are moving from the higher-cost to the lower-cost systems and that systems with higher satisfaction scores have also had higher enrollment gains.

Two notable elements of this approach are its focus on the care system and consumer involvement. The focus on the care system places responsibility at the level at which processes of care can be modified to improve quality. Providing comparative information to consumers at this level of the care system gives them information about care delivery and not just health coverage. This information is perceived as being more valuable for patients.

Adapting Shared-Risk (Budget) Arrangements

Dr. Brent James of Intermountain Health Care described the organization's recent experience in moving toward shared-risk arrangements in which partnerships are established with purchasers, and risk is shared around a budget based on the expectations of caring for a population. Costs are typically projected on the basis of a particular set of disease entities in clinical programs that represent the work of smaller groups. These are referred to as care processes. These groups do not manage just one activity (e.g., mammography), but rather a number of processes for a single condition (e.g., breast cancer). The price is negotiated among the partners. If Intermountain is able to produce care for the population below budget, all the partners share in the savings.

Intermountain perceives several advantages to this approach. First, it permits the organization to share in the benefits of quality improvement. Second, care can be organized around processes that are meaningful to health professionals, patients, and purchasers, which helps align incentives and work priorities. Third, the approach uses a budgeted target to impose financial discipline, but does not rely on capitation, which means it can be applied to smaller groups of practitioners and patients that would not assume actuarial risk. The challenge is the need for good data to set budgets fairly and monitor clinical processes of care.

NEED FOR A NEW APPROACH

Although incentives to improve quality could be strengthened through incremental improvements in existing payment methods, more significant reform of the payment system will be needed over the long term. All health care organizations face serious barriers in pursuing broad-based efforts at quality improvement, and providers face a mix of incentives from different payment methods. Conceptually, a provider group could manage effectively in an environment that was entirely fee for service or entirely capitation, but the present environment is a mix of both. An organization that manages to succeed predominantly under fee-for-service payment will fail under the incentives of capitation. On the other hand, an organization that manages to succeed under capitation will fail on the portion of care that is paid through fee for service. Thus, health care organizations are faced with a financial situation in which it is almost impossible to manage for quality.

There are several ways to improve the way payment methods reward quality care. One option is to refine existing payment methods to provide greater rewards for quality. As noted in the preceding discussion, all existing payment methods can be improved to reward quality better. However, although these incremental improvements are important to pursue, a more fundamental restructuring of the payment system is needed. One of the common threads that runs through most of the recent innovations in payment is greater attention to subpopulations with common clinical needs.

Chapter 4 describes the need for a classification system around priority conditions to facilitate the provision of care based on the common reasons for which people seek care. Although it would be premature to recommend payment based on priority conditions, it is appropriate to study their feasibility as a tool for aligning the scope of services provided with the scope of payment. For example, a patient with a chronic condition may be seeking the acute care services traditionally covered under insurance, but may also need, for example, services related to counseling and behavior change, support groups, e-mail access for communication between visits, strongly managed and continuous coordination with other health professionals, and medical supplies. However, today's payment approaches offer a chronically ill patient face-to-face office visits as the primary mechanism for receiving care and rarely encompass the range of services needed across the continuum of care. Furthermore, the fragmentation of payment by service can make it difficult for care to be coordinated efficiently across multiple settings. There is a misalignment among what the patient needs, the services provided, and how needed services are paid for. Organizing care and payment around priority conditions could offer a framework for aligning payment incentives around a common clinical purpose that is consistent with meeting patient needs as completely and efficiently as possible.

The committee recognizes that such redesign could require significant changes in the purpose and structure of the insurance function. The role of health plans could shift toward a heavy emphasis on obtaining information from various configurations of providers and, in turn, releasing information to the public. Consumers' responsibilities could also shift if they are to become more directly involved in comparing options for care and the arrangements through which they wish to receive care. Despite the challenges, however, the committee believes good-quality care can be recognized and rewarded through payment policies.

Although this chapter focuses on current payment policy and its shortcomings, the committee also discussed a set of larger economic issues. The committee recognizes that the recommendations in this report will reduce costs in some areas and increase costs in others. In general, correcting problems of overuse and misuse is likely to result in cost reductions, whereas correcting problems of underuse is likely to increase costs (Chassin et al., 1998). Quality problems related to overuse increase costs through the provision of services from which patients do not benefit. Patients may also be exposed to unnecessary risks associated with treatment (Fisher and Welch, 1999). Quality problems related to misuse increase costs when tests and procedures have to repeated or when avoidable complications increase treatment needs. On the other hand, quality problems related to underuse represent artificial "savings," as patients do not receive beneficial services, such as immunizations.

In terms of the specific recommendations in this report, there are several potential areas in which cost savings may be produced. Greater use of information technology (see Chapter 7) should result in costs savings in several ways. First, automation of certain functions may reduce some labor costs. This has happened in other industries, such as manufacturing. Second, information technology may permit substitution of less costly alternatives of care. For example, to the extent that monitoring of patients can occur partly through e-mail, some office visits may be eliminated, as in the case of patients with controlled chronic conditions who may be able to visit their physician's office twice a year instead of quarterly, relying on electronic communication between visits. Third, use of computerized drug prescribing has been shown to reduce medication errors, which are known to increase costs (Bates et al., 1997, 1998, 1999).

Cost reductions may also be possible with better application of the evidence base (see Chapter 6). Standardizing care around best practices and reducing variation in treatment patterns should result in reduced and/or more predictable costs of care. The use of effective decision support systems can reduce variation in practice through improved compliance with practice guidelines (Balas et al., 2000; Shea et al., 1996).

Finally, cost savings may be achieved through greater use of multidisciplinary teams (see Chapter 5). When teams are well coordinated and are able to sufficiently plan care and share information, it may become possible to substitute less-costly personnel for higher-cost personnel. Developing and using care teams properly can improve coordination across settings and over time to reduce inefficiencies associated with handoffs among members of the care team.

The committee recognizes, however, that not all activities to improve quality will be cost-reducing. In addition to cost increases associated with correcting problems of underuse, as noted above, there will also be costs associated with implementing changes in the organization and delivery of care. Even if a change ultimately reduces cost, the process of evolving from the current system to the system of the 21st century may incur significant costs. Although some public support can help move such a process forward, health care organizations themselves will need to invest in change, just as other industries (e.g., banking) have invested in transforming their business procedures. Key transitional areas that are likely to increase costs in the short- to mid-term time frame include (1) the need to train people for new jobs in health care (or in other fields) as some workers are displaced by new approaches to organizing and delivering care,

(2) investment in information technology and associated training costs, (3) the need to maintain duplicative systems temporarily while redesigning care processes (i.e., retaining the old process while the new process is being implemented and refined), and (4) capital investment to support redesign and reengineering of the current system.

It is not known how cost increases and decreases will ultimately balance over time. Regardless of the final calculus, however, what can be obtained is better value for the resources expended. Good value does not lie in spending over $1 trillion on health care that leaves some people receiving care they do not need and others not receiving the care they need. There should be a strong commitment to evaluating the economic and other impacts associated with improving the quality of care. However, such evaluations may not be amenable to existing measurement approaches. For example, benefits from information technology have included easier access to medical histories, improved access to summary patient details, support for protocols or guidelines, and quicker reporting of results of treatment (Lock, 1996). These benefits are difficult to quantify and to incorporate into a traditional return-on-investment analysis. Therefore, assessing the impact of new approaches and innovative programs designed to improve quality may require new measurement approaches.

REFERENCES

Aas, I. H. Monrad. Incentives and Financing Methods. *Health Policy* 34:205–20, 1995.

Anderson, Craig A. and Robin D. Daigh. Quality Mind-Set Overcomes Barriers to Success. *Healthcare Financial Management* 45(2):21–32, 1991.

Anderson, Gerard F. and Wendy E. Weller. Methods of Reducing the Financial Risk of Physicians Under Capitation. *Archives of Family Medicine* 8:149–55, 1999.

Anonymous. Top-Priority Actions for Preventing Adverse Drug Events in Hospitals. Recommendations of an Expert Panel. *Am J Health Syst Pharm* 53(7):747–51, 1996.

Averill, Richard F., Norbert I. Goldfield, Jon Eisenhandler, et al. 1999. "3M HIS Research Report 9–99: Development and Evaluation of Clinical Risk Groups (CRGs)." Online. Available at http://www.3M.com/market/healthcare/his/us/documents/reports/crg-article999.pdf [accessed Aug. 23, 2000].

Balas, E. Andrew, Scott Weingarten, Candace T. Garb, et al. Improving Preventive Care by Prompting Physicians. *Arch Int Med* 160(3):301–8, 2000.

Barnum, Howard, Joseph Kutzin, and Helen Saxenian. Incentives and Provider Payment Methods. *International Journal of Health Planning and Management* 10:23–45, 1995.

Bates, David W., Lucian L. Leape, David J. Cullen, et al. Effect of Computerized Physician Order Entry and a Team Intervention on Prevention of Serious Medication Errors. *JAMA* 280(15):1311–6, 1998.

Bates, David W., Nathan Spell, David J. Cullen, et al. The Costs of Adverse Drug Events in Hospitalized Patients. *JAMA* 277(4):307–11, 1997.

Bates, David W., Jonathan M. Teich, Joshua Lee, et al. The Impact of Computerized Physician Order Entry on Medication Error Prevention. *J Am Med Inform Assoc* 6(4):313–21, 1999.

Berk, Marc L. and Alan C. Monheit. The Concentration of Health Expenditures: An Update. *Health Affairs* 11(4):145–9, 1992.

Bowen, Bruce. The Practice of Risk Adjustment. *Inquiry* 32(Spring):33–40, 1995.

Chassin, Mark R., Robert W. Galvin, and the National Roundtable on Health Care Quality. The Urgent Need to Improve Health Care Quality. *JAMA* 280(11):1000–5, 1998.

Christianson, Jon, Roger Feldman, Jonathan P. Weiner, and Patricia Drury. Early Experience With A New Model of Employer Group Purchasing in Minnesota. *Health Affairs* 18(6):100–14, 1999.

Classen, David C., Stanley L. Pestotnik, Scott Evans, et al. Adverse Drug Events in Hospitalized Patients: Excess Length of Stay, Extra Costs, and Attributable Mortality. *JAMA* 277(4):301–6, 1997.

Clemmer, Terry P., Vicki J. Spuhler, Thomas A. Oniki, and Susan D. Horn. Results of a Collaborative Quality Improvement Program on Outcomes and Costs in a Tertiary Critical Care Unit. *Crit Care Med* 27(9):1768–74, 1999.

Cleverley, William O. *Essentials of Health Care Finance.* Gaithersburg, MD: Aspen Publications, 1992.

Conrad, Douglas, Thomas Wickizer, Charles Maynard, et al. Managing Care, Incentives and Information: An Exploratory Look Inside the "Black Box" of Hospital Efficiency. *Health Services Research* 31(3):235–59, 1996.

Cromwell, Jerry, Debra A. Dayhoff, and Armen H. Thoumaian. Cost Savings and Physician Responses to Global Bundled Payments for Medicare Heart Bypass Surgery. *Health Care Financing Review* 19(1):41–57, 1997.

Cunningham, Peter J. and Linda Kohn. Health Plan Switching: Choice Or Circumstance? *Health Affairs* 19(3):158–64, 2000.

Demers, David, Nathaniel Clark, Geoff Tolzmann, et al. Computer Simulated Cost Effectiveness of Care Management Strategies on Reduction of Long-Term Sequelae in Patients with Non-Insulin Dependent Diabetes Mellitus. *Quality Mgmt in Hlth Care* 6(1):1–13, 1997.

Dudley, R. Adams, Lisa V. Bowers, and Harold S. Luft. Reconciling Quality Measurement with Financial Risk Adjustment in Health Plans. *Journal on Quality Improvement* 26(3):137–46, 2000.

Dudley, R. Adams, Robert H. Miller, Tamir Korenbrot, and Harold S. Luft. The Impact of Financial Incentives on Quality of Health Care. *The Milbank Quarterly* 76(4):649–86, 1998.

Ellis, Randall P., Gregory C. Pope, Lisa I. Iezzoni, et al. Diagnosis-Based Risk Adjustment for Medicare Capitation Payments. *Health Care Financing Review* 17(3):101–28, 1996.

Fisher, Elliott S. and H. Gilbert Welch. Avoiding the Unintended Consequences of Growth in Medical Care. How Might More Be Worse? *JAMA* 281(5):446–53, 1999.

Gauthier, Anne K., Jo Ann Lamphere, and Nancy L. Barrand. Risk Selection in the Health Care Market: A Workshop Overview. *Inquiry* 32(Spring):14–22, 1995.

Hallam, Kristen. HCFA to Go Ahead with Medicare PPS. *Modern Healthcare* 30(31):2–3, 2000.

Hillman, Alan L. Managing The Physician: Rules Versus Incentives. *Health Affairs* 10(4):138–46, 1991.

Hornbrook, Mark C. and Michael J. Goodman. Chronic Disease, Functional Health Status, and Demographics: A Multi-Dimensional Approach to Risk Adjustment. *Health Services Research* 31(3):283–307, 1996.

Jarlier, Agnes and Suzanne Charvet-Protat. Can Improving Quality Decrease Hospital Costs? *International Journal for Quality in Health Care* 12(2):125–31, 2000.

Kane, Carol K., David W. Emmons, and Gregory D. Wozniak. Physician Managed Care Contracting. *Socioeconomic Characteristics of Medical Practice 1997/98.* Martin L. Gonzalez and Puling Zhang, eds. Chicago, IL: American Medical Association, 1998.

Lave, Judith R. and Lester B. Lave. Hospital Cost Functions. *Annual Review of Public Health* 5:193–213, 1984.

Lee, A. James. The Role of Financial Incentives in Shaping Clinical Practice Patterns and Practice Efficiency. *American Journal of Cardiology* 80(88):28H–32H, 1997.

Lesser, Cara S. and Paul B. Ginsburg. Update on the Nation's Health Care System: 1997–1999. *Health Affairs* 19(6):206–16, 2000.

Lock, Chris. What Value Do Computers Provide to NHS Hospitals? *BMJ* 312(7043):1407–10, 1996.

Luft, Harold S. Potential Methods to Reduce Risk Selection and Its Effects. *Inquiry* 32(Spring):23–32, 1995.

Maguire, Ann M., Neil R. Powe, Barbara Starfield, et al. "Carving out" Conditions from Global Capitation Rates: Protecting High-Cost Patients, Physicians, and Health Plans in a Managed Care Environment. *The American Journal of Managed Care* 4(6):797–806, 1998.

Medicare Payment Advisory Commission. Chapter 1: Recent Changes in the Medicare Program. *Report to the Congress: Selected Medicare Issues.* Washington, D.C.: MedPAC, 2000a.

———. Chapter 2: Assessing the design and impact of the hospital prospective payment system. *Report to Congress: Selected Medicare Issues.* Washington, D.C.: MedPAC, 2000b.

———. Chapter 7: Reviewing the estimated payment update for physician services. *Report to Congress: Selected Medicare Issues.* Washington, D.C.: MedPAC, 2000c.

Newhouse, Joseph P., Melinda Beeuwkes Buntin, and John D. Chapman. Risk Adjustment and Medicare: Taking A Closer Look. *Health Affairs* 16(5):26–43, 1997.

Rauber, Chris. De-Capitating Managed Care Contracts. *Modern Healthcare* 29(36):52–7, 1999.

Schmitz, Richard B. Building Global Billing and Payment Systems. *Managed Care Quarterly* 7(1):16–28, 1999.

Shea, Steven, William DuMouchel, and Lisa Bahamonde. A Meta-Analysis of 16 Randomized Controlled Trials to Evaluate Computer-Based Clinical Reminder Systems for Preventive Care in the Ambulatory Setting. *J Am Med Inform Assoc* 3(6):399–409, 1996.

Shulkin, David. Comments at IOM "Workshop on the Effects of Financing Policy on Quality of Care." April 24, 2000.

Simon, Carol J. and David W. Emmons. Physician Earnings at Risk: An Examination of Capitated Contracts. *Health Affairs* 16(3):120–6, 1997.

Starfield, Barbara, Jonathan Weiner, Laura Mumford, and Donald Steinwachs. Ambulatory Care Groups: A Categorization of Diagnoses for Research and Management. *Health Services Research* 26(1):53–74, 1991.

The Diabetes Control and Complications Trial Research Group. The Effect of Intensive Treatment of Diabetes on the Development and Progression of Long-Term Complications of Insulin-Dependent Diabetes Mellitus. *N Engl J Med* 329(14):977–86, 1993.

Trude, Sally. *Who Has a Choice of Health Plans?* Washington, D.C.: Center for Studying Health System Change, Issue Brief Number 27 , 2000.

Welch, W. Pete. Bundled Medicare Payment For Acute and Postacute Care. *Health Affairs* 17(6):69–81, 1998.

Williams, Robert M. The Costs of Visits to Emergency Departments. *N Engl J Med* 334(10):642–6, 1996.

9

Preparing the Workforce

Health care is not just another service industry. Its fundamental nature is characterized by people taking care of other people in times of need and stress. Patients are ill, families are worried, and the ultimate outcome may be uncertain. Stable, trusting relationships between a patient and the people providing care can be critical to healing or managing an illness. The people who deliver care are the health system's most important resource.

All of the issues raised in the previous chapters of this report have important implications for the health care workforce, potentially requiring different work in new types of organizations that may use fewer people. Accountabilities and standards of care may change; relationships between patients and health professionals are certain to do so.

The health care workforce is large, having employed almost 6 million people in 1998 (Occupational Employment Statistics, 2000) with a wide variety of educational backgrounds, specialization, and skills. Professional hierarchies are well established and reinforced by training, laws, and regulations, as well as culture and history. In general, health professionals are also conservative, stressing the application of precedent and risk avoidance in clinical practice, particularly relative to changes that may affect the quality of care for patients. As a result, any change can be exceedingly slow and difficult to accomplish, especially if there is not a clear understanding of why the change may be needed or of its impact on current practices.

The importance of appropriately preparing the workforce for the changes in health care delivery that will be necessitated by the recommendations in this report cannot be underestimated. There are many serious challenges facing the health care workforce, including difficulties in retention of personnel, the impending crisis in nursing supply, and the need for strong leadership within the health care system to guide and support what will be a very difficult transition. When clinicians are under stress themselves, it is difficult to take care of patients who are ill and stressed. Indeed, this was one of the key transitional issues identified during the committee's deliberations. It is a broad topic that can only be introduced here, but the committee emphasizes the need for additional study to understand the effects of the changes recommended herein on how the workforce is prepared for practice, how it is deployed, and how it is held accountable.

> **Recommendation 12: A multidisciplinary summit of leaders within the health professions should be held to discuss and develop strategies for (1) restructuring clinical education to be consistent with the principles of the 21st-century health system throughout the continuum of undergraduate, graduate, and continuing education for medical, nursing, and other professional training programs; and (2) assessing the implications of these changes for provider credentialing programs, funding, and sponsorship of education programs for health professionals.**

> **Recommendation 13: The Agency for Healthcare Research and Quality should fund research to evaluate how the current regulatory and legal systems (1) facilitate or inhibit the changes needed for the 21st-century health care delivery system, and (2) can be modified to support health care professionals and organizations that seek to accomplish the six aims set forth in Chapter 2.**

This chapter briefly examines three specific issues: clinical training and education, regulation of the health professions, and legal liability issues. Clinical training and education is seen as particularly important for changing the culture of health care practice to support achievement of the aims set forth in Chapter 2. Greater understanding is needed of why prior efforts at modifying clinical education have not had the desired impact and of the supportive strategies needed to overcome such barriers.

CLINICAL EDUCATION AND TRAINING

To achieve the six aims proposed in Chapter 2, additional skills may be required of health professionals—not just physicians, but all clinicians who care for patients. Prior chapters have identified a number of changes affecting health care delivery, including a shift from acute to chronic care, the need to manage a continually expanding evidence base and technological innovations, more clinical practice occurring in teams and complex delivery arrangements, and changing patient–clinician relationships. The need to balance cost, quality, and access in health care will put pressures on clinical education programs, particularly given the outlay of public dollars for clinical education.

The types of new or enhanced skills required by health professionals might include, for example, the ability to:

• Use a variety of approaches to deliver care, including the provision of care without face-to-face visits (e.g., using electronic communications to provide follow-up care and routine monitoring) (see Chapter 3).

• Synthesize the evidence base and communicate it to patients (see Chapter 6).

• Combine the evidence base, knowledge about population outcomes, and patient preferences to tailor care for an individual patient (Weed and Weed, 1999a) (see Chapter 6).

• Communicate with patients in a shared and fully open manner to support their decision making and self-management (to the extent they so desire), including the potential for unfettered access to the information contained in their medical records (see Chapter 3).

• Use decision support systems and other tools to aid clinical decision making in order to minimize problems of overuse and underuse and reduce waste (Weed and Weed, 1999a) (see Chapter 6).

• Identify errors and hazards in care; understand and implement basic safety design principles, such as standardization and simplification (Institute of Medicine, 2000) (see Chapter 5).

• Understand the course of illness and a patient's experience outside of the hospital (where most training is conducted).

• Continually measure quality of care in terms of both process and outcomes; develop and implement best practices (Berwick et al., 1992) (see Chapter 5).

• Work collaboratively in teams with shared responsibility (Chassin, 1998) (see Chapter 5).

• Design processes of care and measure their effectiveness, even when the members of the team that cares for a patient are not in the same physical locale (Berwick et al., 1992).

• Understand how to find new knowledge as it continually expands, evaluate its significance and claims of effectiveness, and decide how to incorporate it into practice (Chassin, 1998) (see Chapter 6).

• Understand determinants of health, the link between medical care and healthy populations, and professional responsibilities.

Teaching these skills will likely require changes in curriculum. Although some schools have added courses that are consistent with the desired skills, the needed content is likely to evolve over time. For example, many schools now have courses in patient communications, information systems, and biostatistics.

However, communicating with patients to improve adherence to a recommended treatment is different from communicating with patients who are key decision makers and full partners in their care. Using information technology to do a MEDLINE search is important, but not the same as using the technology as a central component in delivering care and using decision support as an aid to clinical decision making. Knowing biostatistics aids in understanding the published literature, but is not the same as using statistics to design processes of care to reduce variations in practice. Likewise, care provided by multidisciplinary teams involves more than knowing the responsibilities of people in a clinical department; it should involve knowing how to form and use teams to customize care across settings and over time, even when the members of the team are in entirely different physical locations.

Although curriculum changes are essential in providing new skills to health professionals, they are not sufficient by themselves. It is also necessary to address how health professional education is approached, organized, and funded to better prepare students for real practice in an information rich environment. Two examples are teaching evidence-based practice and training in multidisciplinary teams.

The traditional emphasis in clinical education, particularly medical education, is on teaching a core of knowledge, much of it focused on the basic mechanisms of disease and pathophysiological principles. Given the expansiveness and dynamic nature of the science base in health care, this approach should be expanded to teach how to manage knowledge and use effective tools that can support clinical decision making (Evidence-Based Medicine Working Group, 1992; Weed and Weed, 1999c). Effective teaching of evidence-based practice requires faculty role models, an emphasis on teaching the application of critical appraisal skills in actual patient care settings, and experience in conducting literature searches and applying methodological rules to the evaluation and understanding of evidence (Evidence-Based Medicine Working Group, 1992). In a survey of 269 internal medicine residency programs, it was found that only 99 offered a freestanding program in evidence-based medicine (Green, 2000). The curricula for these 99 programs varied greatly: 77 included critical appraisal of the literature; 52 provided information on how to search for evidence; 44 covered issues related to the articulation of a focused clinical question; 35 covered the application of evidence to individual decision making; and 23 included integration of the evidence into decision making in actual practice. Nearly all programs provided access to MEDLINE, while only about one-third provided access to the Cochrane Library (see Chapter 6).

Similarly, as more care is provided by teams, more opportunities for multidisciplinary training should be offered (Institute of Medicine, 1996a). People should be trained in the kinds of teams in which they will provide care, starting with initial professional training and continuing through graduate training and ongoing professional development. Multidisciplinary training is difficult to implement because of professional boundaries, the traditional hierarchical structure of health care, clinical specialization, faculty experience, and educational isolation. Changing the situation will require an examination of clinical curricula, funding for education, and faculty preparation. Although there was great interest and innovation in multidisciplinary training during the 1960s, little lasting change resulted (Pew Health Professions Commission, 1993). The ability to plan care and practice effectively using multidisciplinary teams takes on increasing importance as the proportion of the population with chronic conditions grows, requiring the provision of a mix of services over time and across settings.

A changing relationship between clinicians and their patients also calls for new skills in communication and support for patient self-management, especially for patients with chronic conditions. Collaborative management requires collaboration between clinicians and patients in defining problems, setting goals, and planning care; training and support in self-management; and continuous follow-up (Von Korff et al., 1997). Patients with chronic conditions who are provided with knowledge and skills for self-management have been shown to experience improvements in health status and reduced hospitalizations (Lorig et al., 1999). Clinicians need to have skills to train patients in techniques of good self-management.

Teaching a different set of skills also has implications for the capabilities of health care organizations that conduct training programs if these skills and behaviors are to be reinforced in training beyond basic coursework. For example, training can emphasize the importance of information technology in clinical care, but that message is not reinforced if students continue their training in health care organizations that are not equipped with such systems or where the faculty are not prepared to use the skills themselves. This is a particular challenge for training in ambulatory settings and physician offices. Although many would agree that more training needs to be offered in such settings, additional support may be required for this purpose.

Although improved methods of training the next generation of clinicians are important, efforts must also be made to retool practicing clinicians. Traditional methods of continuing education for health professionals, such as formal conferences and dissemination of educational materials, have been shown to have little effect by themselves on changing clinician behaviors or health outcomes (Davis et al., 1995). Continuing education needs to emphasize a variety of interventions, particularly reminder systems, academic detailing, and patient-mediated methods, and use a mix of approaches, including Web-based technologies. Reorientation of credentialing processes to assess a clinician's proficiency in evidence-based practice and the use of decision support tools may be necessary to provide strong incentives for clinicians to undertake this important learning process. The development of clinical leadership is another area that needs attention. Clinical leadership will be required to direct the changes discussed, but there will also be a need for new leaders who are able to function effectively in and lead complex delivery systems.

Finally, there are implications for the training and development of nonclinical administrative and management personnel, as well as governance. By making budgetary and resource decisions for health care organizations, these groups, with input from and in collaboration with the clinical community, influence priorities and the pace at which they are implemented. For example, the administration of a hospital can provide sufficient resources to support the implementation of medication order/entry systems that help clinicians provide safer care, or they can slow the pace at which such systems are implemented by not ensuring sufficient resources or training. Training and development for both management and governance should recognize the important role these groups play in collaborating with clinicians to make possible the types of changes needed for the health system of the 21st century.

There have been many prior examinations of clinical education, particularly medical education. The structure and form of medical education were set through the Flexner report of 1910. That report called for a 4-year curriculum comprising 2 years of basic sciences and 2 years of clinical teaching, university affiliation (instead of proprietary schools), entrance requirements, encouragement of active learning and limited use of lectures and learning by memorization, and emphasis on the importance of problem solving and critical thinking (Ludmerer, 1999; Regan-Smith, 1998).

More than 20 different reports followed Flexner's, each calling for the reform of medical and clinical education. The striking feature of these reports is their similarity in the problems identified and proposed solutions. Christakis (1995) reviewed 19 reports and found eight objectives of reform among them: serve changing public interest, address physician workforce needs, cope with burgeoning knowledge, foster generalism and decrease fragmentation, apply new educational methods, address the changing nature of illness, address the changing nature of practice, and improve the quality and standards of education. Enarson and Burg (1992) reviewed 13 studies of medical education and summarized the recommended changes under the categories of (1) methods of instruction and curriculum content (including the need for a broad general education, definition of educational objectives, acquisition of lifelong learning skills, and expansion of training sites); (2) internal structure of medical school (including integration of medical education across the continuum of preparation, control of education programs in multidisciplinary and interdepartmental groups, and definition of budget for teaching); and (3) the relationship between medical schools and external organizations (including integration of accreditation processes, assessment of readiness for graduate training, and use of licensing exams).

Many believe that changes in medical education are needed. In their survey of medical school deans, Cantor et al. (1991) found that 68 percent believed fundamental change in medical education was needed. This was true for their own institutions as well as medical education overall. Petersdorf and Turner (1995) report that the education given to students is "dated and arcane" and not in tune with societal needs. In interpreting their survey of young physicians, Cantor et al. (1993) found that "while medical training has remained largely unchanged, the demands placed on practicing physicians have changed dramatically."

Some believe that the premises of the current apprenticeship model of medical education are so faulty in today's complex health care environment that they need drastic overhaul (Chassin, 1998). Others have suggested that "research's stranglehold on medical education reform needs to be broken by separating researchers from medical student teaching and from curriculum decision making" (Regan-Smith, 1998). Teaching should be an explicit and compensated part of one's job. Still others have called for new relationships between medical schools and academic health centers that would permit the latter to focus on making the best decisions for patient care and allow medical schools to control education and its location (Thier, 1994). In such a circumstance, academic health centers might be affiliated with several medical schools and medical schools might be affiliated with multiple health centers to allow for greater flexibility by the partners.

Medical curriculum has not been static over the years, but has undergone extensive changes (Anderson, 2000; Milbank Memorial Fund and Association of American Medical Colleges, 2000). However, many believe that in general, the current curriculum is overcrowded and relies too much on memorizing facts, and that the changes implemented have not altered the underlying experience of educators and student (Ludmerer, 1999; Regan-Smith, 1998). Despite the changes that have been made, the fundamental approach to clinical education has not changed since 1910. A number of reasons have been cited for so little response to so many calls for reform:

- Lack of funding to review curriculum and teaching methods and of resources to make changes in them (Griner and Danoff, 2000; Meyer et al., 1997)
- Emphasis on research and patient care, with little reward for teaching (Cantor et al., 1991; Griner and Danoff, 2000; Ludmerer, 1999; Petersdorf and Turner, 1995; Regan-Smith, 1998)
- Need for faculty development to ensure that faculty are available at training sites and able to teach students effectively (Griner and Danoff, 2000; Weed, 1981)
- Decentralized structure in medical schools, with powerful department chairs (Cantor et al., 1991; Marston, 1992; Petersdorf and Turner, 1995; Regan-Smith, 1998)
- No coordinated oversight across the continuum of education, and fragmented responsibilities for undergraduate and graduate education, licensing, certification, etc. (Enarson and Burg, 1992; Ludmerer, 1999)

• Difficulty in assessing the impact of changes in teaching methods or curriculum (Ludmerer, 1999)

Although much has been written on medical education, future work on the clinical preparation of the workforce should include examining issues related to the education of all health professionals individually and the way they interact with each other. Separation of clinical training programs and dispersed oversight of training programs, especially across the continuum of initial training, graduate training, and continuing development, inhibit the types and magnitude of change in clinical education. For example, various aspects of medical education are affected by the policies of the Liaison Committee on Medical Education, the Association of American Medical Colleges, the Accreditation Council for Graduate Medical Education, 27 residency review committees, the American Board of Medical Specialties and its 24 certifying boards, the Bureau of Health Professions at the Department of Health and Human Services, the American Medical Association, the American Osteopathic Association and its 18 certifying boards, the American Association of Colleges of Osteopathic Medicine, and various professional societies involved in continuing medical education. Similarly, nursing education is influenced by the policies of the American Association of Colleges of Nursing, the National League for Nursing, the American Nurses Credentialing Center, the National Council of State Boards of Nursing, the American Nurses Association, and various specialty nursing societies. Academic health centers and faculty also play a strong role in shaping the education experience of their students. Such diffusion of responsibilities for clinical education makes it difficult to create a vision for health professional education in the 21st century.

REGULATION OF THE PROFESSIONS

If innovative programs are to flourish, they will require regulatory environments that foster innovation in organizational arrangements, staffing and work relationships, and use of technology. The 21st-century health care system described in this report cannot be achieved without substantial change in the current environment of regulation and oversight.

In general, regulation in this country can be characterized as a dense patchwork that is slow to adapt to change. It is dense because there is a forest of laws, regulations, agencies, and accreditation processes through which each care delivery system must navigate at the local, state, and federal levels. It is a patchwork system because the regulatory and accreditation frameworks at the state level are often inconsistent, contradictory, and duplicative, in part because the needs, priorities, and available resources of the states are not equal. And the regulating process is slow in that it is unable to keep pace with changes in health care. The health care delivery system is under great pressure to innovate and change to incorporate new knowledge and technologies. Regulatory and accreditation requirements can, at times, be at odds with needed innovations (Pew Health Professions Commission, 1993). Statutes and regulations, while not the only factors that influence the practices of nonphysician clinicians, are powerful determinants of their authority and independence (Cooper et al., 1998).

A key regulatory issue that affects the health care workforce and the way it is used is scope-of-practice acts, implemented at the state level. The general public does not have adequate information to judge provider qualifications or competence, so professional licensure laws are enacted to assure the public that practitioners have met the qualifications and minimum competencies required for practice (Pew Health Professions Commission, 1993; Safriet, 1994). Along with licensure, such state laws that define the scope of practice for specific types of caregivers serve as an important component of the overall system of health care quality oversight.

One effect of licensure and scope-of-practice acts is to define how the health care workforce is deployed. In general, medical practice acts are defined broadly so that individual practitioners are licensed for medicine (not a specific specialty), and are thereby permitted to perform all activities that fall within medicine's broad scope of practice. Although a dermatologist would not likely perform open-heart surgery, doing so is not restricted by licensure. However, patients often seek out information about a physician's reputation and credentials, and professional societies also monitor the activities of their members. Other health professions have more narrowly defined scopes of practice, having to carve out their responsibilities from the medical practice act in each state (Safriet, 1994).

Although scope-of-practice acts are motivated by the desire to establish minimum standards to ensure the safety of patients, they also have implications for the changes to the health care system recommended in this report. Since, any change can potentially affect scope-of-practice acts, it can be difficult to use alternative approaches to care, such as telemedicine, e-visits, nonphysician providers, and multidisciplinary teams, all of which can help in caring for patients across settings and over time (see Chapter 3).

Current systems of licensure raise both jurisdictional and liability issues for some clinical applications of telemedicine, such as centralized consultation services to support primary care (Institute of Medicine, 1996b) or the provision of online, continuous, 24-hour monitoring and clinical management of patients in intensive care units for hospitals that have no or too few critical care intensivists on staff to provide this coverage (Janofsky, 1999; Rosenfeld et al., 2000). Integrated delivery systems that cross state lines and telemedicine have rendered geographic boundaries obsolete (Finocchio et al., 1998), making it more difficult for those charged by statute to protect the public.

Scope-of-practice acts can include provisions that inhibit the use of nonphysician practitioners, such as advanced practice nurses and physician assistants, for primary care (Pew Health Professions Commission, 1993; Safriet, 1994).

In some states, advanced practice nurses can diagnose, treat, and prescribe; in others they work only under the direction of a physician (Cooper et al., 1998). Inconsistencies are exacerbated by variation in the scope of practice by setting of care. For example, advanced practice nurses may be permitted a broader scope of practice in rural areas or community health clinics than in other settings (Safriet, 1994). Such policies are enacted to address problems of underservice that exist in certain areas. Although patient needs do not necessarily differ in rural versus urban areas of a state, the available resources of talent, capital, and personnel often vary considerably.

Scope-of-practice acts can also affect the ability to form cohesive care teams that draw on individuals from different disciplines to complement one another in patient care. The skills of some nonphysician providers may overlap with a subset of physician services, often creating tensions among clinicians (Cooper et al., 1998). For example, although there is a difference in their knowledge and training for practice, certified registered nurse anesthetists and anesthesiologists have a subset of skills that overlap (Cromwell, 1999). Separate governance structures and standards are maintained for different types of health professionals even though they may perform a subset of overlapping functions, practice together in the same state and at the same health care institutions, and serve the same population of patients (Finocchio et al., 1998). The complexity of rules across disciplines and settings makes it a challenge to form multidisciplinary teams and establish best practices, especially those that draw on caregivers based in different settings (e.g., hospital, physician's office, and home). Scope-of-practice laws are not the only barrier to greater use of multidisciplinary teams (Sage and Aiken, 1997), but are an important one.

Because licensure and scope-of-practice acts are implemented at the state level, there is a great deal of variation among the states in who is licensed and what standards for licensure and practice are applied. State licensure is not constitutionally based, but rather founded in tradition (Safriet, 1994). On the one hand, state licensure permits regulations to be tailored to meet local needs, resources, and patient expectations. On the other hand, the resulting state-by-state variation is not always logical given the growth of the Internet and the formation of large, multistate provider groups that cut across geographic boundaries. Even with new technologies and organizational arrangements, however, public protections must still be ensured. In response, some have proposed nationally uniform scopes of practice (O'Neil and the Pew Health Professions Commission, 1998) or, at least, more coordinated, publicly accountable policies (Grumbach and Coffman, 1998). The National Council of State Boards of Nursing has endorsed a mutual recognition model for interstate nursing practice that retains state licensure authority, but provides a mechanism for practice across state lines (similar to a driver's license that is granted by one state and recognized in other states) (Finocchio et al., 1998). Still others have argued the relative merits of state-based versus national licensing systems (Federation of State Medical Boards, 1998).

The committee does not recommend one approach over another, but does call for greater coordination and communication among professional boards both within and across states as this issue is resolved over time.

Although the preceding examples suggest that some regulations may be duplicative or outdated for today's clinical practice, gaps exist in other areas as well. For example, current licensure and scope-of-practice laws offer no assurance of continuing competency. In a field with a continually expanding knowledge base, there is no mechanism for ensuring that practitioners remain up to date with current best practices. Responsibility for assessing competence is dispersed among multiple authorities. For example, a licensing board may question competence only if it receives a complaint, but does not routinely assess competency after initial licensure. A health care organization may assess competence when an individual applies for privileges or employment. Professional societies and organizations may require examination for certification, but are just beginning to assess competence in addition to knowledge for those health professionals who voluntarily seek certification. There are no consistent methods for ensuring the continued competence of health professionals within current state licensing functions or other processes.

At least two approaches have been suggested to address this gap. First, some researchers have suggested that licensure be based on a professional's demonstrated ability to perform certain functions or on a certain level of practice (Cooper et al., 1998; Weed and Weed, 1999b). In aviation, for example, pilots are granted a private, commercial, or air transport license by the Federal Aviation Administration. Generally, pilots first obtain a private, single-engine license and then progressively add multi-engine and instrument qualifications to obtain a commercial license. They can then accumulate flying hours and experience to qualify for an air transport license, subsequently obtaining particular types of ratings for specific aircraft (Bisgard, 2000). In addition, professional pilots are recertified at regular intervals throughout their flying career. Taking such an approach in health care would represent a profound paradigm shift, with a gradation of licensure being based on the services in which a health professional has demonstrated competence to serve patients.

A second approach has been suggested, involving an additional level of oversight in which teams of practitioners, in addition to individuals, would be licensed or certified to perform certain tasks (Pew Health Professions Commission, 1993). For example, an individual receiving care for diabetes could go to a "certified" diabetes team that would ensure specific competencies and resources within the delivery team. The team could be collocated or comprise a dispersed network of individual providers practicing and communicating with each other as a team. The certification requirements could be used as a measure of quality by consumers and as a tool for quality improvement by teams seeking to obtain such certification.

It would be premature for the committee to offer a recommendation related to licensure, scope-of-practice, or other regulations. In raising these issues, however, we recognize their importance in supporting or hindering the types of changes recommended in this report. Thus we call for additional, in-depth study aimed at understanding the areas and forms of regulation that are most beneficial for patients and in which modification may be needed to achieve the 21st-century health care system envisioned in this report. Properly conceived and executed, regulation can both protect the public's interest and support the ability of health care professionals and organizations to innovate and change to meet the needs of their patients.

LEGAL LIABILITY ISSUES

The recommendations in this report represent, in many instances, a very different way of delivering services to patients. Achieving the aims set forth in Chapter 2 will require significant innovations in the delivery of care, innovations that may also raise concerns associated with traditional forms of accountability, especially liability issues. Delivering care that is patient-centered, evidence-based, and systems-minded has implications for traditional methods of accountability, particularly with regard to patients' participation in their care, efforts to define standards of care consistent with the evidence base rather than local traditions, and the responsibilities of individual practitioners who deliver care within larger systems that have the capacity for improvement.

Innovations in care can contribute to increased threats of litigation because, by definition, innovation implies a change from previous practice, and medical advances are often imperfect when first applied in clinical practice. Mohr (2000) cites an early example of compound fractures. Through a change in treatment, patients may have avoided an amputation, but they did not always regain full functioning of the limb and pursued litigation against the physician. Significant innovation in health care will occur in many areas with the use of new processes of care and new technologies that will alter how and by whom services are delivered to patients. It is not yet clear how these new processes and technologies, such as e-mail, will affect the liability of health professionals in the future.

Although less studied, changes in organizational approaches raise similar issues. For example, patients may receive care from members of a care team other than a physician or be counseled by e-mail rather than in a face-to-face visit. Such changes can be disorienting to patients if not well understood and in the short run, and create new hazards and new risks of litigation. Thus there is a need for good educational efforts and communication with patients about the changes taking place. It is also necessary, however, to examine the extent to which current liability approaches inhibit the kinds of changes needed to improve the quality and safety of care. For example, liability concerns can affect the willingness of physicians and other clinicians to share information about areas in which quality improvement is needed if they believe the information may subsequently be used against them (Institute of Medicine, 2000). The committee's previous report on patient safety calls for peer review protection of data that are used inside health care organizations or shared with others solely for purposes of improving safety and quality, as well as an improved climate for identifying areas needing improvement (Institute of Medicine, 2000).

Legal issues are also likely to influence the development of evidence-based practice. The legal system influences health care through two types of decisions—medical malpractice and benefits coverage—both of which involve judgments about the quality of care (Rosoff, 2001). Should the legal system fail to incorporate evidence-based thinking into its decision-making processes (whether related to medical malpractice or other decisions), clinicians and health care organizations will be subject to confusing and conflicting incentives and demands.

Legal decisions that involve determining whether care provided was consistent with the "standard practice in the relevant medical community" (Rosoff, 2001) often rely on expert testimony. It is unclear how courts will incorporate clinical evidence and clinical practice guidelines into legal decision making. To date, clinical practice guidelines have had little effect on litigation. In a legal search covering the period January 1980 to May 1994, Hyams et al. (1996) found only 37 cases involving clinical practice guidelines. But clinical practice guidelines probably have had some effect on prelitigation decisions, since surveys show that medical malpractice attorneys consider guidelines in making decisions about whether to take on malpractice cases and conducting settlement negotiations (Hyams et al., 1996).

Alternative approaches to liability, such as enterprise liability or no-fault compensation, could produce a legal environment more conducive to uncovering and resolving quality problems. Enterprise liability shifts liability from individual practitioners to responsible organizations (Abraham and Weiler, 1994; Sage et al., 1994). For example, workplace injuries to employees are handled through a form of no-fault, enterprise liability. Although analysis of such approaches is beyond the scope of the present study, the committee believes they merit a focused, in-depth analysis.

RESEARCH AGENDA FOR THE
FUTURE HEALTH CARE WORKFORCE

Modifying training, regulatory, and legal environments is not a quick strategy for changing practice. These environments are closely interrelated with the delivery setting. Training programs are not likely to change unless the delivery setting does so, but the setting cannot change if people are not trained to practice differently. Similarly, the delivery setting cannot change without modifications in regulation and legislation, but adjustments in practice often prompt additional regulation to protect against unwanted consequences.

A comprehensive approach is needed for the many aspects of health care workforce planning. Many prior efforts in such planning have focused on attempting to determine an appropriate supply of clinicians. Previous studies have examined the adequacy of supply for selected disciplines (e.g., physicians) or the mix of providers within a discipline (e.g., primary care and specialty mix of physicians), or have assumed a specific organizational model (e.g., supply of physicians needed given extensive enrollment in HMOs). Although a comprehensive workforce agenda should address issues of supply, it would be difficult to conduct any such studies meaningfully without first addressing how clinicians might be deployed given different approaches to training, regulation, and liability. It is not sufficient to ask how many health professionals are needed; one must also ask what types are needed (Pew Health Professions Commission, 1993). Ultimate assessments of supply depend on how responsibility for patients is divided among licensed clinicians, as well as on society's expectations (Cromwell, 1999). Workforce planning should shift from determining the supply of clinicians in specific disciplines who continue to perform the same tasks using the same methods toward assessing the adequacy of supply given that care is provided through processes that rely on multidisciplinary approaches, modern technological support, and continuous care. The starting point for addressing workforce issues should not be the present environment of licensure, reimbursement, and organization of care, but a vision of how care ought to be delivered in the 21st century. A comprehensive agenda on workforce planning should cover the following key issues:

- Training and Education Issues

    – What is the vision for the education and training of health professionals for the 21st century? What is the relationship between the education of health care providers and quality of care?
    – How is the vision relayed throughout the continuum of education? How can new health professionals learn most effectively the basic skills related to patient-centeredness, evidence-based practice, and systems thinking? How can such skills be reinforced in graduate training programs? How can they be meaningfully relayed to professionals already in practice?
    – What are the implications of changes in clinical education for the health care organizations that serve as training sites? What is the potential effect on the role and mission of academic health centers?
    – What are the implications of changes in clinical education for licensing and accreditation processes? For funding approaches to support clinical education?

- Legal and Regulatory Issues

  – How can regulatory and other oversight processes be coordinated to reinforce the principles of patient-centeredness, evidence-based practice, and systems thinking? What specific legal and regulatory constraints inhibit changes in processes of care? Where are different types of regulations needed? In what areas can existing regulations be streamlined or reduced?
  – How can greater coordination among licensing boards within an individual state and across states be facilitated? How can the continuing competence of health professionals be assessed and ensured?
  – Can liability reform support the principles of patient-centeredness, evidence-based practice, and systems thinking? Are alternative models, such as enterprise liability, desirable?
  – What is the link between regulation of health professions and quality of care?
  – What are the appropriate links among licensure, accountability, and liability?

- Workforce Supply

  – Given a greater understanding of the previous issues (e.g., what training is provided, the need for greater flexibility in deploying human resources, and alternative approaches to accountability), what are the implications for the needed supply and mix of health professionals?

REFERENCES

Abraham, Kenneth S. and Paul C. Weiler. Enterprise Medical Liability and the Choice of the Responsible Enterprise. *American Journal of Law and Medicine* 20(1 & 2):29–36, 1994.

Anderson, Brownell M., ed. A Snapshot of Medical Students' Education at the Beginning of the 21st Century: Reports from 130 Schools. *Academic Medicine* 75(9, Suppl), 2000.

Berwick, Donald M., A. Enthoven, and J. P. Bunker. Quality Management in the NHS: The Doctor's Role—II. *BMJ* 304:304–8, 1992.

Bisgard, J. Cris, Delta Airlines, Oct. 26, 2000. Personal communication: e-mail.

Cantor, Joel C., Laurence C. Baker, and Robert G. Hughes. Preparedness for Practice: Young Physicians' Views of Their Professional Education. *JAMA* 270(9):1035–40, 1993.

Cantor, Joel C., Alan B. Cohen, Dianne C. Barker, et al. Medical Educators' Views on Medical Education Reform. *JAMA* 265(8):1002–6, 1991.

Chassin, Mark R. Is Health Care Ready for Six Sigma Quality? *Milbank Quarterly* 76(4):575–91, 1998.

Christakis, Nicholas A. The Similarity and Frequency of Proposals to Reform U.S. Medical Education: Constant Concerns. *JAMA* 274(9):706–11, 1995.

Cooper, Richard A., Tim Henderson, and Craig L. Dietrich. Roles of Nonphysician Clinicians as Autonomous Providers of Patient Care. *JAMA* 280(9):795–802, 1998.

Cromwell, Jerry. Barriers to Achieving a Cost-Effective Workforce Mix: Lessons from Anesthesiology. *Journal of Health Politics, Policy and Law* 24(6):1331–61, 1999.

Davis, David A., Mary Ann Thomson, Andrew D. Oxman, and Brian Haynes. Changing Physician Performance: A Systematic Review of the Effect of Continuing Medical Education Strategies. *JAMA* 274(9):700–5, 1995.

Enarson, Cam and Frederic D. Burg. An Overview of Reform Initiatives in Medical Education: 1906 Through 1992. *JAMA* 268(9):1141–3, 1992.

Evidence-Based Medicine Working Group. Evidence-Based Medicine: A New Approach to Teaching the Practice of Medicine. *JAMA* 268(17):2420–5, 1992.

Federation of State Medical Boards. 1998. "Maintaining State-Based Medical Licensure and Discipline: A Blueprint for Uniform and Effective Regulation of the Medical Profession." Online. Available at http://www.fsmb.org/uniform.htm [accessed Jan. 12, 2001].

Finocchio, L. J., C. M. Dower, N. T. Blick, C. M. Gragnola, and the Taskforce on Health Care Workforce Regulation. *Strengthening Consumer Protection: Priorities for Health Care Workforce Regulation.* San Francisco, CA: Pew Health Professions Commission, 1998.

Green, Michael L. Evidence-Based Medicine Training in Internal Medicine Residency Programs: A National Survey. *J Gen Intern Med* 15(3):129–33, 2000.

Griner, Paul F. and Deborah Danoff. Sustaining Change in Medical Education. *JAMA* 283(18):2429–31, 2000.

Grumbach, Kevin and Janet Coffman. Physicians and Nonphysician Clinicians. Complements or Competitors? *JAMA* 280(9):825–6, 1998.

Hyams, Andrew L., David W. Shapiro, and Troyen A. Brennan. Medical Practice Guidelines in Malpractice Litigation: An Early Retrospective. *Journal of Health Politics, Policy and Law* 21(2):289–313, 1996.

Institute of Medicine. *Primary Care: America's Health in a New Era.* Molla S Donaldson, Karl D. Yordy, Kathleen N. Lohr, and Neal A. Vanselow, eds. Washington, D.C.: National Academy Press, 1996a.

———. *Telemedicine: A Guide to Assessing Telecommunications for Health Care.* Marilyn J. Field, ed. Washington, D.C.: National Academy Press, 1996b.

———. *To Err Is Human: Building a Safer Health System.* Linda T. Kohn, Janet M. Corrigan, and Molla S. Donaldson, eds. Washington, D.C.: National Academy Press, 2000.

Janofsky, Michael. Finding Value in Intensive Care, From Afar. *The New York Times.* Health and Fitness, July 27, 1999.

Lorig, Kate R., David S. Sobel, Anita L. Steward, et al. Evidence Suggesting that a Chronic Disease Self-Management Program Can Improve Health Status While Reducing Hospitalization: A Randomized Trial. *Medical Care* 37(1):5–14, 1999.

Ludmerer, Kenneth. *Time to Heal: American Medical Education from the Turn of the Century to the Era of Managed Care.* New York, NY: Oxford University Press, 1999.

Marston, Robert Q. *Medical Education in Transition.* Princeton, NJ: The Robert Wood Johnson Foundation, 1992.

Meyer, Gregg S., Allison Potter, and Nancy Gary. A National Survey to Define a New Core Curriculum to Prepare Physicians for Managed Care Practice. *Academic Medicine* 72(8):669–76, 1997.

Milbank Memorial Fund and Association of American Medical Colleges. *The Education of Medical Students: Ten Stories of Curriculum Change.* New York, NY: Milbank Memorial Fund, 2000.

Mohr, James C. American Medical Malpractice Litigation in Historical Perspective. *JAMA* 283(13):1731–7, 2000.

O'Neil, E. H. and the Pew Health Professions Commission. *Recreating Health Professional Practice for a New Century.* San Francisco, CA: Pew Health Professions Commission, 1998.

Occupational Employment Statistics. 2000. "1998 National Occupational Employment and Wage Estimates: Professional, Paraprofessional, and Technical Occupations." Online. Available at http://stats.bls.gov/oes/national/oes_prof.htm [accessed Jan. 12, 2001].

Petersdorf, Robert G. and Kathleen S. Turner. Medical Education in the 1990s—and Beyond: A View from the United States. *Academic Medicine* 70(7, Suppl):S41–7, 1995.

Pew Health Professions Commission. *Contemporary Issues in Health Professions Education and Workforce Reform.* San Francisco, CA: University of California, San Francisco - Center for Health Professionals, 1993.

Regan-Smith, Martha G. "Reform without Change": Update, 1998. *Academic Medicine* 73(5):505–7, 1998.

Rosenfeld, Brian A., T. Dorman, M. J. Breslow, et al. Intensive Care Unit Telemedicine: Alternate Paradigm for Providing Continuous Intensivist Care. *Crit Care Med* 28(12):3925–31, 2000.

Rosoff, Arnold J. Evidence-Based Medicine in the Law: The Courts Confront Clinical Practice Guidelines. *Journal of Health Politics, Policy and Law* 327–68, forthcoming April 2001.

Safriet, Barbara J. Impediments to Progress in Health Care Workforce Policy: License and Practice Laws. *Inquiry* 31(3):310–7, 1994.

Sage, William M. and Linda H. Aiken. Chapter 4: Regulating Interdisciplinary Practice. *Regulation of Healthcare Professions.* Timothy S. Jost. Chicago, IL: Health Administration Press, 1997.

Sage, William M., Kathleen E. Hastings, and Robert A. Berenson. Enterprise Liability for Medical Malpractice and Health Care Quality Improvement. *American Journal of Law and Medicine* 20(1 & 2):1–28, 1994.

Thier, Samuel O. Academic Medicine's Choices in an Era of Reform. *Academic Medicine* 69(3):185–9, 1994.

Von Korff, Michael, Jessie Gruman, Judith Schaefer, Susan J. Curry, and Edward H. Wagner. Collaborative Management of Chronic Illness. *Ann Int Med* 127(12):1097–102, 1997.

Weed, Lawrence L. Physicians of the Future. *N Engl J Med* 304(15):903–7, 1981.

Weed, Lawrence L. and Lincoln Weed. Opening the Black Box of Clinical Judgment. Part I: A Micro Perspective on Medical Decision-Making. *eBMJ.* November 13, 1999a. Online. Available at http://www.bmj.com/cgi/content/full/319/7220/1279/DC2 [accessed Jan. 24, 2001].

———. Opening the Black Box of Clinical Judgment. Part II: Consumer Protection and the Patient's Role. *eBMJ.* November 13, 1999b. Online. Available at http://www.bmj.com/cgi/content/full/319/7220/1279/DC2 [accessed Jan. 24, 2001].

———. Opening the Black Box of Clinical Judgment. Part III: Medical Science and Education. *eBMJ.* November 13, 1999c. Online. Available at http://www.bmj.com/cgi/content/full/319/7220/1279/DC2 [accessed Jan. 24, 2001].

Appendix A

Report of the Technical Panel on the State of Quality to the Quality of Health Care in America Committee

Millions of Americans receive high-quality health care in the United States. Our capacity to provide the most sophisticated and effective care is unrivaled, and there is no evidence that any other system achieves better quality. Yet there is abundant evidence that serious and extensive quality problems exist throughout the U.S. health care system, resulting in harm to many Americans. Opportunities for improvement exist in all areas of clinical practice, across the continuum of care.

As a result of overuse, underuse, and misuse of health care services, our society pays a substantial price. The opportunity costs of poor quality include years of life lost or spent with major or minor impairments, pain and suffering, disability costs, and lost productivity. In many areas, especially those involving overuse and misuse of health care services, that improving quality is also likely to lower health care costs.

BACKGROUND

The Quality of Health Care in America (QHCA) Project, a part of the Institute of Medicine's Special IOM Initiative on Quality, was established in June 1998 and charged with developing a strategy to produce a significant improvement in quality over the coming decade.

The Committee on the Quality of Health Care in America, chaired by William C. Richardson, Ph.D., was responsible for this 2-year project.

Four advisory groups were established to assist the QHCA Committee in carrying out its charge. To provide a broad base of expertise, these advisory groups consisted of both committee members and other distinguished leaders within the health care arena. Each advisory group was chaired by a member(s) of the QHCA Committee. One of these four groups, the Technical Advisory Panel on the State of Quality, chaired by Mark Chassin, M.D., was asked to review and synthesize literature on the state of quality in the health care industry. Other members of this panel included: Arnold Epstein, M.D., M.A.; Brent James, M.D.; James P. Logerfo, M.D.; Harold Luft, Ph.D.; R. Heather Palmer, M.B., B.Ch.; Kenneth B. Wells, M.D. This appendix presents the panel's findings.

REVIEW OF THE LITERATURE

In developing its approach to this effort, the State of Quality Panel reviewed an earlier synthesis of the literature on quality that was carried out by investigators at the RAND Corporation (Schuster et al., 1998). This earlier review covered papers that, for the most part, were published between 1993 and mid-1997. To extend that earlier work, the IOM commissioned an updated synthesis from the investigators at RAND. This update covered the literature included in the earlier review with the addition of (1) papers published between July 1997 and August 1998, and (2) selected publications identified by members of the State of Quality Panel. A draft of this commissioned paper was reviewed by the State of Quality Panel at its November 1998 meeting, and subsequently revised in accordance with the panel's suggestions. The final version, provided at the end of this appendix, was completed in January 1999.

DISCUSSION OF FINDINGS

A synthesis of findings from the literature on the quality of health care provides abundant evidence of poor quality. There are examples of exemplary care, but the quality of care is not consistent. Thus, the average American cannot assume that he or she will receive the best care modern medicine has to offer.

There are many examples of overuse, underuse, and misuse of health care services. Overuse refers to the provision of health services for which the potential risks outweigh the potential benefits. Underuse indicates that a health care service for which the potential benefits outweigh the potential risks was not provided. Misuse occurs when otherwise appropriate care is provided, but in a manner that does or could lead to avoidable complications.

Overuse of health care services is common. Examples include the following:

• performance of major surgery (e.g., hysterectomy, coronary artery bypass graft) without appropriate reasons;
• provision of antibiotics for the common cold and other viral upper respiratory tract infections for which they are ineffective;

• insertion of tubes in children's eardrums in the absence of clinically appropriate indications; and
• performance of chiropractic spinal manipulation for certain back conditions for which there is no evidence of benefit.

Lack of insurance is a major contributing factor to *underuse*. Even with comprehensive insurance coverage, however, much of the population fails to receive recommended preventive services, and many patients do not receive the full range of clinically indicated services for acute and chronic conditions. Examples include the following:

• *Cardiac care* In a study of 3,737 Medicare patients with a diagnosis of heart attack who were eligible for treatment with beta blockers, only 21 percent were found to have received beta blockers within 90 days of discharge. The adjusted mortality rate for patients with treatment was 43 percent below that of patients without treatment (Soumerai et al., 1997).
• *Pneumococcal vaccine* In 1989, the U.S. Preventive Services Task Force recommended that people 65 years and older receive a one-time vaccination for pneumonia, and in 1996, this recommendation was modified to apply to all immunocompetent people aged 65 and older. Yet studies of the proportion of elderly who had been vaccinated produced estimates in the range of only 28 to 36 percent (CDC, 1995; Kottke et al., 1997).
• *Acute care for pneumonia* Two studies of hospitalized patients with pneumonia found serious shortcomings in the proportion of patients receiving appropriate components of care (Kahn et al., 1990; Meehan et al., 1997).

In recent years, increased attention has been focused on *misuse*. Studies of misuse are particularly challenging because actual or potential adverse events often go undocumented and unreported. But studies of preventable deaths and adverse drug events point to frequent and sometimes serious errors. For example, one study of over 4,000 hospitalized patients found that there were 19 preventable or potential adverse drug events per 1,000 patient days in intensive care units and 10 preventable or potential adverse drug events per 1,000 patient days in general care units (Cullen et al., 1997).

LEVEL OF HARM CAUSED BY POOR QUALITY

The existing literature does not allow a comprehensive estimate of the burden of harm due to poor quality. The literature on health care quality covers only a portion of the full range of quality concerns. For the most part, published studies focus on individuals who come into contact with the health care system. From a population perspective, the opportunity cost of poor quality must also include the health benefits lost as a result of limited access due to financial or other barriers and poor patient adherence to therapeutic advice. These opportunity costs include years of life lost or spent with major or minor impairments, pain and suffering, disability costs, and lost productivity.

The literature also does not reveal how frequently the various types of quality problems occur. For example, some kinds of overuse problems may have a greater likelihood of being documented than some types of misuse or underuse problems because the data necessary to document overuse are more likely to reside in administrative datasets or medical records.

From the available literature, it is also not possible to produce estimates of the costs of eliminating certain types of quality problems or the benefits likely to be derived. But there is no doubt that major improvements are possible in many clinical areas and health care settings, across the full continuum of care.

NEED FOR FURTHER WORK

The panel's work represents a modest effort to review the state of health care quality. Specifically, the literature review was commissioned for this study limited in the following ways:

• It focused only on publications in leading peer-reviewed journals. Other sources of information, such as the data and analyses of Medicare Peer Review Organizations (PROs) or analyses using malpractice data, were not included. The Medicare PRO program is a particularly promising source of information on quality because the PROs have been conducting quality review projects involving physicians, hospitals, and health plans for over 10 years.
• The review did not focus in depth on specific clinical areas. An intensive review by clinical area would provide a more complete picture of the full spectrum of quality problems and their frequency of occurrence.
• The review did not include the many publications based on reports of patient experience or satisfaction.
• The review did not include the body of studies reporting the impact of quality improvement activities. Thus it permits only anecdotal observations on the effectiveness of various of attempts to improve quality.
• Although the publications included in the review appeared in peer-reviewed journals, the panel made no attempt to assess the scientific rigor of the methodologies employed.

Despite the above limitations, the panel believes that more in-depth reviews would not change its general conclusions that there are many areas in which quality of care can be improved. At the same time, additional research might be helpful for several reasons:

- A fuller understanding of quality problems would be useful in identifying specific areas in which those problems are greatest, as well as the most promising opportunities for improvement.
- Condition-specific analyses would provide better estimates of the potential benefits foregone as a result of poor quality and the best strategies for improvement.
- Additional work focused in particular clinical areas might also be helpful in raising awareness of practitioners and others who are skeptical about the existence of quality problems in their areas of expertise. Condition-specific analyses of quality that employ rigorous and valid measures could help build stronger support for quality improvement initiatives.
- Additional reviews of the literature should be conducted to identify factors that contribute to poor quality and effective strategies for improvement. For example, review of the literature on quality substantiates that for certain complex procedures, higher volume leads to better outcomes. But we do not know whether this result is attributable to the greater skill of an experienced surgeon, the greater standardization of processes in high-volume settings, or some other factor. Abundant evidence exists that quality can be improved, and there is much to be learned from the review of various improvement strategies about the roles of patients, clinicians, and systems and the use of various types of incentives.
- Additional conceptual work, literature and data analysis, and development of measures are needed to improve capacities for quality-of-care assessment in certain key areas of medicine. An example is quality assessment in the areas of mental health, substance abuse, and neurologic disorders, and quality assessment for special populations, such as the frail elderly, poor children, and ethnic minorities.

REFERENCES

Centers for Disease Control and Prevention. 1995. Influenza and Pneurnococcal Vaccination Coverage Levels among Persons Aged > 65 Years—United States, January–December 1995. *Morbidity and Mortality Weekly Report* 46:176–82.

Cullen D.J., et al. 1997. Preventable Adverse Drug Events in Hospitalized Patients: a Comparative Study of Intensive Care and General Care Units. *Critical Care Medicine* 8:1289–97.

Kahn, K.L., W.H. Rogers, L.V. Rubenstein, et al. 1990. Measuring Quality of Care with Explicit Process Criteria before and after Implementation of the DRG-Based Prospective Payment System. *Journal of the American Medical Association* 264:1969–73.

Kottke, T.E., L.I. Solberg, ML. Brekke, et al. 1995, Aspirin in the Treatment of Acute Myocardial Infarction in Elderly Medicare Beneficiaries: Patterns of Use and Outcomes. *Circulation* 92:2841–7.

Meehan, T.P., M.J. Fine, H.M. Krumholz, et al. 1997. Quality of Care, Process and Outcomes in Elderly Patients with Pneumonia. *Journal of the American Medical Association* 278:2080–4

Schuster, Mark A., Elizabeth A. McGlynn, and Robert H. Brook. 1998. "How Good Is the Quality of Health Care in the United States?" 1998. 76 (4) *Milbank Quarterly* 517–563.

Soumerai, S.B., T.D. McLaughlin, E. Hertzmark, G. Thibault, and L. Goldman. 1997. Adverse Outcomes of Underuse of Beta-Blockers in Elderly Survivors of Acute Myocardial Infarction. *Journal of the American Medical Association* 277:115–21.

The Quality of Health Care
in the United States:
A Review of Articles Since 1987

Mark A. Schuster, M.D., Ph.D.;[1]   Elizabeth A. McGlynn, Ph.D.;[2]
Cung B. Pham, B.A.;[3]   Myles D. Spar, M.D.;[4]   and Robert H.
Brook, M.D., Sc.D.[5]

Submitted January 1999

Quality of health care is on the national agenda. In September 1996, President Clinton established the Advisory Commission on Consumer Protection and
Quality in the Health Care Industry, which has released its final report on how to
define, measure, and promote quality of health care (Advisory Commission on
Consumer Protection and Quality in the Health Care Industry, 1998).

Much of the interest in quality of care has developed in response to the
dramatic transformation of the health care system in recent years. New organizational structures and reimbursement strategies have created incentives that may
affect quality of care. Although some of the systems are likely to improve quality,
concerns about potentially negative consequences have prompted a movement to
assure that quality will not be sacrificed to control costs.

The concern about quality arises more from fear and anecdote than from
facts; there is little systematic evidence about quality of care in the United States.
The nation has no mandatory national system and few local systems to track the
quality of care delivered to the American people. More information is available
on the quality of airlines, restaurants, cars, and VCRs than on the quality of health
care.

In 1997, the National Coalition on Health Care (NCHC) commissioned us to
review the academic literature for articles that provide evidence of the quality of
care in the United States (Schuster et al., 1998). The Institute of Medicine's

Authors' affiliations: [1]Health Sciences, RAND; Department of Pediatrics, UCLA   [2]Health Sciences, RAND   [3]Department of Pediatrics, UCLA   [4]HSR&D Field Program, Sepulveda Veterans
Administration Medical Center; and   [5]Health Sciences, RAND; Department of Medicine, UCLA.

Technical Advisory Panel on the State of Quality commissioned an update to include studies published between January 1997 and July 1998. In this report, we summarize our findings from both the original study and the update. In the absence of a national quality tracking system, we believe such a summary is the best way to provide an overview of the quality of care delivered in the United States. We provide examples to illustrate quality in diverse settings, for diverse conditions, and for diverse demographic groups, and to offer insight into the quality that exists nationwide.

DEFINING QUALITY

The Institute of Medicine has defined *quality* as "the degree to which health services for individuals and populations increase the likelihood of desired health outcomes and are consistent with current professional knowledge" (Lohr, 1990). Good quality means providing patients with appropriate services in a technically competent manner, with good communication, shared decision making, and cultural sensitivity.

Quality can be evaluated based on structure, process, and outcomes (Donabedian, 1980). *Structural quality* evaluates health system capacities, *process quality* assesses interactions between clinicians and patients, and *outcomes* offer evidence about changes in patients' health status. The best process measures are those for which there is research evidence that better processes lead to better outcomes. For example, controlling blood pressure reduces mortality from stroke and heart disease; performing routine mammography identifies breast cancer at an earlier stage so that a cure is more likely; prescribing inhaled corticosteroids reduces the likelihood and severity of asthma flare-ups. Similarly, the best outcome measures are those which are tied to processes of care, in other words, those over which the health care system has influence. For example, the survival rate for pancreatic cancer would not be a good outcome measure because we do not yet have treatments that meaningfully affect survival. By contrast, pain level in patients with pancreatic cancer is a reasonable outcome measure.

All three dimensions can provide valuable information for measuring quality, but most of the quality-of-care literature focuses on measuring processes of care. Two measurement approaches dominate in the literature: (a) assessing appropriateness of care and (b) adherence to professional standards.

(a) An intervention or service (e.g., a lab test, procedure, medication) is considered *appropriate* if, for individuals with particular clinical and personal characteristics, its expected health benefits (e.g., increased life expectancy, pain relief, decreased anxiety, improved functional capacity) exceed its expected health risks (e.g., mortality, morbidity, anxiety anticipating the intervention, pain caused by the intervention, inaccurate diagnoses) by a wide enough margin to make the intervention or service worth doing (Brook et al., 1986). A subset of appropriate care is *necessary* or crucial care. Care is considered necessary if there is a reasonable chance of a nontrivial benefit to the patient and if it would be improper not to provide the care—in other words, if it might be considered ethically unacceptable not to provide this care (Kahan et al., 1994; Laouri et al., 1997).

(b) Another way to measure process quality is to determine whether care meets or adheres to professional standards. This assessment can be done by creating a list of *quality indicators* that describe a process of care that should occur for a particular type of patient or clinical circumstance and by evaluating whether patients' care is consistent with the indicators. Quality indicators are based on standards of care, which are either found in the research literature and in statements of professional medical organizations or determined by an expert panel. Current performance can be compared against a physician's or a plan's own prior performance, against the performance of other physicians and plans, or with reference to a benchmark that establishes a goal. Indicators can cover a specific condition (e.g., children with sickle cell disease should be prescribed daily penicillin prophylaxis starting by no later than six months of age, until at least five years of age), or they can cover general aspects of care regardless of condition (e.g., patients prescribed a medication should be asked about medication allergies).

HOW WE CONDUCTED OUR LITERATURE SEARCHES

This report draws on two searches of the scientific literature. The original NCHC report was based on a search for quality-of-care articles from the MEDLINE PLUS database (1993 to present) conducted in June 1997 and on relevant studies identified from the bibliographies of these articles. This database incorporates both the National Library of Medicine (NLM)'s MEDLINE database and the Health Planning and Administration's HEALTH database. The NCHC report excluded articles published before 1987. In conducting our literature search, we did not aim to be exhaustive, but rather to find examples that encompass a broad range of conditions and settings. (The inclusion criteria are described in the next section.)

For this update, we conducted a systematic search of articles published between January 1, 1997, and July 31, 1998, using the NLM's Medical Subject Headings (MeSH) to search for appropriate articles. This system is designed so that each MeSH term corresponds to a single concept appearing in the biomedical literature. Trained NLM indexers assign relevant MeSH terms to each database entry (usually about 10–12 per entry) (NLM, 1997a). The more than 17,000 MeSH terms are organized in a tree format, with multiple hierarchical layers of subheadings (NLM, 1997b)(Our search terms appear at the end of the report).

We conducted our search on August 24, 1998, and obtained 2,402 entries. Two authors reviewed each entry and its abstract to determine whether the study had potential for inclusion in our summary tables. Based on this initial screening, we retrieved more than 200 articles. Each was reviewed by two authors to determine whether the article was eligible for inclusion in this report. Some articles identified in the literature search were not available from the library by the completion date of the report.

Because we did not find any studies of misuse in our update search, we conducted a supplemental search using key words such as "adverse," "event#," and "preventable" that produced additional relevant articles. In addition, several studies were recommended by members of the Institute of Medicine's Technical Advisory Panel on the State of Quality.

Criteria for Including Studies

We include only data from large or diverse U.S. populations—for example, the nation, an entire state, an entire city, or several hospitals. Studies from multiple offices of a single managed care organization are also considered eligible, but we do not include data from studies that cover only a single hospital or clinic. Although such studies are informative and the cumulative weight of their findings compelling, they are especially subject to concerns that they provide evidence of isolated problems rather than insight into the quality of care delivered more broadly.

We include baseline data from quality improvement interventions as well as data for comparison/control/nonintervention groups from such interventions. We report baseline rather than follow-up data because the former are more likely to be representative of the quality of care provided around the country. Quality measurement conducted after a specific intervention shows the potential for interventions to improve quality, but until such interventions are commonplace, these post-intervention results are unlikely to represent what is taking place in most parts of the country. In addition, even the post-intervention results from such studies virtually always show room for further improvement.

We report results only from studies for which we can identify a standard of good quality and exclude those for which there is no standard. For example, some studies show variations in practices that may reflect variations in quality. However, the studies cannot determine which hospital or clinic or group of physicians is providing better or worse quality care.

Types of Studies Not Included

There are several ways to measure quality of care that are not represented among the studies listed in our summary tables. Although these approaches are valuable components of the quality-of-care toolbox, they have not been used in a way that provides an overview of quality in the United States.

Studies often *compare outcomes across multiple institutions* to show which have better and which have worse outcomes, but the studies do not always present a standard against which to compare outcomes. As a consequence, we do not know if the institution with the best outcomes is not nearly as good as it should be, or if the institution with the worst outcomes is nonetheless doing quite well. We only know how they compare with each other. If the outcomes are not risk-adjusted, it can be even more difficult to interpret them. This does not mean that studies cannot use outcomes to shed light on variations in quality. For example, prescription of beta blockers after a heart attack is a frequently used measure of quality. One study found that only about one in five eligible patients with a heart attack received beta blockers within 90 days of hospital discharge and also that those who received the treatment were much less likely to die than those who did not (Soumerai et al., 1997). Another study showed that poorer quality of care for children with asthma was associated with more hospitalizations (Homer et al., 1996).

We found a similar limitation with using *satisfaction ratings*, which some consider a type of outcome. We do not report on levels of satisfaction because it is difficult to determine what is an acceptable level of satisfaction. There is generally no standard to which to compare the results, and we do not know whether the institution with the best satisfaction ratings could and should be doing much better.

Studies of *access to care* are not typically classified as quality-of-care studies, but a person who is unable to obtain health care could hardly be said to be receiving good quality care. Access studies are beyond the scope of this report. However, we need to keep in mind that quality-of-care studies often measure quality only for people who have interacted with the health care system and so tend to overstate quality of care received by the population as a whole (Franks et al., 1993a, 1993b; Lurie et al., 1984, 1986; Sorlie et al., 1994).

In general, *structural measures* have not been consistently shown to relate either to process quality or outcomes, but there are exceptions. For example, volume of care provided (in other words, the number of procedures performed or the number of patients cared for) by an institution or clinician has often been found to relate to quality (Hannan et al., 1989, 1995; Kelly and Hellinger, 1986; Kitahata et al., 1996; Luft et al., 1979; Phibbs et al., 1996; Riley and Lubitz, 1985; Stone et al., 1992).

Another type of study does not provide direct evidence of quality of health care but is useful for identifying reasons for poor quality. Studies in which *physicians report* what they generally do or what they would do for a particular scenario can be informative, especially when physicians report practices that indicate poor quality. Although these studies do not describe care provided to individual patients, they can indicate a need for further education or other efforts to improve clinical practices.

Finally, we note that our search mechanism almost certainly missed articles with relevant data. Many studies not intended as quality-of-care studies provide data that shed light on quality of care. Some of these were identified through our search, but it is likely that many others were not.

PROFILE OF QUALITY OF CARE IN THE UNITED STATES

We divided our review of quality in the United States into three categories: underuse (Table A-1), overuse (Table A-2), and misuse (Table A-3). Underuse indicates that a health care service for which the potential *benefits* outweigh the potential *risks* (i.e., necessary care) is not provided. Overuse indicates the reverse—a health care service is provided when the potential *risks* outweigh the potential *benefits* (i.e., inappropriate care). Misuse occurs when otherwise appropriate care is provided in a way that leads to or could lead to avoidable complications. Examples of misuse include when an antibiotic appropriate to the patient's infection is prescribed despite the fact that the patient has a documented allergy to the antibiotic, or when two drugs, each of which is appropriate for a patient's condition, are prescribed despite contraindications to prescribing them together. An incorrect dose or dosing schedule is also considered misuse.

In each summary table, we list (and sometimes describe) the health care service for which quality is reported, the sample on which the report is based, the data source for the sample, the findings, and the reference. The tables report data from 73 articles.

Perhaps the most striking revelation to emerge from this review is the surprisingly small amount of systematic knowledge available on the quality of health care delivered in the United States. Even though health care is a huge industry that affects the lives of most Americans, we have only snapshots of information about particular conditions, types of surgery, and locations of care.

Gaps Between Ideal Care and Actual Care

The dominant finding of our review is that there are large gaps between the care people should receive and the care they do receive. This is true for preventive, acute, and chronic care, whether one goes for a checkup, a sore throat, or diabetic care. It is true whether one looks at overuse, underuse, or misuse. It is true in different types of health care facilities and for different types of health insurance. It is true for all age groups, from children to the elderly. And it is true whether one is looking at the whole country or a single city.

A few examples emphasize this point. An annual influenza vaccine is recommended as a preventive measure for all adults 65 years or older, a group at especially high risk for complications and death from influenza (U.S. Preventive Services Task Force, 1989, 1996). However, in 1993, only 52 percent of people in this age group in the United States received the vaccine; among people who had been to the doctor at least once that year, the percentage was slightly higher at 56 percent (Centers for Disease Control and Prevention, 1995b).

A major issue in acute care is the overuse of antibiotics, which has led to the development of strains of bacteria that are resistant to available antibiotics (Centers for Disease Control and Prevention, 1994a). Antibiotics are almost never an appropriate treatment for people with a common cold because almost all colds are caused by a virus, for which antibiotics are not effective. However, in a study of Medicaid beneficiaries diagnosed with a cold in Kentucky during a one-year period from 1993 to 1994, 60 percent filled a prescription for an antibiotic (Mainous et al., 1996). In a national study of patient visits in 1992, 51 percent of adult patients and 44 percent of patients younger than 18 years old diagnosed with a common cold were treated with antibiotics (Gonzales et al., 1997; Nyquist et al., 1998).

Other types of medications are also not always used in the most appropriate manner. Among hospitalized elderly patients with depression who were discharged on antidepressant medication, 33 percent were on a dose below the recommended level (Wells et al., 1994b). In a study of 634 patients with depression or depressive symptoms in Boston, Chicago, and Los Angeles, 19 percent were treated with minor tranquilizers and no antidepressants (Wells et al., 1994a), despite the lack of evidence that tranquilizers work for depression and the risk that they will cause side effects or addiction (Depression Guideline Panel, 1993).

Patients with chronic conditions, for which certain routine examinations and tests are crucial in order to prevent complications, do not all get the care they need. Diabetes mellitus causes several complications that are less likely to occur with good care. One of these complications is an eye condition called diabetic retinopathy, which is the leading cause of new blindness among persons aged 20 to 74 in the United States. It is recommended that patients with insulin-dependent diabetes mellitus have an annual dilated eye examination (the clinician uses drops to enlarge the pupil to see behind it more easily) starting five years after diagnosis and that patients with non-insulin-dependent diabetes mellitus have the exam annually starting at the time of diagnosis. In a national study in 1989, only 49 percent of adults with either type of diabetes had undergone a dilated eye examination in the past year (66 percent in the past two years), and 61 percent had undergone any type of eye exam in the past year (79 percent in the past two years). Twenty percent of diabetics had no eye exam in the past two years. Among diabetics who were at particularly high risk for vision loss because they already had retinopathy or because they had had diabetes for a long time, 61 percent and 57 percent, respectively, had a dilated examination in the past year (Brechner et al., 1993).

Sometimes surgery is performed on people who do not need it. A study of seven managed care organizations revealed that about 16 percent of hysterectomies performed during a one-year period from 1989 to 1990 were carried out for inappropriate reasons. An additional 25 percent were done for reasons of uncertain clinical benefit (Bernstein et al., 1993b). There are also examples of patients who need surgery but do not receive it. In a study of four hospitals, 43 percent of patients with a positive exercise stress test demonstrating the need for coronary angiography had received it within 3 months; 56 percent had received it within 12 months (Laouri et al., 1997).

Adverse events are injuries caused by medical management of a disease rather than by the disease itself. A review in New York State in 1984 found that 1.0 percent of hospitalizations had an adverse event due to negligence (Brennan et al., 1991). A study of two Boston hospitals found an adjusted rate of preventable adverse drug events of 1.8 per 100 non-obstetric hospital admissions; 20 percent of these events were life-threatening (Bates et al., 1995).

Not all studies have found such poor quality. In a study of patients from 10 academic medical centers who had cataract surgery, 2 percent had the surgery for inappropriate reasons (Tobacman et al., 1996). In a study of patients in New York State who underwent coronary artery bypass graft surgery, 1.6 percent had surgery for inappropriate reasons (Leape et al., 1996). Nonetheless, the majority of studies described in the tables show much room for improving quality.

How Managed Care Affects Quality

Many have been quick to conclude that managed care is responsible for much of the poor quality care found in the U.S. health care system. However, studies published in the research literature neither clearly confirmed nor refuted this conclusion. Some studies find that managed care organizations provide better care than fee-for-service; some find that fee-for-service provides better care; still others find that the care is about the same (Miller and Luft, 1993, 1994). Results vary depending on the setting, the type of care assessed, and the methodology.

Examining how managed care affects quality is complicated by the research approach, which has generally lumped together managed care organizations without distinguishing them by type (e.g., group- and staff-model health maintenance organizations, independent practice associations, preferred provider organizations, point-of-service plans) or by features (e.g., comprehensiveness of the benefits package, nonprofit versus for-profit status). For purposes of examining quality, it would be more useful to assess the effect of specific characteristics of managed care organizations. For example, including immunizations in a benefits package may have a larger impact on immunization rates than whether the care is offered by a managed care organization or a fee-for-service provider.

A final important constraint on examining managed care's affect on quality is the pace of change in this industry. Indeed, managed care is changing so rapidly (Landon et al., 1998) that most currently available studies are already out of date. We do not have a quality measurement system that enables timely assessment of the rapid changes occurring in the health care marketplace. Even the most widely used systems (e.g., the Health Plan Employer Data and Information Set, described below) are far from universal and do not include both managed care and fee-for-service.

Trends in Quality-of-Care Assessment

Because the Technical Advisory Panel specifically requested an update on studies published in 1997–1998, we examined these studies as a group. There are several notable findings. First, few of these later studies reported on overuse of care. By contrast, our original review produced many examples of overuse. These early studies were based principally on the UCLA/RAND appropriateness method (Brook, 1994), which was one of the key methods used for quality assessment in the late 1980s and early 1990s. We do not know why the number of appropriateness studies has declined in recent years. Perhaps the many studies published throughout the prior decade convinced researchers that a great deal of inappropriate care is being provided, and they saw no need to make the same point over and over again. Or perhaps researchers now prefer other types of research questions and methodologies.

Most of the recent studies provided examples of underuse. The findings are similar to those in the original review. For most types of care that researchers choose to study, we find that although many people do receive high quality care, many others do not. For example, a national study found that smoking status of adult patients was known by about two-thirds of primary care physicians after seeing their adult patients (Thorndike et al., 1998). Most preventive screening tests in the various studies were performed on more than half of the studied population but far from all. Blood pressure screening was particularly high (88 percent at last visit in one study [Kottke et al., 1997]), and in at least one study, cholesterol screening was high as well (84 percent) (Davis et al., 1998). Papanicolaou tests also appear to be provided to a large percentage of eligible women (Kottke et al., 1997). Quality continues to vary for acute care as well. The vast majority of hospitalized patients with pneumonia had timely oxygenation measurements (89 percent), but a lower percentage received blood cultures before antibiotics (57 percent) (Meehan et al., 1997).

Most of the studies of underuse were in chronic care. Mental health care falls below standards, with 70 percent of schizophrenics in one study receiving poor symptom management, and 79 percent of those experiencing medication side effects receiving poor management of them (Young et al., 1998). Cardiac care was the major area in which quality-of-care studies were conducted over the past decade, and the care patterns documented in the earlier studies continue among the recent ones. Excellent clinical research has shown repeatedly that certain medications should and should not be used for people with myocardial infarctions or unstable angina, yet several quality-of-care studies show that many patients are still not getting proper treatments (e.g., Berger et al., 1998; Krumholz et al., 1998; Simpson et al., 1997; Soumerai et al., 1998). As mentioned above, one study with particularly striking results found that only 21 percent of eligible patients with a heart attack received beta blockers within 90 days of hospital discharge (Soumerai et al., 1997). Although patients with cardiovascular disease—a subset of the population that unambiguously needs cholesterol testing—had very high rates of cholesterol testing (96 percent), a much lower percentage of these patients received comprehensive treatment when their tests were abnormal (McBride et al., 1998).

Other Sources of Information About Quality of Care

In this paper, we have described reports of quality that have appeared in the research literature. There are also some systems that measure quality in select sectors of the United States, most notably the National Committee for Quality Assurance's (NCQA) Health Plan Employer Data and Information Set (HEDIS). HEDIS is a performance measurement tool designed to help purchasers and consumers evaluate managed care plans and to hold plans accountable for the quality of their services. In 1996, more than 330 plans—over half the U.S. plans representing more than three-quarters of all commercial managed care enrollees—were reporting HEDIS measures on their commercial enrollees. Average adherence rates for select indicators made publicly available by NCQA fell primarily in the 60 to 70 percent range, with the extremes at 38 percent for diabetic eye exams (past year) and 84 percent for initiation of prenatal care in the first trimester (Thompson et al., 1998). Thus, HEDIS's findings are consistent with those of the studies we have reported. Whether assessing quality as part of a research study or as part of a marketplace tool, the evidence repeatedly shows that quality falls short of standards.

CONCLUSIONS

There is good reason to be proud of the U.S. health care system, and evidence from international studies does not show consistent superiority elsewhere in the world (Gray et al., 1990; Pilpel et al., 1992; McGlynn et al., 1994; Froehlich et al., 1997; Meijler et al., 1997; Tamblyn et al., 1997; Wong et al., 1997). The United States is responsible for many important advances in health care technology, and state-of-the-art care is available in both large and small communities throughout the country. However, just because outstanding care is available does not mean that it is always provided or that everyone has access to such care. Most people in the studies reported here did receive excellent care. What is notable is that many did not.

The quality of health care provided in the United States varies among hospitals, cities, and states. Whether the care is preventive, acute, or chronic, it frequently does not meet professional standards. We can do much better. The solution is not simply a matter of spending more money on health care. A large part of our quality problem is the amount of inappropriate care provided in this country. Eliminating such nonbeneficial and potentially harmful care would generate large savings in human and financial costs. However, there are also many examples of people who receive either too little or technically poor care; fixing these problems may increase expenditures.

Some people might conclude that quality is good enough based on the evidence we have presented in this report—in other words, that the standards used in the various studies are too high. We would disagree with such a conclusion.

Clinicians and health plans that are motivated to improve the quality of care they deliver can use information on quality to focus their improvement efforts. For example, a group of all cardiothoracic surgeons practicing in Maine, New Hampshire, and Vermont, using continuous quality improvement and other techniques to improve their practices, reduced their combined mortality rates by 24 percent (O'Connor et al., 1996). Government action also has the potential to spur improvement. In New York State (NYS), risk-adjusted mortality for coronary artery bypass graft (CABG) surgery decreased 41 percent from 4.17 percent in 1989 (when the NYS Department of Health began disseminating information regarding the outcomes of CABG surgery) to 2.45 percent in 1992 (Hannan et al., 1994). Between 1987 (before the NYS reporting program began) and 1992, unadjusted 30-day mortality rates following CABG declined by 33 percent in NYS Medicare patients, compared with a 19 percent decline nationwide, giving NYS the lowest statewide risk-adjusted CABG mortality rate in the country (Peterson et al., 1998).

If quality-of-care information is made available regularly and in an interpretable form, consumers and large purchasers can use it to make informed decisions when choosing among clinicians and plans, which will, in turn, give providers an added incentive to improve quality. Policy makers can also use information about quality of care to determine the impact of public and private changes in the health care marketplace. We are currently experiencing a dramatic shift in the organization and financing of health services delivery in the United States. The private sector has been the driving force behind this transformation, but the public sector is beginning to use its market power as well. Incentives to move Medicaid and Medicare beneficiaries into managed care represent one of many examples of public sector change.

Although quality assessment organizations, accreditation organizations, and government agencies are currently doing work to measure quality of care, most of this activity has begun during the past decade. The rapid development of the field is encouraging, but it is confined to organizations that cover specific sections of the country or restrict themselves to certain segments of the health care marketplace. Their work, as well as the findings of individual studies such as those listed in Tables A-1 to A-3, provides some evidence of the situation throughout the country.

But changes in the U.S. health care delivery system are occurring more rapidly than evaluations of them can be performed. Much of the information concerning the relation between the organization of the health care system and quality of care is already outdated. At present, the United States has only a patchwork of systems that measure quality, with little uniformity, breadth, or ability to produce rapid results. Furthermore, these systems do not yet assess most providers of health care in the United States. There is no system that provides a comprehensive assessment of quality of care for the nation—including how quality varies by population subgroups (e.g., gender, age, race/ethnicity, income, region of country, size of community) and how quality is changing over time. Efforts such as HEDIS could eventually lead to development of a comprehensive, national quality assessment system, but such a system may not develop rapidly unless there is an organized effort to ensure that it does.

The United States cannot afford to let this situation continue. A systematic strategy for routine monitoring and reporting on quality, as well as the information systems needed to support such activities, will be essential if we are to preserve the best of the American health care system while striving to improve the efficiency with which high-quality services are provided.

This strategy could be organized by the federal government, the private sector, or a public–private partnership. It could involve coordination among all three. But in any case, the strategy will need to cover the aspects of quality that patients, purchasers, and providers care about; it will need to collect data in a way that is manageable, reasonable, and affordable; and it will need to produce information in a format that is useful for making a variety of decisions.

The United States is capable of implementing a quality measurement system that can provide the multiple participants in the health care system with the information they need to ensure delivery of high-quality care. In light of the changes that the health care system has been experiencing, a strategy to measure and consequently to improve quality is needed now.

ACKNOWLEDGMENTS

Partial funding was provided by the National Coalition on Health Care and the Institute of Medicine. We are indebted to Allison L. Diamant, M.D., M.S.P.H., Mark Chassin, M.D., M.P.P., M.P.H., Janet Corrigan, Ph.D., Molla Donaldson, D.Ph., Rachel Spilka, Ph.D., and Joseph H. Triebwasser, M.D., for comments on drafts of this paper. We are also indebted to James Tebow, Ph.D., Lauren N. Nguyen, M.P.H., Yuko Sano, A.B., Sinaroth Sor, M.D., and Myra Wong, A.B., for document and research assistance.

REFERENCES

Advisory Commission on Consumer Protection and Quality in the Health Care Industry. 1998. *Quality First: Better Health Care for All Americans. Final Report to the President of the United States.* Washington, D.C.

Agency for Health Care Policy and Research. 1994. Acute Low Back Problems in Adults. *Clinical Practice Guideline #14.*

Agency for Health Care Policy and Research. 1996. Helping Smokers Quit, Guide for Primary Care Clinicians, Number 18, AHCPR Publication Number 96-0693.

American Academy of Pediatrics. 1988. *Guidelines for Health Supervision II.* Elk Grove Village, Ill.

———. 1994. *1994 Red Book. Report of the Committee on Infectious Diseases.* Elk Grove Village, Ill.

American College of Obstetricians and Gynecologists Committee on Obstetric Practice. 1996. Prevention of Early-Onset Group B Streptococcal Disease in Newborns. Washington, D.C.: American College of Obstetricians and Gynecologists.

American College of Obstetricians and Gynecologists. Technical Bulletin Number 170–July 1992. 1993. *International Journal of Gynecology and Obstetrics* 42:55-9.

Bates, D.W., D.J. Cullen, N. Laird, et al. 1995. Incidence of Adverse Drug Events and Potential Adverse Drug Events. *Journal of the American Medical Association* 274:29–34.

Berger, A.K., D.W. Edris, J.A. Breall, et al. 1998. Resource Use and Quality of Care for Medicare Patients with Acute Myocardial Infarction in Maryland and the District of Columbia: Analysis of Data from the Cooperative Cardiovascular Project. *American Heart Journal* 135: 349–56.

Bernstein, S.J., L.H. Hilborne, L.L. Leape, et al. 1993a. The Appropriateness of Use of Coronary Angiography in New York State. *Journal of the American Medical Association* 269:766–9.

Bernstein, S.J., E.A. McGlynn, A.L. Siu, et al. 1993b. The Appropriateness of Hysterectomy: A Comparison of Care in Seven Health Plans. *Journal of the American Medical Association* 269:2398–402.

Brechner, R.J., C.C. Cowie, L.J. Howie, W.H. Herman, J.C. Will, and M.I. Harris. 1993. Ophthalmic Examination among Adults with Diagnosed Diabetes Mellitus. *Journal of the American Medical Association* 270:1714–8.

Brennan, T.A., L.L. Leape, N.M. Laird, et al. 1991. Incidence of Adverse Events and Negligence in Hospitalized Patients. *New England Journal of Medicine* 324:370–6.

Bronstein, J.M., V.A. Johnson, C.A. Fargason, Jr. 1997. Impact of Care Setting on Cost and Quality under Medicaid. *Journal of Health Care for the Poor and Underserved* 8: 202–16.

Brook, R.H., M.R. Chassin, and A. Fink. 1986. A Method for Detailed Assessment of the Appropriateness of Medical Technologies. *International Journal Technology Assessment in Health Care* 2:53–63.

Brook, R.H. 1994 The RAND/UCLA Appropriateness Method. In: McCormick KA, Moore SR, Siegel RA, eds. *Clinical Practice Guideline Development: Methodology Perspectives,* AHCPR Pub. No. 95-0009, Rockville, MD: U.S. Public Health Service 59–70.

Carey, T.S., K. Weis, and C. Homer. 1991. Prepaid versus Traditional Medicaid Plans: Lack of Effect on Pregnancy Outcomes and Prenatal Care. *Health Services Research* 26(2):165–81.

Centers for Disease Control and Prevention. 1993a. Mammography and Clinical Breast Examinations among Women Aged 50 Years and Older-Behavioral Risk Factor Surveillance System, 1992. *Morbidity and Mortality Weekly Report* 42:737–41.

———. 1993b. Physician and Other Health-Care Professional Counseling of Smokers to Quit—United States, 1991. *Morbidity and Mortality Weekly Report* 42:854–7.

———. 1993c. State-Specific Changes in Cholesterol Screening-Behavioural Risk Factor Surveillance System, 1988–91. *Morbidity and Mortality Weekly Reports* 42:663–7.

———. 1994a. Addressing Emerging Infectious Disease Threats: A Prevention Strategy for the United States. *Morbidity and Mortality Weekly Report* 43(RR-5):1–18.

———. 1994b. Adults Taking Action to Control Their Blood Pressure-United States, 1990. *Morbidity and Mortality Weekly Report* 43:509–17.

———. 1995a. Recommended Childhood Immunization Schedule-United States, 1995. *Morbidity and Mortality Weekly Report* 44(RR-5):1–9.

———. 1995b. Influenza and Pneumococcal Vaccination Coverage Levels among Persons Aged > 65 Years—United States, 1973–1993. *Morbidity and Mortality Weekly Report* 44:506–15.

———. 1996. Trends in Cancer Screening–United States, 1987 and 1992. *Morbidity and Mortality Weekly Report* 45:57–61.

———. 1997. National, State, and Urban Area Vaccination Coverage Levels among Children Aged 19–35 Months–United States, January–December 1995. *Morbidity and Mortality Weekly Report* 46:176–82.

Chassin, M.R., J. Kosecoff, R.E. Park, et al. 1987. Does Inappropriate Use Explain Geographic Variations in the Use of Health Care Services? A Study of Three Procedures. *Journal of the American Medical Association* 258:2533–7.

Cullen, D.J., B.J. Sweitzer, D.W. Bates, E. Burdick, A. Edmondson, L.L. Leape. 1997. Preventable Adverse Drug Events in Hospitalized Patients: A Comparative Study of Intensive Care and General Care Units. *Critical Care Medicine.* 25:1289–97.

Davis, K.C., M.E. Cogswell, S. Lee, R. Rothenberg, J.P. Koplan. 1998. Lipid Screening in a Managed Care Population. *Public Health Services* 113:346–50.

Depression Guideline Panel. 1993. *Depression in Primary Care.* Volume 2: *Treatment of Major Depression. Clinical Practice Guideline Number 5.* Pub. no. (PHS) 93-0551. Rockville, Md.: U.S. Department of Health and Human Services.

Donabedian, A. 1980. *Explorations in Quality Assessment and Monitoring,* Volume 1: *The Definition of Quality and Approaches to Its Assessment.* Ann Arbor, Mich.: Health Administration Press.

Dowell, S.F., and B. Schwartz. 1997. Resistant Pneumococci: Protecting Patients through Judicious Use of Antibiotics. *American Family Physician* 55:1647–54.

Draper, D., K.L. Kahn, E.J. Reinisch, et al. 1990. Studying the Effects of the DRG-Based Prospective Payment System on Quality of Care. Design, Sampling, and Fieldwork. *Journal of the American Medical Association* 264:1956–61.

Dubois, R.W., and R.H. Brook. 1988. Preventable Deaths: Who, How Often, and Why? *Annals of Internal Medicine* 109:582–9.

Ellerbeck, E.F., S.F. Jencks, M.J. Radford, et al. 1995. Quality of Care for Medicare Patients with Acute Myocardial Infarction: A Four-State Pilot Study from the Cooperative Cardiovascular Project. *Journal of the American Medical Association* 273:1509–14.

Franks, P., C.M. Clancy, M.R. Gold. 1993a. Health Insurance and Mortality: Evidence from a National Cohort. *Journal of the American Medical Association* 270:737–41.

Franks, P., C.M. Clancy, M.R. Gold, P.A. Nutting. 1993b. Health Insurance and Subjective Health Status: Data from the 1987 National Medical Expenditure Survey. *American Journal of Public Health* 83:1295–9.

Froehlich, F., I. Pache, B. Bumand, et al. 1997. Underutilization of Upper Gastrointestinal Endoscopy. *Gastroenterology* 112:690–7.

Gonzales, R., J.F. Steiner, and M.A. Sande. 1997. Antibiotic Prescribing for Adults With Colds, Upper Respiratory Tract Infections, and Bronchitis by Ambulatory Care Physicians. *Journal of the American Medical Association* 278:901–4.

Gray, D., J.R. Hampton, S.J. Bernstein, J. Kosecoff, and R.H. Brook. 1990. Audit of Coronary Angiography and Bypass Surgery. *Lancet* 335:1317–20.

Greenfield, S., D.M. Blanco, R.M. Elashoff, and P.A. Ganz. 1987. Patterns of Care Related to Age of Breast Cancer Patients. *Journal of the American Medical Association* 257:2766–70.

Greenspan, A.M., H.R. Kay, B.C. Berger, R.M. Greenberg, A.J. Greenspon, and M.S. Gaughan. 1988. Incidence of Unwarranted Implantation of Permanent Cardiac Pacemakers in a Large Medical Population. *New England Journal of Medicine* 318:158–63.

Guadagnoli, E., C.L. Shapiro, J.C. Weeks, et al. 1998. The Quality of Care for Treatment of Early Stage Breast Carcinoma: Is It Consistent with National Guidelines? *Cancer* 83:302–9.

Hand, R., S. Sener, J. Imperato, et al. 1991. Hospital Variables Associated With Quality of Care for Breast Cancer Patients. *Journal of the American Medical Association* 266:3429–32.

Hannan, E.L. H. Kilburn, M. Racz, E. Shields, and M.R. Chassin. 1994. Improving the Outcomes of Coronary Artery Bypass Surgery in New York State. *Journal of the American Medical Association* 271:761–6.

Hannan, E.L., J.F. O'Donnell, H. Kilburn, Jr., H.R. Bernard, A. Yazici. 1989. Investigation of the Relationship between Volume and Mortality for Surgical Procedures Performed in New York State Hospitals. *Journal of the American Medical Association* 262:503–10.

Hannan, E.L., A.L. Siu, D. Kumar, H. Kilburn, Jr., M.R. Chassin. 1995. The Decline in Coronary Artery Bypass Graft Surgery Mortality in New York State: The Role of Surgeon Volume. *Journal of the American Medical Association* 273:209–13.

Hilborne, L.H., L.L. Leape, S.J. Bernstein, et al. 1993. The Appropriateness of Use of Percutaneous Transluminal Coronary Angioplasty in New York State. *Journal of the American Medical Association.* 269:761–5.

Hillner, B.E., M.K. McDonald, L. Penberthy, et al. 1997. Measuring Standards of Care for Early Breast Cancer in an Insured Population. *Journal of Clinical Oncology* 15:1401–8.

Homer, C.J., P. Szilagyi, L. Rodewald, et al. 1996. Does Quality of Care Affect Rates of Hospitalization for Childhood Asthma? *Pediatrics* 98:18–23.

Joint National Committee on Detection, Evaluation, and Treatment of High Blood Pressure. 1993. The Fifth Report of the Joint National Committee on Detection, Evaluation, and Treatment of High Blood Pressure (JNC V). *Archives of Internal Medicine* 153:154–83.

Kahan, J.P., S.J. Bernstein, L.L. Leape, et al. 1994. Measuring the Necessity of Medical Procedures. *Medical Care* 32:357–65.

Kahn, K.L., W.H. Rogers, L.V. Rubenstein, et al. 1990. Measuring Quality of Care with Explicit Process Criteria before and after Implementation of the DRG-Based Prospective Payment System. *Journal of the American Medical Association* 264:1969–73.

Kelly, J.V., F.J. Hellinger. 1986. Physician and Hospital Factors Associated with Mortality of Surgical Patients. *Medical Care* 24:785–800.

Kitahata, M.M., T.D. Koepsell, R.A. Deyo, C.L. Maxwell, W.T. Dodge, and E.H. Wagner. 1996. Physicians' Experience with the Acquired Immunodeficiency Syndrome as a Factor in Patients' Survival. *New England Journal of Medicine* 334:701–6.

Kleinman, L.C., J. Kosecoff, R.W. Dubois, and R.H. Brook. 1994. The Medical Appropriateness of Tympanostomy Tubes Proposed for Children Younger than 16 Years in the United States. *Journal of the American Medical Association* 271:1250–5.

Klinkman, M.S., D.W. Gorenflo, and T.S. Ritsema. 1997. The Effects of Insurance Coverage on the Quality of Prenatal Care. *Archives of Family Medicine* 6:557–66.

Kogan, M.D., G.R. Alexander, M. Kotelchuck, D.A. Nagey, and B.W. Jack. 1994. Comparing Mothers' Reports on the Content of Prenatal Care Received with Recommended National Guidelines for Care. *Public Health Reports* 109:637–46.

Kottke, T.E., L.I. Solberg, M.L. Brekke, et al. 1997. Delivery Rates for Preventive Services in 44 Midwestern Clinics. *Mayo Clinic Proceedings* 72: 515–23.

Krumholz, H.M., M.J. Radford, E.F. Ellerbeck, et al. 1995. Aspirin in the Treatment of Acute Myocardial Infarction in Elderly Medicare Beneficiaries: Patterns of Use and Outcomes. *Circulation* 92:2841–7.

———. 1996. Aspirin for Secondary Prevention after Acute Myocardial Infarction in the Elderly: Prescribed Use and Outcomes. *Annals of Internal Medicine* 124:292–8.

Krumholz, H.M., D.M. Philbin, Y. Wang, et al. 1998. Trends in the Quality of Care with Medicare Beneficiaries Admitted to the Hospital with Unstable Angina. *Journal of the American College of Cardiology* 31: 957–63.

Landon, B.E., I.B. Wilson, and P.D. Cleary. 1998. A Conceptual Model of the Effects of Health Care Organizations on the Quality of Medical Care. *Journal of the American Medical Association* 279:1377–82.

Laouri, M., R.L. Kravitz, S.J. Bernstein, et al. 1997. Underuse of Coronary Angiography: Application of a Clinical Method. *International Journal for Quality in Health Care* 9:5–22.

Lazovich D., E. White, D.B. Thomas, R.E. Moe. 1991. Underutilization of Breast-Conserving Surgery and Radiation Therapy Among Women With Stage I or II Breast Cancer. *Journal of the American Medical Association* 266:3433–8.

Leape, L.L., T.A. Brennan, N. Laird, et al., 1991. The Nature of Adverse Events in Hospitalized Patients: Results of the Harvard Medical Practice Study II. *New England Journal of Medicine* 324:377–84.

Leape, L.L., L.H. Hilbome, R.E. Park, et al. 1993. The Appropriateness of Use of Coronary Artery Bypass Graft Surgery in New York State. *Journal of the American Medical Association* 269:753–60.

Leape, L.L., L.L. Hilbome, J.S. Schwartz, et al. 1996. The Appropriateness of Coronary Artery Bypass Graft Surgery in Academic Medical Centers. *Annals of Internal Medicine* 125:8–18.

Legorreta. A.P., J. Christian-Herman, R.D. O'Connor, et al. 1998. Compliance with National Asthma Management Guidelines and Specialty Care: A Health Maintenance Organization Experience. *Archives of Internal Medicine* 158: 457–64.

Lieu, T.A., J.C. Mohle-Boetani, G.T. Ray, L.M. Ackerson, D.L. Walton. 1998. Neonatal Group B Streptococcal Infection in a Managed Care Population. *Obstetrics and Gynecology* 92: 21–7.

Liu, Z., K.L. Shilkret, L. Finelli. 1998. Initial Drug Regimens for the Treatment of Tuberculosis: Evaluation of Physician Prescribing Practices in New Jersey. *Chest* 113:1446-51.

Lohr, K.N. Ed. 1990. *Medicare: A Strategy for Quality Assurance.* Washington D.C.: National Academy Press.

Luft, H.S., J.P. Bunker, A.C. Enthoven. 1979. Should Operations Be Regionalized? The Empirical Relation between Surgical Volume and Mortality. *New England Journal of Medicine* 301:1364–9.

Lurie, N., N.B. Ward, M.F. Shapiro, R.H. Brook. 1984. Termination of Medical Benefits: Does it Affect Health? *New England Journal of Medicine* 311:480–4.

Lurie, N., N.B. Ward, M.F. Shapiro, et al. 1986. Termination of Medical Benefits: A Follow-Up Study One Year Later. *New England Journal of Medicine* 314:1266–8.

Mainous, A.G., W.J.-Hueston, and J.R. Clark. 1996. Antibiotics and Upper Respiratory Infection: Do Some Folks Think There Is a Cure for the Common Cold? *Journal of Family Practice* 42:357–61.

McBride, P.M., H.G. Schrott, M.B. Plane, G. Underbakke, R.L. Brown. 1998. Primary Care Practice Adherence to National Cholesterol Education Program Guidelines for Patients with Coronary Heart Disease. *Archives of Internal Medicine* 158:1238–44.

McCaig, L.F., and J.M. Hughes. 1995. Trends in Antimicrobial Drug Prescribing among Office-Based Physicians in the United States. *Journal of the American Medical Association* 273:214–9.

McGlynn, E.A., C.D. Naylor, G.M. Anderson, et al. 1994. Comparison of the Appropriateness of Coronary Angiography and Coronary Artery Bypass Surgery between Canada and New York State. *Journal of the American Medical Association* 272:934–40.

Meehan, T.P., J. Hennen, M.J. Radford, M.K. Petrillo, P. Elstein, and D.J. Ballard. 1995. Process and Outcome of Care for Acute Myocardial Infarction among Medicare Beneficiaries in Connecticut: A Quality Improvement Demonstration Project. *Annals of Internal Medicine* 122:928–36.

Meehan, T.P., M.J. Fine, H.M. Krumholz, et al. 1997. Quality of Care, Process and Outcomes in Elderly Patients with Pneumonia. *Journal of the American Medical Association* 278:2080–4

Meijler, A.P., H. Rigter, S.J. Bernstein, et al. 1997. The Appropriateness of Intention to Treat Decisions for Invasive Therapy in Coronary Artery Disease in the Netherlands. *Heart* 77:219–24.

Miller, R.H., and H.S. Luft. 1993. Managed Care: Past Evidence and Potential Trends. *Frontiers of Health Services Management* 9:3–37.

————. 1994. Managed Care Plan Performance since 1980: A Literature Analysis. *Journal of the American Medical Association* 271:1512–9.

Murata, P.J., E.A. McGlynn, A.L. Siu, et al. 1994. Quality Measures for Prenatal Care: A Comparison of Care in Six Health Care Plans. *Archives of Family Medicine* 3:41–9.

NIH Consensus Conference Treatment of Early-Stage Breast Cancer. 1991. *Journal of the American Medical Association* 265:391–5.

National Library of Medicine. 1997a. Medical subject headings, Annotated Alphabetic List, 1998. Bethesda, Md.: U.S. Dept. of Health and Human Services, Public Health Service, National Institutes of Health, National Library of Medicine; Washington, D.C.

————. 1997b. Medical Subject Headings, Tree Structures, 1998. Bethesda, Md.: U.S. Dept. of Health and Human Services, Public Health Service, National Institutes of Health, National Library of Medicine; Washington, D.C.

Nyquist, A., R. Gonzales, J.F. Steiner, and M.A. Sande. 1998. Antibiotic Prescribing for Children With Colds, Upper Respiratory Tract Infections, and Bronchitis. *Journal of the American Medical Association* 279:875–7.

O'Connor, G.T., S.K. Plume, E.M. Olmstead, et al. 1996. A Regional Intervention to Improve the Hospital Mortality Associated With Coronary Artery Bypass Graft Surgery. *Journal of the American Medical Association* 275:841–6.

Payne, S.M., C. Donahue, P. Rappo, et al. 1995. Variations in Pediatric Pneumonia and Bronchitis/Asthma Admission Rates. Is Appropriateness a Factor? *Archives of Pediatrics and Adolescent Medicine* 149:162–9.

Peterson, E.D., E.R. DeLong, J.G. Jollis, L.H. Muhlbaier, and D.B. Mark. 1998. The Effects of New York's Bypass Surgery Provider Profiling on Access to Care and Patient Outcomes in the Elderly. *Journal of the American College of Cardiology* 32:993–9.

Phibbs, C.S., J.M. Bronstein, E. Buxton, and R.H. Phibbs. 1996. The Effects of Patient Volume and Level of Care at the Hospital of Birth on Neonatal Mortality. *Journal of the American Medical Association* 276:1054–9.

Pilpel, D., G.M. Fraser, J. Kosecoff, S. Weitzman, and R.H. Brook. 1992. Regional Differences in Appropriateness of Cholecystectomy in a Prepaid Health Insurance System. Public *Health Review* 20:61–74.

Retchin, S.M., and J. Preston. 1991. Effects of Cost Containment on the Care of Elderly Diabetics. *Archives of Internal Medicine* 151:2244–8.

Regier, D.A., W.E. Narrow, D.S. Rae, R.W. Maderscheid, B.Z. Locke, and F.K. Goodwin. 1993. The de facto US Mental and Addictive Disorders Service System. *Archives of General Psychiatry* 50:85–94.

Riley, G., J. Lubitz. 1985. Outcomes of Surgery among the Medicare Aged: Surgical Volume and Mortality. *Health Care Financing Review* 7:37–47.

Schucker, B., J.T. Wittes, N.C. Santanello, et al. 1991. Change in Cholesterol Awareness and Action. *Archives of Internal Medicine* 151:666–73.

Schuster, M.A., E.A. McGlynn, R.H. Brook. 1998. How Good Is the Quality of Health Care in the United States? *Milbank Quarterly* 76:517–63.

Shekelle, P.G., I. Coulter, E.L. Hurwitz, et al. 1998. Congruence Between Decisions to Initiate Chiropractic Spinal Manipulation for Low Back Pain and Appropriateness Criteria in North America. *Annals of Internal Medicine* 129:9–17.

Simon, G.E., and M. VonKorff. 1995. Recognition, Management, and Outcomes of Depression in Primary Care. *Archives of Family Medicine* 4:99–105.

Simpson, R.J. Jr., R.R. Weiser. S. Naylor, C.A. Sueta, A.K. Metts. 1997. Improving Care for Unstable Angina Patients in a Multiple Hospital Project Sponsored by a Federally Designated Quality Improvement Organization. *American Journal of Cardiology.* 80(8B):80H–4H.

Sorlie, P.D., N.J. Johnson, E. Backlund, D.D. Bradham. 1994. Mortality in the Uninsured Compared with that in Persons with Public and Private Insurance. *Archives of Internal Medicine* 154:2409–16.

Soumerai, S.B., T.D. McLaughlin, E. Hertzmark, G. Thibault, and L. Goldman. 1997. Adverse Outcomes of Underuse of Beta-Blockers in Elderly Survivors of Acute Myocardial Infarction. *Journal of the American Medical Association* 277:115–21.

Soumerai, S.B., T.J. McLauglin, J.H. Gurwitz, et al. 1998. Effect of Local Medical Opinion Leaders on Quality of Care for Acute Myocardial Infarction: A Randomized Controlled Trial. *Journal of the American Medical Association* 279:1358–63.

Starfield, B., N.R. Powe, J.R. Weiner, et al. 1994. Costs vs Quality in Different Types of Primary Care Settings. *Journal of the American Medical Association* 272:1903–8.

Stone, V., G. Seage, T. Hertz, and A. Epstein. 1992. The Relation between Hospital Experience and Mortality for Patients with AIDS. *Journal of the American Medical Association* 268:2655–61.

Stoner, T.J., B. Dowd, W. P.Carr, G. Maldonado, T.R. Church, J. Mandel. 1998. Do Vouchers Improve Breast Cancer Screening Rates? Results from a Randomized Trial. *Health Services Research.* 33:11–28.

Summary of the Second Report of the National Cholesterol Education Program Expert Panel on Detection, Evaluation, and Treatment of High Blood Cholesterol in Adults (Adult Treatment Panel II). 1993. *Journal of the American Medical Association* 626: 3015–23.

Tamblyn, R., L. Berkson, W.D. Dauphinee, et al. 1997. Unnecessary Prescribing of NSAIDs and the Management of NSAID-Related Gastropathy in Medical Practice. *Annals of Internal Medicine* 127:429–38.

Thamer, M., N.F. Ray, S.C. Henderson, et al. 1998. Influence of the NIH Consensus Conference on *Helicobacter Pylori* on Physician Prescribing Among a Medicaid Population. *Medical Care* 36:646–60.

Thompson, J.W., J. Bost, F. Ahmed, C.E. Ingalls and C. Sennett. 1998. The NCQA's Quality Compass: Evaluating Managed Care in the United States. *Health Affairs* 17:152–8.

Thorndike, AX, N.A. Rigotti, R.S. Stafford, and D.E. Singer. 1998. National Patterns in the Treatment of Smokers by Physicians. *Journal of the American Medical Association* 279:604–8.

Tobacman, J.K., P. Lee, B. Zimmerman, H. Kolder, L. Hilborne, and R.H. Brook. 1996. Assessment of Appropriateness of Cataract Surgery at Ten Academic Medical Centers in 1990. *Ophthalmology* 103:207–15.

Udvarhelyi, I.S., K. Jennison, R.S. Phillips, and A.M. Epstein. 1991. Comparison of the Quality of Ambulatory Care for Fee-for-Service and Prepaid Patients. *Annals of Internal Medicine* 115:394–400.

U.S. Preventive Services Task Force. 1989. *Guide to Clinical Preventive Services.* Baltimore: William & Wilkins.

———. 1996. *Guide to Clinical Preventive Services.* Baltimore: William & Wilkins.

Weiner, J.P., S.T. Parente, D.W. Garnick, J. Fowles, A.G. Lawthers, and H. Palmer. 1995. Variation in Office-Based Quality: A Claims-Based Profile of Care Provided to Medicare Patients with Diabetes. *Journal of the American Medical Association* 273:1503–8.

Wells, K.B., R.D. Hays, M.A. Burnam, et al. 1989. Detection of Depressive Disorder for Patients Receiving Prepaid or Fee-for-Service Care: Results from the Medical Outcomes Study. *Journal of the American Medical Association* 262:3298–302.

Wells, K., W. Katon, B. Rogers, and P. Camp. 1994a. Use of Minor Tranquilizers and Antidepressant Medications by Depressed Outpatients: Results from the Medical Outcomes Study. *American Journal of Psychiatry* 151:694–700.

Wells, K.B., G. Norquist, B. Benjamin, W. Rogers, K. Kahn, and R. Brook. 1994b. Quality of Antidepressant Medications Prescribed at Discharge to Depressed Elderly Patients in General Medical Hospitals before and after Prospective Payment System. *General Hospital Psychiatry* 16:4–15.

Wells, K.B., W.H. Rogers, L.M. Davis, et al. 1993. Quality of Care for Hospitalized Depressed Elderly Patients before and after Implementation of the Medicare Prospective Payment System. *American Journal of Psychiatry* 150:1799–805.

Winslow, C.M., J.B. Kosecoff, M. Chassin, D.E. Kanouse, and R.H. Brook. 1988. The Appropriateness of Performing Coronary Artery Bypass Surgery. *Journal of the American Medical Association* 260:505–9.

Wong, J.H., J.M. Findlay, and M.E. Suarez-Almazor. 1997. Regional Performance of Carotid Endarterectomy: Appropriateness, Outcomes, and Risk Factors for Complications. *Stroke* 28:891–8.

Young, A.S., G. Sullivan, M.A. Bumam, R.H. Brook. 1998. Measuring the Quality of Outpatient Treatment for Schizophrenia. *Archives of General Psychiatry* 55:611–7.

TABLE A-1 Examples of Quality of Health Care in the United States—Underuse: Did Patients Receive the Care They Should Have Received?

Health Care Service[a]	Sample Description	Data Source	Quality of Care	Reference[b]
PREVENTIVE CARE				
Immunizations				
Childhood Vaccines				
Three Polio; four Diphtheria, Tetanus, Pertussis; one Measles, Mumps, Rubella; and three Haemophilus influenzae type b (Hib) by 18 months old. (Three to four doses of Hib are recommended, depending on formulation; three Hepatitis B virus vaccines [HBV] are also recommended but were not included in this particular study.) (American Academy of Pediatrics [AAP], 1994; Centers for Disease Control and Prevention [CDC], 1995a).	Children 19–35 months old in 31,997 households from a nationally representative sample of the United States (U.S.).	National Immunization Survey (NIS), 1995.	74% received all the vaccines. (If three doses of Hib are not included, the percentage is 76%.)	CDC, 1997
Influenza Vaccine				
Annual vaccination of all people ≥ 65 years old is recommended (U.S. Preventive Services Task Force [USPSTF], 1989). This recommendation has since been reiterated (USPSTF,1996).	Approximately 8,000 adults ≥ 65 years old from a sample of people representative of the U.S. civilian, noninstitutionalized population.	National Health Interview Survey (NHIS), 1993.	52% received annual influenza vaccine.	CDC, 1995b
Same as above.	From a sample of 7,997 randomly selected patients ≥ 20 years old who had visited a clinic during the	Mailed surveys with phone follow-up of patients who visited one of 44 clinics from August 1, to	72% of people ≥ 65 years had an influenza vaccine in the prior year.	Kottke et al., 1997

	study period, 6,830 (85%) completed surveys.	September 9, 1994, in the Minneapolis-St. Paul metropolitan area with contracts with one of two managed care companies.	CDC, 1995b
Pneumococcal Vaccine One-time vaccination for all people ≥ 65 years old is recommended (USPSTF, 1989). In 1996, the recommendation was modified to specify one-time vaccination for all immunocompetent individuals ≥ 65 years old (USPSTF, 1996).	Approximately 8,000 adults ≥ 65 years old from a sample of people representative of the U.S. civilian, noninstitutionalized population. NHIS, 1993	28% received pneumococcal vaccine.	
Same as above.	From a sample of 7,997 randomly selected patients ≥ 20 years old who had visited a clinic during the study period, 6,830 (85%) completed surveys. Mailed surveys with phone follow-up of patients who visited one of 44 clinics from August 1, to September 9, 1994, in the Minneapolis-St. Paul metropolitan area with contracts with one of two managed care companies.	36% of people ≥ 65 years old had ever had a pneumococcal vaccine.	Kottke et al., 1997
Cancer Screening *Breast Cancer Screening* Recommendations vary. In 1989, the USPSTF recommended an annual clinical breast exam (CBE) for women ≥ 40 years old and mammography every 1–2 years for women 50–75 years old (USPSTF, 1989).	21,601 women ≥ 50 years old from a sample of people representative of the U.S. population (excluding Arkansas and Wyoming, Behavioral Risk Factor Surveillance System, 1992.	58% had clinical breast exam in the prior year; 46% had mammography in the prior year; 40% had both examinations in the	CDC, 1993a

continues

TABLE A-1 Continued

Health Care Service[a]	Sample Description	Data Source	Quality of Care	Reference[b]
In 1996, it recommended mammography every 1–2 years with or without annual clinical breast exam for women 50–69 years old (USPSTF, 1996).	and including the District of Columbia).		prior year.	
Same as above.	From a sample of 7,997 randomly selected patients ≥ 20 years old who had visited a clinic during the study period, 6,830 (85%) completed surveys.	Mailed surveys with phone follow-up of patients who visited one of 44 clinics from August 1, to September 9, 1994, in the Minneapolis-St. Paul metropolitan area with contracts with one of two managed care companies.	72% of women ≥ 50 years old had a breast examination in the prior two years; 68% of women 50 years or older had a mammogram in the prior two years.	Kottke et al., 1997
Same as above.	221 women > 50 years old.	Interview survey of women in farm households randomly sampled from six southern Minnesota counties, 1992.	38% of women had not received a mammogram in the prior 18 months.	Stoner et al., 1998
Cervical Cancer Screening Women with an intact uterus (having a cervix) should have a Papanicolaou (Pap) smear after initiation of sexual intercourse and every 1–3 years thereafter. Some organizations recommend starting Pap smears for all women who have reached 18 years old, regardless of sexual history (USPSTF, 1989). These recommendations	Women ≥ 18 years old with an intact uterus from a sample of 128,412 people representative of the U.S. civilian, noninstitutionalized population.	NHIS, 1992.	67% had a Pap smear in the prior 3 years.	CDC, 1996

have since been reiterated (USPSTF, 1996).				
Same as above.	Mailed surveys with phone follow-up of patients who visited one of 44 clinics from August 1, to September 9, 1994, in the Minneapolis-St. Paul metropolitan area with contracts with one of two managed care companies.	From a sample of 7,997 randomly selected patients ≥ 20 years old who had visited a clinic during the study period, 6,830 (85%) completed surveys.	84% of women had a Pap smear in the prior two years.	Kottke et al., 1997
Colon Cancer Screening Recommendations vary. In 1980, the American Cancer Society recommended annual fecal occult blood testing (FOBT) starting at 50 years old. Some other organizations made similar recommendations. In 1989, the USPSTF did not make recommendations (USPSTF, 1989), but in 1996, it recommended annual FOBT, sigmoidoscopy (periodicity unspecified), or both starting at 50 years old (USPSTF, 1996).	NHIS, 1992	Adults ≥ 40 years old from a sample of 128,412 people representative of the U.S. civilian, noninstitutionalized population.	14% of men and 15% of women had FOBT in the prior year; 44% of men and 43% of women had ever had FOBT; 11% of men and 7% of women had proctosigmoidoscopy in the prior 3 years.	CDC, 1996
Same as above.	Medical records for patients from four group practices in Massachusetts, November 1, 1985, to October 31, 1987.	250 women 40-65 years old who had no major illnesses, who received primary care at one of the group practices, and who were eligible for preventive care.	51%–59% of women had FOBT every 2 years or flexible sigmoidoscopy every 5 years.	Udvarhelyi et al., 1991

continues

TABLE A-1 Continued

Health Care Service[a]	Sample Description	Data Source	Quality of Care	Reference[b]
Cardiac Risk Factors *Smoking Counseling* The USPSTF recommends a complete history of tobacco use as well as tobacco cessation counseling on a regular basis (USPSTF, 1989, 1996). The Agency for Health Care Policy and Research (AHCPR) recommends that primary care physicians identify patients' smoking status and counsel smokers at every visit (AHCPR, 1996).	8,778 smokers ≥ 18 years old from a sample of 43,732 people representative of the U.S. civilian, noninstitutionalized population.	NHIS, 1991.	37% of smokers who had a visit with a physician or other health care professional during the prior year had been advised to quit smoking.	CDC, 1993b
Same as above.	From a sample of 7,997 randomly selected patients ≥ 20 years old who had visited a clinic during the study period, 6,830 (85%) completed surveys.	Mailed surveys with phone follow-up of patients who visited one of 44 clinics from August 1, to September 9, 1994, in the Minneapolis-St. Paul metropolitan area with contracts with one of two managed care companies.	53% of smokers were asked their smoking status. 47% of smokers were advised to quit.	Kottke et al., 1997
Same as above.	A nationally representative sample of 3,254 physicians representing 145,716 adult patient ambulatory care visits.	National Ambulatory Medical Care Survey (NAMCS), 1991–1995.	Physicians knew the patient's smoking status at 66% of all patient visits. (The percentage for primary care physicians ranged from about 61% to	Thorndike et al., 1998

		67%, depending on the year.) Smoking counseling was provided at 22% of visits of known smokers. (The percentage for primary care physicians ranged from 20% to 38%.)	Schucker et al., 1991
Blood Cholesterol Screening In 1988, the National Heart, Lung, and Blood Institute recommended routine cholesterol screening at least every 5 years starting at 20 years old. In 1989, the USPSTF recommended periodic screening for middle-aged men (USPSTF, 1989), and in 1996, it recommended periodic screening for men 35–65 years old and women 45–65 years old. Treatment includes dietary therapy, physical activity, or lipid-lowering medications depending on the patient (National Cholesterol Education Program [NCEP], 1993).	3,700 adults ≥ 18 years old from a representative sample of the non-African American U.S. population.	Telephone survey by the National Heart, Lung, and Blood Institute, 1990.	65% of adults had ever had a blood cholesterol test; 51% had the test in the prior year; and an additional 14% had it prior to that. 35% had never had a blood cholesterol test.	
Same as above.	Adults ≥ 20 years old from a sample of people representative of the U.S. population (excluding Wyoming, Kansas, and	CDC's Behavioral Risk Factor Surveillance System, 1991.	The state-specific rates of adults who had cholesterol screening in the prior 5 years ranged from 57% to 70%.	CDC, 1993c

continues

TABLE A-1 Continued

Health Care Service[a]	Sample Description	Data Source	Quality of Care	Reference[b]
	Nevada, and including the District of Columbia) (sample sizes for individual states range from 670 to 3,190 people).			
Same as above.	From a sample of 7,997 randomly selected patients ≥ 20 years old who had visited a clinic during the study period, 6,830 (85%) completed surveys.	Mailed surveys with phone follow-up of patients who visited one of 44 clinics from August 1, to September 9, 1994, in the Minneapolis-St. Paul metropolitan area with contracts with one of two managed care companies.	68% had had their cholesterol measured during the prior 5 years.	Kottke et al., 1997
Blood Cholesterol Screening and Treatment				
Same as above.	1,004 people 40–64 years old from a sample that had been enrolled continuously for at least 5 years and had at least one outpatient visit during the study period.	Medical records from three sites of a managed care plan (South Florida; Jacksonville, Florida; and Atlanta, Georgia), January 1, 1988, to December 31, 1993.	84% were screened for elevated cholesterol levels at least once during the 6-year period. 86% with a diagnosis of hypercholesterolemia were treated with diet therapy, cholesterol-lowering drugs, or both.	Davis et al., 1998

Blood Pressure Screening

In 1989, the USPSTF recommended blood pressure measurements for normotensive patients ≥ 21 years old every 2 years if their last diastolic and systolic blood pressures were below 85 mm Hg and 140 mm Hg, respectively, and annually if their last diastolic was 85–89 mm Hg (USPSTF, 1989). In 1996, these recommendations were modified to specify *apparently* normotensive patients (USPSTF, 1996).

From a sample of 7,997 randomly selected patients ≥ 20 years old who had visited a clinic during the study period, 6,830 (85%) completed surveys.

Mailed surveys with phone follow-up of patients who visited one of 44 clinics from August 1, to September 9, 1994, in the Minneapolis-St. Paul metropolitan area with contracts with one of two managed care companies.

88% had blood pressure measured at the most recent visit.

Kottke et al., 1997

General Preventive Care

Well-Child Care

The AAP recommends routine history, physical examination, screening tests, and anticipatory guidance throughout childhood (AAP, 1988).

All children who had their second birthday during the first half of the study year, and all 2-year-olds with otitis media or asthma, from a sample of 2,024 patients of 135 providers.

Medical records from physicians' offices, community health centers, and hospital outpatient facilities sampled from Maryland Medicaid claims data, 1988.

For each type of clinical setting, the study reports the average percentage of technical quality indicators for well-child care that were not met. Each average fell in the 35%–65% range.

Starfield et al., 1994

Well-Adult Care

Patients should have preventive health visits every 1–3 years when 19–64 years old and every year when ≥ 65 years old (USPSTF, 1989).

All adults with asthma, hypertension, and diabetes from a sample of 2,024 patients of 135 providers.

Same as above.

For each type of clinical setting, the study reports the average percentage of technical quality indicators for well-adult care that were not met. Each average fell in the 45%–55% range.

Starfield et al., 1994

continues

TABLE A-1 Continued

Health Care Service[a]	Sample Description	Data Source	Quality of Care	Reference[b]
ACUTE CARE **Pneumonia** *Pneumonia: Hospital Care* Includes documentation of tobacco use/ nonuse and lower-extremity edema; blood pressure readings; oxygen therapy or intubation for hypoxic patients.	1,408 patients hospitalized with pneumonia from a nationally representative sample of 7,156 patients hospitalized with any of five conditions (congestive heart failure, acute myocardial infarction, pneumonia, stroke, hip fracture) (Draper et al., 1990).	Medical records for Medicare patients from 297 hospitals in five states (California, Florida, Indiana, Pennsylvania, Texas), July 1, 1985, to June 30, 1986.	52%–90% of patients with pneumonia received appropriate components of care.	Kahn et al., 1990
Includes various components of pneumonia care consistent with prevailing standards of care.	1,343 patients ≥ 65 years old hospitalized with pneumonia.	National Medicare claims data and medical records, October 1, 1994, to September 30, 1995	89% had oxygenation assessment within 24 hours of hospital arrival, 76% received antibiotics within 8 hours of arrival, 69% had blood cultures within 24 hours of arrival, and 57% had blood cultures collected before initial antibiotic administration.	Meehan et al., 1997

Otitis Media

Otitis Media: Treatment

Indicator	Sample	Data Source	Findings	Reference
Includes various components of otitis media care consistent with prevailing standards of care.	464 children ≥ 3 years old diagnosed with otitis media from a sample of 2,024 patients of 135 providers.	Medical records from physicians' offices, community health centers, and hospital outpatient facilities sampled from Maryland Medicaid claims data, 1988.	For each type of clinical setting, the study reports the average percentage of technical quality indicators for otitis media that were not met. Each average fell in the 10%–40% range.	Starfield et al., 1994

Hip Fractures

Hip Fracture: Hospital Care

Indicator	Sample	Data Source	Findings	Reference
Includes documentation of mental status and pedal or leg pulse, serum potassium level, electrocardiogram.	1,404 patients hospitalized with hip fracture from a nationally representative sample of 7,156 patients hospitalized with any of five conditions (congestive heart failure, acute myocardial infarction, pneumonia, stroke, hip fracture) (Draper et al., 1990).	Medical records for Medicare patients from 297 hospitals in five states (California, Florida, Indiana, Pennsylvania, Texas), July 1, 1985, to June 30, 1986.	67%–94% of patients with hip fracture received appropriate components of care.	Kahn et al., 1990

Urinary Tract Infections

Urinary Tract Infections: Diagnosis

Indicator	Sample	Data Source	Findings	Reference
The provision of a urine culture in diagnosing a urinary tract infection (UTI) is consistent with prevailing standards of care.	535 episodes of UTI from 465 children who received ambulatory care for UTIs out of a sample of 147,356 children < 8 years old with	Medicaid claims from Alabama, July 1, 1989, to June 30, 1993.	52% received a urine culture.	Bronstein et al., 1997

continues

TABLE A-1 Continued

Health Care Service[a]	Sample Description	Data Source	Quality of Care	Reference[b]
continuous Medicaid coverage (exclusive of children with Medicaid because of Supplemental Security Income) for all 12 months of 1992.				

Pregnancy and Delivery

Prenatal Care: Medical History, Physical Examination, and Laboratory Tests

| Includes various components of prenatal care consistent with prevailing standards of care. | 9,924 women who had live births in 1988 from a nationally representative sample of the U.S. population (excluding South Dakota and Montana, and including the District of Columbia). | National Maternal and Infant Health Survey (NMIHS), 1988. | 80% were asked about health history during the first or second visit. 98% had their weight and height measured, 96% had blood pressure measured, and 86% received a physical or pelvic examination during the first or second visit. 79% received blood tests and 93% received urinalysis during the first or second visit. 56% received all of the evaluations listed above during the first or second visit. | Kogan et al., 1994 |

Prenatal Care: Counseling About Nutrition, Weight Gain, Substance Use, and Breastfeeding

Includes various components of prenatal care consistent with prevailing standards of care.	Same as above.	97% were counseled about vitamins, 93% were counseled about diet, and 72% were counseled about proper weight gain during pregnancy during at least one prenatal visit. 68% were counseled to reduce or eliminate alcohol consumption, 69% to reduce or eliminate smoking, and 65% to stop use of illegal drugs during at least one prenatal visit. 53% were counseled about breastfeeding during at least one prenatal visit. 32% received all of the counseling listed above during at least one prenatal visit.	Kogan et al., 1994

Prenatal Care: Screening Tests

Includes tests to screen for anemia, asymptomatic bacteriuria, syphilis, gonorrhea, hepatitis B, rubella immunity, and Rh factor and antibody.	Random sample of 586 women who had a live birth from 24,170 births that occurred during the study period.	Medical records for patients from six HMOs in six states (Arizona, California, Colorado, Massachusetts, Minnesota, Oregon), August 1, 1989, to July 31, 1990.	Among six HMOs, women received 64%–95% (average 82%) of seven recommended routine prenatal screening tests.	Murata et al., 1994

TABLE A-1 Continued

Health Care Service[a]	Sample Description	Data Source	Quality of Care	Reference[b]
Prenatal Care: Other Routine Prenatal Care Includes first prenatal visit during first trimester, accurate determination of gestational age, screening for inherited disorders, measurement of symphysis-fundal height, and blood pressure measurement.	Same as above.	Same as above.	Among six HMOs, women received 78%–87% (average 84%) of five processes of routine prenatal care.	Murata et al., 1994
Prenatal Care: Pregnancy Complications Includes diagnostic and treatment interventions after abnormal screening test results, and care to mitigate effects of pregnancy-induced hypertension and gestational diabetes.	Same as above.	Same as above.	Among six HMOs, women received 54%–77% of care for complications of pregnancy.	Murata et al., 1994
Prenatal Care: Proteinuria Urine is checked for protein to evaluate for the presence of preeclampsia, a serious complication of pregnancy.	Inpatient records for 2,336 women from a sample of 2,878 births in 1985; prenatal care records for 823 of these women.	Medical records for patients sampled from Medicaid claims files for women and children enrolled in Aid to Families with Dependent Children (AFDC) in two communities in California and two communities in Missouri, 1985.	Testing was provided at 75%–83% of visits. Follow-up was performed for 41%–65% of patients with proteinuria.	Carey et al., 1991

Prenatal Care: Recording of Gestational Age

Includes a component of prenatal care consistent with prevailing standards of care.	Same as above.	Gestational age was recorded at 78%–95% of visits.	Carey et al., 1991

Prenatal Care: Assessment of Fetal Heart Tones after 18 Weeks of Gestation

Includes a component of prenatal care consistent with prevailing standards of care.	Same as above.	Fetal heart tones were assessed at 81%–93% of visits.	Carey et al., 1991

Prenatal Care: Follow-up for Low Hematocrit

Low hematocrit indicates anemia.	Same as above.	Follow-up was performed for 32%–51% of patients with low hematocrit.	Carey et al., 1991

Prenatal Care: Follow-up for High Blood Pressure

Includes a component of prenatal care consistent with prevailing standards of care.	Same as above.	Follow-up was performed for 31%–53% of patients with high blood pressure.	Carey et al., 1991

Prenatal Care: Physical Examination

Includes various components of prenatal care consistent with prevailing standards of care.	267 women receiving routine, low-risk prenatal care were randomly selected, with stratification by insurance type (Medicaid, health maintenance organization, fee-for-service). Medical records from seven private and hospital-based prenatal care sites in Washtenaw County, Michigan, for women receiving care between January 1, 1991, and December 31, 1992.	99% had blood pressure assessed at each visit. 93% had fundal height assessed at each visit after 20 weeks gestation.	Klinkman et al., 1997

continues

TABLE A-1 Continued

Health Care Service[a]	Sample Description	Data Source	Quality of Care	Reference[b]
Prenatal Care: Laboratory Screening Tests				
Includes various components of prenatal care consistent with prevailing standards of care.	Same as above.	Same as above.	Patients received an average of 81%–83% (depending on insurance type) of recommended laboratory screening tests.	Klinkman et al., 1997
Delivery: Neonatal Group B Streptococcal (GBS) Disease				
The American College of Obstetricians and Gynecologists recommends intrapartum antibiotics for women with rupture of membranes (ROM) for 18 hours or more to prevent neonatal Group B Streptococcal (GBS) infection (ACOG, 1993, 1996).	81 women with ROM ≥ 18 hours from among all women with deliveries during the study period.	Medical records from two HMO hospitals (in which protocols similar to ACOG guidelines had been adopted) in San Francisco and Oakland, California, for women who delivered from January to June 1995.	88% received an antibiotic effective against GBS, 37% received antibiotics within 20 hours of ROM (median duration of ROM was 31 hours).	Lieu et al., 1998
CHRONIC CARE **Asthma** *Adult Asthma Care*				
Includes various components of asthma care consistent with prevailing standards of care.	Adults ≥ 18 years old in a group of 393 adults and children diagnosed with asthma, from a sample of 2,024 patients of 135 providers.	Medical records from physicians' offices, community health centers, and hospital outpatient facilities sampled from Maryland Medicaid claims data, 1988.	For each type of clinical setting, the study reports the average percentage of technical quality indicators for adult asthma that were not met. Each of the averages was located in the 40%–45% range. Between 5% and 35% of care was inappropriate.	Starfield et al., 1994

Childhood Asthma Care Includes various components of asthma care consistent with prevailing standards of care.	Children < 18 years old in a group of 393 adults and children diagnosed with asthma, from a sample of 2,024 patients of 135 providers.	Same as above.	For each type of clinical setting, the study reports the average percentage of technical quality indicators for childhood asthma that were not met. Each of the averages was located in the 30%–40% range. Between 0% and 20% of care was inappropriate.	Starfield et al., 1994
Asthma Care Includes various components of asthma care consistent with prevailing standards of care.	5,580 patients ≥ 14 years old who were prescribed asthma medications.	Survey of patients from multiple sites of a health maintenance organization in California, 1996.	72% of patients with severe asthma had a steroid inhaler, 26% of patients needing daily medications had a peak flow meter at home, and 42% were advised about self-management tools.	Legorreta et al., 1998
Diabetes Mellitus *Diabetes Mellitus: Dilated Eye Examination* Annual dilated eye examination to screen for retinopathy starting at time of diagnosis of non-insulin-dependent diabetes mellitus (NIDDM) and 5 years after diagnosis of insulin-dependent diabetes mellitus (IDDM).	2,392 adults ≥ 18 years old with IDDM (124 patients), NIDDM treated with insulin (922 patients), and NIDDM not treated with insulin (1,346 patients) from a sample of 84,572 people	NHIS, 1989.	49% had a dilated eye examination in the prior year; 66% had an examination in the prior 2 years; 61% and 57% of patients at high risk of vision loss because of a	Brechner et al., 1993

continues

TABLE A-1 Continued

Health Care Service[a]	Sample Description	Data Source	Quality of Care	Reference[b]
	representative of the U.S. civilian, noninstitutionalized population.		history of retinopathy or of long duration of diabetes, respectively, had an examination in the prior year.	
Diabetes Mellitus: Any Eye Examination Dilated eye examination is recommended, as described above, but any eye examination is also reported to determine whether there was any effort to assess for retinopathy.	Same as above.	Same as above.	61% had an eye examination in the prior year; 79% had an examination in the prior 2 years.	Brechner et al., 1993
Diabetes Mellitus: Eye Exam by Ophthalmologist Dilated eye examination is recommended, as described above, but an examination by an ophthalmologist serves as a proxy for a dilated eye examination.	97,388 Medicare patients ≥ 65 years old diagnosed with diabetes mellitus.	All Medicare claims data (Parts A and B) from three states (Alabama, Iowa, Maryland), submitted from July 1, 1990, to June 30, 1991.	54% did not have an examination by an ophthalmologist during the prior year.	Weiner et al., 1995
Diabetes Mellitus: Physical Examination Includes various components of diabetes care consistent with prevailing standards of care.	292 patients ≥ 65 years old with diabetes mellitus.	National Medicare Competition Evaluation, with medical records from 8 HMOs and 113 fee-for-service providers for patients drawn from	92%–96% had their weight recorded at least once after diagnosis. 70% (for both HMO and FFS providers) had a peripheral vascular examination. 94%–96% had	Retchin and Preston, 1991

	enrollment lists of patients with start-up dates between January 1983, and May 1984; records were abstracted from the start-up date to March 31, 1986.	blood pressure recorded at least annually. 30%–48% had a funduscopic examination or referral to an ophthalmologist within 2 years of diagnosis. 58%–63% had tonometry performed.	Weiner et al., 1995
Diabetes Mellitus: Hemoglobin A1C Hemoglobin A1C (or glycosylated hemoglobin) is a blood test that reflects the metabolic control of diabetes. The test should be performed at least once a year for diabetics.	97,388 Medicare patients ≥ 65 years old diagnosed with diabetes mellitus.	84% did not receive a hemoglobin A1C test during the prior year.	Weiner et al., 1995
Diabetes Mellitus: Cholesterol Screening It is recommended that total cholesterol be measured at least once a year for diabetics.	All Medicare claims data (Parts A and B) from three states (Alabama, Iowa, Maryland), submitted from July 1, 1990, to June 30, 1991.	45% did not receive blood cholesterol screening during the prior year	Weiner et al., 1995
Diabetes Mellitus: Laboratory Studies and Follow-ups Includes various components of diabetes care consistent with prevailing standards of care.	Same as above.		
	292 patients ≥ 65 years old with diabetes mellitus.	74%–89% had urinalysis performed. 75%–95% had creatinine or serum urea nitrogen determined at least annually after diagnosis. 82%–83% had an electrocardiogram performed within 6 months of diagnosis. 91%–95% had at least one repeated blood	Retchin and Preston, 1991

continues

TABLE A-1 Continued

Health Care Service[a]	Sample Description	Data Source	Quality of Care	Reference[b]
		abstracted from the start-up date to March 31, 1986.	glucose within 12 months of diagnosis. 84%–90% who were not taking insulin had blood glucose recorded at least every 12 months. 74% (for both HMO and FFS providers) who were taking insulin had blood glucose recorded at least every 6 months.	
Diabetes Mellitus: Influenza Vaccine Includes diabetes care consistent with prevailing standards of care.	Same as above.	Same as above.	19%–62% received an influenza vaccination.	Retchin and Preston, 1991
Diabetes Mellitus Includes various components of diabetes care consistent with prevailing standards of care.	368 adults ≥ 18 years old diagnosed with diabetes, from a sample of 2,024 patients of 135 providers.	Medical records from physician offices, community health centers, and hospital outpatient facilities sampled from Maryland Medicaid claims data, 1988.	For each clinical setting, the study reports the average percentage of technical quality indicators for diabetes that were not met. Each average was located in the 40%–60% range.	Starfield et al., 1994

Peptic Ulcer Disease

Peptic Ulcer Disease: Treatment

People with *H. pylori* peptic ulcer disease (PUD) should be prescribed antimicrobial therapy for the infection, as strongly recommended by the National Institutes of Health Consensus Development Conference in February 1994.	About 3,571 Medicaid beneficiaries ≥ 18 years old who received care for PUD and who were not receiving nonsteroidal antiinflammatory drugs.	Computerized inpatient, outpatient, and pharmaceutical claims files of the Pennsylvania Medicaid Program, March 1994, to February 1996.	11% of patients received antimicrobials within five days of a PUD encounter.	Thamer et al., 1998

Hypertension

Hypertension: Treatment

Hypertension (high blood pressure) is a leading risk factor for coronary heart disease, congestive heart failure, stroke, ruptured aortic aneurysm, renal disease, and retinopathy, all of which contribute to high morbidity and mortality (U.S. Preventive Services Task Force, 1989). This was reiterated in 1996 (U.S. Preventive Services Task Force, 1996).	246 patients > 30 years old with chronic uncomplicated hypertension.	Medical records for patients from four group practices in Massachusetts, November 1, 1985, to October 31, 1987.	41%–54% of patients had their hypertension controlled (mean blood pressure < 150/90).	Udvarhelyi et al., 1991
Same as above.	Nationally representative sample of U.S. adults with hypertension (sample size not available).	National Health and Nutrition Examination Survey III, 1988–1991.	55% of people with hypertension had blood pressure under control (blood pressure < 160/95 on one occasion and reported currently taking antihypertensive medications); 21% when using strict criteria (blood pressure < 140/90 and reported currently taking antihypertensive medications).	Joint National Committee on Detection, 1993

continues

TABLE A-1 Continued

Health Care Service[a]	Sample Description	Data Source	Quality of Care	Reference[b]
Same as above.	8,697 adults ≥ 18 years old diagnosed with hypertension from a sample of 36,610 people representative of the U.S. population.	NHIS, 1990.	89% of adults with hypertension received advice from a physician about controlling hypertension (i.e., taking antihypertensive medication, decreasing salt intake, losing weight, or exercising); 80% reported taking at least one action to control hypertension.	CDC, 1994b
Same as above.	593 adults ≥ 18 years old diagnosed with hypertension, from a sample of 2,024 patients of 135 providers.	Medical records from physician offices, community health centers, and hospital outpatient facilities sampled from Maryland Medicaid claims data, 1988.	For each type of clinical setting, the study reports the average percentage of technical quality indicators for hypertension that were not met. Each average fell in the 40%–55% range.	Starfield et al., 1994
Mental Health *Depression: Detection* Includes diagnostic criteria consistent with prevailing standards of care.	650 patients with current depressive disorder from a sample of 22,462 adult patients who visited one large HMO; several	Medical Outcomes Study in three cities (Boston, Chicago, Los Angeles); questionnaires completed February to October 1986;	44%–51% of depressed patients who visited general medical clinicians had their depression detected during the visit. 78%–94% of	Wells et al., 1989

			depressed patients who visited mental health specialists had their depression detected during the visit.	Wells et al., 1989
Depression: Treatment Includes various components of depression care consistent with prevailing standards of care.	Same as above.	multispecialty, mixed-group practices; single-specialist small group practices; or solo practice providers in each city during the study period.	phone interviews completed May to December 1986.	
	Same as above.		50%–58% of depressed patients who visited general medical clinicians received appropriate care (the depression was detected, and they were counseled or referred to a mental health specialist or another clinician was noted to be providing the majority of the patient's care). 83%–93% of depressed patients who visited mental health specialists received appropriate care.	
Depression: Admission Assessment Includes various components of depression care consistent with prevailing standards of care.	1,198 patients hospitalized with depression, representative of all Medicare elderly patients hospitalized in general medical hospitals with a discharge diagnosis of	Medical records for Medicare patients from 297 hospitals in five states (California, Florida, Indiana, Pennsylvania, Texas), July 1, 1985, to June 30, 1986.	As part of admission assessment, 23% of patients did not have adequate psychological assessment, 26% did not have cognitive assessment, 50% did not have assessment of	Wells et al., 1993

continues

TABLE A-1 Continued

Health Care Service[a]	Sample Description	Data Source	Quality of Care	Reference[b]
	depression.		psychosis, 19% did not have documentation of psychiatric history, 47% did not have documentation of whether patient had a history of suicide attempts or ideation, 24% did not have documentation of prior or current medication use, and 45% did not have documentation that heart sounds were examined. Mean number of components of neurologic examination (assessment of pupils, deep tendon reflexes, and gait) performed was 1.4.	
Mental/Addictive Disorder Includes diagnostic criteria and treatment consistent with prevailing standards of care.	People with mental or addictive disorder from a sample of 20,291 adults ≥ 18 years old.	National Institute of Mental Health's Epidemiologic Catchment Area study interviews, 1980–1985.	29% of people with any mental or addictive disorder received some professional or voluntary mental health service during the prior 12 months, as did 32% of people with any disorder except	Regier et al., 1993

Condition and guideline	Study sample	Methods	Findings	Reference
			substance use, 37% of people with any mental disorder with comorbid substance use, 24% of people with substance use (e.g., alcohol), 64% of people with schizophrenia, 46% of people with any affective disorder (e.g., depression), 33% of people with any anxiety disorder (e.g., obsessive-compulsive), 70% of people with somatization, 31% of people with antisocial personality disorder, and 17% of people with severe cognitive impairment.	
Schizophrenia: Treatment Includes various components of schizophrenia care consistent with prevailing standards of care.	224 patients from a random sample of patients 18–65 years old with schizophrenia or schizoaffective disorder who had been treated at the clinic for >3 months, had been hospitalized < 21 days during the prior 3 months, and had >1 visit with a psychiatrist during the sampling period.	Patient interviews and medical records from a Veterans Affairs Medical Center clinic and a community mental health center clinic during a 3-month period in early 1996.	70% of patients with significant psychotic symptoms received poor management of their symptoms, and 79% of patients with significant medication side effects (akathisia, parkinsonism, tardive dyskinesia) received poor management of the side effects. 35% of patients with severe	Young et al., 1998

continues

TABLE A-1 Continued

Health Care Service[a]	Sample Description	Data Source	Quality of Care	Reference[b]
			disability were not receiving case management. 57% of patients in close contact with family members had no communication between the clinic and the family.	
Cancer				
Breast Cancer: Diagnosis				
Patients with breast cancer have better outcomes if diagnosis is made at an early stage.	5,766 newly diagnosed patients with histologically confirmed breast cancer.	Data submitted to American Cancer Society, Illinois Division, Chicago, by 99 hospitals out of 104 Illinois hospitals with active cancer registries, 1988.	The average rate across hospitals of patients diagnosed with cancer at a late stage (IIb through IV) was 18%.	Hand et al., 1991
Breast Cancer: Diagnosis				
Patients with breast cancer have better outcomes if hormone receptor levels in tumor tissue are determined.	2,958 newly diagnosed patients with histologically confirmed Stage II–IV breast cancer.	Same as above.	The average rate across hospitals of patients who did not have a hormone receptor test was 11%.	Hand et al., 1991
Diagnosis should be made with fine needle aspiration, cytology, limited incisional biopsy, or definitive wide local excision.	918 insured women ≤ 64 years old with local/ regional invasive breast cancer Stage I or II.	Data collected by Virginia Cancer Registry from 50 hospitals that represented 85% of Virginia hospital beds, and claims data from	92% had initial biopsy prior to total mastectomy.	Hillner et al., 1997

continues

Breast Cancer: Treatment

Includes various components of breast cancer treatment consistent with prevailing standards of care.	199 women 50–69 years old and 175 women ≥ 70 years old with adenocarcinoma of the breast receiving primary cancer management at a participating hospital.	Medical records from seven hospitals in southern California, for women with breast cancer diagnosed in 1980, to 1982.	67% of women ≥ 70 years old received appropriate treatment, compared with 83% of women 50–69 years old. After controlling for comorbidity, hospital, and cancer stage, a difference in appropriateness related to age persisted.	Greenfield et al., 1987
Breast conservation, defined as excision of the tumor and surrounding tissue, with axillary dissection, followed by radiation therapy, was preferable to mastectomy for the majority of women with Stage I or II breast cancer, as supported by clinical trials and a 1990 NIH Consensus Conference (NIH Consensus Conference, 1991).	8,095 women with a first primary breast cancer, Stage I or II.	Data from the Seattle-Puget Sound cancer registry, which covers cancer cases in 13 western Washington counties and is part of the Surveillance, Epidemiology, and End Results (SEER) program of the National Cancer Institute, 1983–1989.	34% had breast-conserving surgery.	Lazovich et al., 1991
Same as above.	2,657 women with complete records out of 2,731 women with a first primary breast cancer, Stage I or II, who underwent breast-conserving surgery.	Same as above.	85% received radiation therapy.	

Trigon Blue Cross Blue Shield of Virginia, 1989–1991.

TABLE A-1 Continued

Health Care Service[a]	Sample Description	Data Source	Quality of Care	Reference[b]
Same as above.	4,311 newly diagnosed patients with histologically confirmed Stage I–II breast cancer.	Data submitted to American Cancer Society, Illinois Division, Chicago, by 99 hospitals out of 104 Illinois hospitals with active cancer registries, 1988.	The average rate across hospitals of patients who did not receive radiotherapy after partial mastectomy was 48%.	Hand et al., 1991
Same as above.	918 insured women ≤ 64 years old with local/regional invasive breast cancer Stage I or II.	Data collected by Virginia Cancer Registry from 50 hospitals that represented 85% of Virginia hospital beds and claims data from Trigon Blue Cross Blue Shield of Virginia, 1989–1991.	86% received local breast radiation following lumpectomy.	Hillner et al., 1997
Patients with breast cancer have better outcomes if adjuvant therapy is given to patients with Stage II neoplasms.	2,248 newly diagnosed patients with histologically confirmed Stage II breast cancer.	Data submitted to American Cancer Society, Illinois Division, Chicago, by 99 out of 104 Illinois hospitals with active cancer registries, 1988.	The average rate across hospitals of patients who did not receive adjuvant therapy was 44%.	Hand et al., 1991
Premenopausal, node-positive women with local/regional breast cancer should receive adjuvant chemotherapy.	918 insured women ≤ 64 years old with local/ regional invasive breast cancer Stage I or II.	Data collected by Virginia Cancer Registry from 50 hospitals that represented 85% of Virginia hospital beds, and claims data from	83% of premenopausal women with at least one positive axillary node received adjuvant chemotherapy.	Hillner et al., 1997

Statement	Population	Data Source	Findings	Reference
		Trigon Blue Cross Blue Shield of Virginia, 1989, to 1991.		
Patients with breast cancer have better outcomes if axillary lymph node dissection is done as part of the surgical treatment with Stage I and II neoplasms.	4,311 newly diagnosed patients with histologically confirmed Stage I-II breast cancer	Data submitted to American Cancer Society, Illinois Division, Chicago, by 99 hospitals out of 104 Illinois hospitals with active cancer registries, 1988	The average rate across hospitals of patients who did not have a lymph node dissection was 9%.	Hand et al., 1991
Same as above.	918 insured women ≤ 64 years old with local/regional invasive breast cancer Stage I or II.	Data collected by Virginia Cancer Registry from 50 hospitals that represented 85% of Virginia hospital beds, and claims data from Trigon Blue Cross Blue Shield of Virginia, 1989–91.	88% underwent axillary node dissection.	Hillner et al., 1997
Women with early stage breast carcinoma (TNM Stages I and II) who undergo breast-conserving surgery should then receive radiation therapy.	1,292 women who underwent breast-conserving surgery from a sample of 2,575 women with early-stage breast carcinoma, excluding patients for whom national recommendations were not likely to apply.	Medical records, patient surveys, and physician surveys for patients from 18 Massachusetts hospitals from a stratified random sample of 20, from September 1993, to September 1995, and from 30 Minnesota hospitals, from January 1993, to December 1993.	84%–86% received radiation therapy after breast-conserving surgery.	Guadagnoli et al., 1998

continues

TABLE A-1 Continued

Health Care Service[a]	Sample Description	Data Source	Quality of Care	Reference[b]
For early-stage breast carcinoma (TNM Stages I and II), axillary lymph node dissection should be performed.	2,559 women who had axillary lymph node dissection from a sample of 2,575 women with early-stage breast carcinoma, excluding patients for whom national recommendations were not likely to apply.	Same as above.	81%–94% underwent axillary lymph node dissection.	Guadagnoli et al., 1998
For early-stage breast carcinoma (TNM Stages I and II), premenopausal women with positive lymph nodes should receive chemotherapy.	228 premenopausal women with positive lymph nodes from a sample of 2,575 women with early-stage breast carcinoma, excluding patients for whom national recommendations were not likely to apply.	Same as above.	94%–97% received chemotherapy.	Guadagnoli et al., 1998
For early-stage breast carcinoma (TNM Stages I and II), postmenopausal women with positive lymph nodes and positive estrogen receptor status should receive hormonal therapy.	168 postmenopausal women with positive lymph nodes and positive estrogen receptor status from a sample of 2,575 women with early-stage breast carcinoma, excluding patients for whom national recommendations were not likely to apply.	Same as above.	59%–63% received hormonal therapy.	Guadagnoli et al., 1998

Breast Cancer: Follow-up

Annual mammography is appropriate for women who have had local/regional breast cancer.	918 insured women ≤ 64 years old with local/regional invasive breast cancer Stage I or II.	Data collected by Virginia Cancer Registry from 50 hospitals that represented 85% of Virginia hospital beds, and claims data from Trigon Blue Cross Blue Shield of Virginia, 1989–1991.	79% of women had a mammogram within the first 18 months postoperatively.	Hillner et al., 1997

Cardiovascular Disease

Cardiovascular Disease: Blood Cholesterol Testing

Clinical trials have shown a 30%–50% reduction in morbidity and mortality rates with management of cholesterol levels for patients with cardiovascular disease (CVD). The Adult Treatment Panel (ATP-II) of the National Cholesterol Education Program recommended management of cholesterol in patients with CVD with goals of LDL level < 100 mg/dL and triglyceride level < 200 mg/dL (NCEP, 1993).	603 patients 27–70 years old with CVD.	Physician survey, patient survey, and medical records from 159 physicians in 45 primary care practices in and around four midwestern cities: Eau Claire, Wisconsin; Iowa City, Iowa; Madison, Wisconsin; Minneapolis, Minnesota; August 1993, to February 1995.	96% had total cholesterol levels, 67% had LDL values, 90% had triglyceride levels, and 75% had HDL levels recorded in the past 5 years. 72% with LDL > 130 mg/dL had received diet counseling, and 42% had received cholesterol-lowering medication; 58% with LDL 100–130 mg/dL had received diet counseling, and 42% had received cholesterol-lowering medication.	McBride et al., 1998

continues

TABLE A-1 Continued

Health Care Service[a]	Sample Description	Data Source	Quality of Care	Reference[b]
Coronary Artery Disease: Coronary Angiography				
Coronary angiography is a method for evaluating coronary artery anatomy to determine whether a patient is a candidate for coronary artery bypass graft surgery or percutaneous transluminal coronary angioplasty.	352 patients who met explicitly defined criteria for necessity of coronary angiography, from among a randomly selected sample of 5,850 stress tests.	Medical records from four teaching hospitals (three public, one private) in Los Angeles, California and patient telephone interviews (with 243 of the 352 patients), January 1, 1990, to June 30, 1991.	43% of patients received coronary angiography within 3 months of the positive exercise stress test; 56% received coronary angiography within 12 months of the positive test.	Laouri et al., 1997
Myocardial Infarction (MI): Treatment with Aspirin				
Aspirin is an effective, inexpensive, and safe treatment for a heart attack. Aspirin therapy reduces short-term mortality in patients with suspected heart attack by 23%. Aspirin should not be given to patients with certain conditions (e.g., hemorrhagic stroke, gastrointestinal bleeding).	7,917 Medicare patients ≥ 65 years old hospitalized with heart attack who were "ideal" candidates for treatment with aspirin, with no possible contraindications to aspirin therapy.	Medical records for Medicare beneficiaries who were hospitalized in four states (Alabama, Connecticut, Iowa, Wisconsin), as part of the Cooperative Cardiovascular Project Pilot, June 1, 1992, to February 28, 1993.	64% received aspirin within the first 2 days of hospitalization.	Krumholz et al., 1995
Same as above.	5,490 Medicare patients ≥ 65 years old hospitalized with heart attack who were alive at discharge and who had no contraindications to aspirin therapy.	Same as above.	76% were discharged with instructions to take aspirin. Patients who were prescribed aspirin at discharge had a 6-month mortality rate of 8.4%, compared with 17% for	Krumholz et al., 1996

Same as above.	7,486 patients who were "ideal" candidates for treatment with aspirin during initial hospitalization from a sample of 16,124 Medicare patients hospitalized with a principal diagnosis of heart attack; 5,841 patients who were alive at discharge and who were "ideal" candidates for treatment with aspirin prior to or at time of discharge, from the same sample.	Same as above.	83% received aspirin during hospitalization; 77% received aspirin prior to or at time of discharge.	Ellerbeck et al., 1995
Same as above.	187 patients with confirmed heart attack who were alive at discharge and who had no contraindications to aspirin therapy from a sample of 300 Medicare patients ≥ 65 years old hospitalized with a principal diagnosis of heart attack.	Medicare mortality data issued by the Health Care Financing Administration (HCFA) and medical records for Medicare patients from six hospitals in Connecticut, as part of the Medicare Hospital Information Project, October 1, 1988, to September 30, 1991.	73% received aspirin at time of discharge.	Meehan et al., 1995

patients not prescribed aspirin.

continues

TABLE A-1 Continued

Health Care Service[a]	Sample Description	Data Source	Quality of Care	Reference[b]
Same as above.	Subset of 2,938 patients with admitting diagnosis of MI.	Medical records from 16 Minnesota hospitals for patients admitted August 1, 1995, to April 30, 1996.	The median percentage of eligible patients ≥ 65 years old receiving aspirin in the first 48 hours of hospitalization was 77%.	Soumerai et al., 1998
Unstable Angina: Treatment with Aspirin				
Same as above.	384 patients who were "ideal" candidates for treatment with aspirin on admission and 321 who were "ideal" candidates for aspirin at discharge, from a sample of 450 patients ≥ 65 years old hospitalized with unstable angina.	Medical records and administrative data for patients with Medicare from three Connecticut hospitals, 1993–1995.	72% received aspirin on admission (66% in 1993–1994 and 82% in 1995). 65% were prescribed aspirin at discharge (66% in 1993–1994 and 79% in 1995).	Krumholz et al., 1998
Unstable Angina: Treatment with Aspirin				
Same as above.	735 patients who were "ideal" candidates for treatment with aspirin during hospitalization and 531 who were "ideal" candidates for aspirin at discharge, from a sample of 882 patients ≥ 65 years old with unstable angina.	Medical records of Medicare beneficiaries discharged from 16 hospitals in North Carolina between October 1, 1993, and September 30, 1994.	76% received aspirin during their hospital stay. 67% were prescribed aspirin at discharge.	Simpson et al., 1997

| Same as above. | 2,392 patients who were "ideal" candidates for aspirin during hospitalization and 1,387 who were "ideal" candidates for aspirin at discharge, from a sample of 4,300 patients with MI. | Medical records from acute care hospitals in Maryland and the District of Columbia in Medicare's National Claims History File sampled during January 1994, to July 1995. | 87% received aspirin during their stay. 77% received aspirin at discharge. | Berger et al., 1998 |

MI: Treatment with Thrombolytics

| Thrombolytics are medications that break down some of the acute blockage in the blood vessels that causes a heart attack, thereby reducing infarct size and limiting left ventricular dysfunction. Thrombolytics have been shown to reduce post-MI mortality by as much as 25%, though they should not be given to patients with certain conditions (e.g., recent hemorrhagic stroke). | 1,105 patients who were "ideal" candidates for treatment with thrombolytic agents from a sample of 16,124 Medicare patients hospitalized with a principal diagnosis of heart attack. | Medical records for Medicare beneficiaries who were hospitalized in four states (Alabama, Connecticut, Iowa, Wisconsin), as part of the Cooperative Cardiovascular Project Pilot, June 1, 1992, to February 28, 1993. | 70% received thrombolytics during hospitalization. | Ellerbeck et al., 1995 |
| Same as above. | 68 patients with confirmed heart attack who had no contraindications to thrombolytic therapy, and who had electrocardiographic indications for thrombolytic therapy, from a sample of 300 Medicare patients ≥ 65 years old | Medicare mortality data issued by HCFA and medical records for Medicare patients from 6 hospitals in Connecticut, as part of the Medicare Hospital Information Project, October 1, 1988, to September 30, 1991. | 43% received thrombolytics during hospitalization | Meehan et al., 1995 |

continues

TABLE A-1 Continued

Health Care Service[a]	Sample Description	Data Source	Quality of Care	Reference[b]
	hospitalized with a principal diagnosis of heart attack.			
Same as above.	245 patients who were "ideal" candidates for thrombolytics in the first hour of arrival from a sample of 4,300 patients with MI.	Medical records from acute care hospitals in Maryland and the District of Columbia in Medicare's National Claims History File sampled during January 1994, to July 1995.	60% received thrombolytics within 1 hour after arrival.	Berger et al., 1998
Same as above.	Subset of 2,938 patients with admitting diagnosis of MI.	Medical records from 16 Minnesota hospitals for patients admitted August 1, 1995, to April 30, 1996.	The median percentage of eligible patients ≥ 65 years old receiving thrombolytics in the first 48 hours of hospitalization was 55%.	Soumerai et al., 1998
MI: Reperfusion (Thrombolysis/Percutaneous Transluminal Coronary Angioplasty [PTCA]) PTCA uses a miniature balloon catheter to decrease stenosis (blockage) in blood vessels supplying the heart. (Thrombolysis is described above.)	398 patients who were considered "ideal" candidates for reperfusion from a sample of 4,300 patients with MI.	Medical records from acute care hospitals in Maryland and the District of Columbia in Medicare's National Claims History File sampled during January 1994, to June 1995.	64% received reperfusion therapy (thrombolysis/ PTCA) within 12 hours of arrival at hospital.	Berger et al., 1998

MI: Treatment with Heparin

Indicator	Sample	Data Source	Findings	Reference
Heparin is beneficial to patients with heart attack, though heparin should not be given to patients with certain conditions (e.g., bleeding disorders, stroke).	9,857 patients who were "ideal" candidates for treatment with heparin from a sample of 16,124 Medicare patients hospitalized with a principal diagnosis of heart attack.	Medical records for Medicare beneficiaries who were hospitalized in four states (Alabama, Connecticut, Iowa, Wisconsin), as part of the Cooperative Cardiovascular Project Pilot, June 1, 1992, to February 28, 1993.	69% received heparin during hospitalization.	Ellerbeck et al., 1995

Unstable Angina: Treatment with Heparin

Indicator	Sample	Data Source	Findings	Reference
Same as above.	369 patients who were "ideal" candidates for treatment with heparin, from a sample of 450 patients $\geq$ 65 years old hospitalized with unstable angina.	Medical records and administrative data for patients with Medicare from three Connecticut hospitals, 1993–1995.	24% received intravenous heparin (20% in 1993 to 1994 and 32% in 1995). Of those receiving heparin, 51% had a therapeutic activated partial thromboplastin time (PTT) within 24 hours.	Krumholz et al., 1998
Same as above.	91 patients who were considered "ideal" candidates for heparin intravenously administered, from a sample of 882 patients $\geq$ 65 years old with unstable angina.	Medical records of Medicare beneficiaries discharged from 16 hospitals in North Carolina between October 1, 1993, and September 30, 1994.	63% received heparin administered intravenously.	Simpson et al., 1997

continues

TABLE A-1 Continued

Health Care Service[a]	Sample Description	Data Source	Quality of Care	Reference[b]
MI: Treatment with Intravenous Nitroglycerin				
Intravenous nitroglycerin is beneficial to patients with heart attack who have persistent chest pain, although intravenous nitroglycerin should not be given to patients with certain conditions (e.g., shock or hypotension on admission).	1,754 patients who were "ideal" candidates for treatment with intravenous nitroglycerin from a sample of 16,124 Medicare patients hospitalized with a principal diagnosis of heart attack.	Medical records for Medicare beneficiaries who were hospitalized in four states (Alabama, Connecticut, Iowa, Wisconsin), as part of Cooperative Cardiovascular Project Pilot, June 1, 1992, to February 28, 1993.	74% received intravenous nitroglycerin during hospitalization.	Ellerbeck et al., 1995
MI: Smoking Cessation Advice				
Smokers with coronary artery disease who stop smoking have a better prognosis than those who keep smoking; at the time of heart attack, these smokers are most susceptible to advice about cessation of smoking.	1,691 smokers who were "ideal" candidates for smoking cessation advice from a sample of 16,124 Medicare patients hospitalized with a principal diagnosis of heart attack.	Same as above.	28% received smoking cessation advice prior to or at time of discharge.	Ellerbeck et al., 1995
Same as above.	551 patients who were smokers from a sample of 4,300 patients with MI.	Medical records from acute care hospitals in Maryland and the District of Columbia in Medicare's National Claims History File sampled during January 1994, to July 1995.	41% received smoking cessation advice.	Berger et al., 1998

Unstable Angina: Smoking Cessation Advice

Same as above.	133 patients who were identified as smokers, from a sample of 882 patients ≥ 65 years old with unstable angina.	Medical records of Medicare beneficiaries discharged from 16 hospitals in North Carolina between October 1, 1993, and September 30, 1994.	23% received smoking cessation counseling.	Simpson et al., 1997

MI: Treatment with Angiotensin-Converting Enzyme (ACE) Inhibitors

ACE inhibitors can reduce post-MI mortality in patients with left ventricular dysfunction, although ACE inhibitors should not be given to patients with certain conditions (e.g., aortic stenosis).	1,473 patients who were "ideal" candidates for treatment with ACE inhibitors from a sample of 16,124 Medicare patients hospitalized with a principal diagnosis of heart attack.	Medical records for Medicare beneficiaries who were hospitalized in four states (Alabama, Connecticut, Iowa, Wisconsin), as part of Cooperative Cardiovascular Project Pilot, June 1, 1992, to February 28, 1993.	59% received ACE inhibitors prior to or at time of discharge.	Ellerbeck et al., 1995
Same as above.	407 patients who were considered "ideal" candidates for ACE inhibitors from a sample of 4,300 patients with MI.	Medical records from acute care hospitals in Maryland and the District of Columbia in Medicare's National Claims History File sampled during January 1994, to July 1995.	65% received ACE inhibitors for low ejection fraction (EF).	Berger et al., 1998

Unstable Angina: Treatment with ACE Inhibitors

Same as above.	177 patients who were considered "ideal" candidates for an ACE	Medical records of Medicare beneficiaries discharged from 16	39% received an ACE inhibitor during hospitalization. 42%	Simpson et al., 1997

continues

TABLE A-1 Continued

Health Care Service[a]	Sample Description	Data Source	Quality of Care	Reference[b]
	inhibitor during hospitalization and 127 who were "ideal" candidates for an ACE inhibitor at discharge, from a sample of 882 patients ≥ 65 years old with unstable angina.	hospitals in North Carolina between October 1, 1993, and September 30, 1994.	received an ACE inhibitor at discharge.	
MI: Treatment with Beta Blockers Beta blocker therapy can reduce post-MI mortality by as much as 25%, although beta blockers should not be given to patients with certain conditions (e.g., low left ventricular ejection fraction, pulmonary edema).	2,976 patients who were "ideal" candidates for treatment with beta blockers from a sample of 16,124 Medicare patients hospitalized with a principal diagnosis of heart attack.	Medical records for Medicare beneficiaries who were hospitalized in four states (Alabama, Connecticut, Iowa, Wisconsin), as part of Cooperative Cardiovascular Project Pilot, June 1, 1992, to February 28, 1993.	45% received beta blockers prior to or at time of discharge.	Ellerbeck et al., 1995
Same as above.	3,737 Medicare patients ≥ 65 years old with principal diagnosis of heart attack who were eligible for treatment with beta blockers, from a statewide cohort of 5,332 people who had survived a heart attack for at least 30 days and	New Jersey Medicare hospital admissions and enrollment data, 1986–1992; New Jersey Medicaid drug utilization and enrollment files, 1986–1991; New Jersey Program of Pharmacy Assistance for the Aged and Disabled drug	21% received beta blockers within 90 days of discharge; adjusted mortality rate for patients with treatment was 43% lower than that of patients without treatment.	Soumerai et al., 1997

Intervention	Population	Data Source	Findings	Reference
	who had prescription drug coverage.	utilization data, 1986–1991.		
Same as above.	104 patients with confirmed heart attack who were alive at discharge and who had no contraindications to beta blockers from a sample of 300 Medicare patients ≥ 65 years old hospitalized with a principal diagnosis of heart attack.	Medicare mortality data issued by HCFA and medical records for Medicare patients from 6 hospitals in Connecticut, as part of the Medicare Hospital Information Project, October 1, 1988, to September 30, 1991.	41% received beta blockers at time of discharge.	Meehan et al., 1995

MI: Treatment with Beta Blockers

Intervention	Population	Data Source	Findings	Reference
Same as above.	Subset of 2,938 patients with admitting diagnosis of MI.	Medical records from 16 Minnesota hospitals for patients admitted August 1, 1995, to April 30, 1996.	The median percentage of eligible patients receiving beta blockers in the first 48 hours of hospitalization was 78%.	Soumerai et al., 1998
Same as above.	302 patients who were considered "ideal" candidates for beta blockers at discharge from a sample of 4,300 patients with MI.	Medical records from acute care hospitals in Maryland and the District of Columbia in Medicare's National Claims History File sampled during January 1994, to July 1995.	60% received beta blockers at discharge.	Berger et al., 1998

Unstable Angina: Treatment with Beta Blockers

Intervention	Population	Data Source	Findings	Reference
Same as above.	815 patients who were "ideal" candidates for beta	Medical records of Medicare beneficiaries	45% received beta blockers during hospitalization.	Simpson et al., 1997

continues

TABLE A-1 Continued

Health Care Service[a]	Sample Description	Data Source	Quality of Care	Reference[b]
	blockers during hospitalization and 589 who were "ideal" candidates for beta blockers at discharge, from a sample of 882 patients ≥ 65 years old with unstable angina.	discharged from sixteen hospitals in North Carolina between October 1, 1993, and September 30, 1994.	38% received beta blockers at discharge.	
MI: Hospital Care Includes documentation of examination of jugular veins and alcoholism/smoking habits.	1,437 patients hospitalized with acute myocardial infarction from a nationally representative sample of 7,156 patients hospitalized with any of five conditions (congestive heart failure, acute myocardial infarction, pneumonia, stroke, hip fracture) (Draper et al., 1990).	Medical records for Medicare patients from 297 hospitals in five states (California, Florida, Indiana, Pennsylvania, Texas), July 1, 1985, to June 30, 1986.	64%–68% of patients with acute myocardial infarction received appropriate components of care.	Kahn et al., 1990
Unstable Angina: Low-Cholesterol Diet Includes care for unstable angina consistent with prevailing standards of care.	637 discharged patients who were "ideal" candidates for a low-cholesterol diet, from a sample of 882 patients ≥ 65 years old with unstable angina.	Medical records of Medicare beneficiaries discharged from 16 hospitals in North Carolina and September 30, 1994.	38% were prescribed a low-cholesterol diet at discharge.	Simpson et al., 1997

Unstable Angina: Lipid-Lowering Drugs Includes care for unstable angina consistent with prevailing standards of care.	637 patients who were "ideal" candidates for a lipid-lowering drug at discharge, from a sample of 882 patients ≥ 65 years old with unstable angina.	Same as above.	16% received lipid-lowering drugs at discharge.	Simpson et al., 1997
Congestive Heart Failure: Hospital Care Includes documentation of past surgery and lung examination, blood pressure readings, electrocardiogram, serum potassium level, oxygen therapy or intubation for hypoxic patients.	1,465 patients hospitalized with congestive heart failure from a nationally representative sample of 7,156 patients hospitalized with any of five conditions (congestive heart failure, acute myocardial infarction, pneumonia, stroke, hip fracture) (Draper et al., 1990).	Same as above.	66%–97% of patients with congestive heart failure received appropriate components of care.	Kahn et al., 1990
Stroke: Hospital Care Includes documentation of previous stroke and gag reflex, blood pressure readings, electrocardiogram, serum potassium level.	1,442 patients hospitalized with stroke from a sample of 7,156 patients hospitalized with any of five conditions (congestive heart failure, acute myocardial infarction, pneumonia, stroke, hip fracture) (Draper et al., 1990).	Same as above.	38%–94% of patients with stroke received appropriate components of care.	Kahn et al., 1990

aIf a description in the first column has no citation, it is covered by the citation in the reference column. bWe contacted the authors of some of the articles to clarify details related to the sample and to the data analysis.

TABLE A-2 Examples of Quality of Acute Health Care in the United States—Overuse: Did Patients Receive Inappropriate Care?

Health Care Service[a]	Sample Description	Data Source	Quality of Care	Reference[b]
Antibiotic Use *Common Cold* Almost all colds are caused by a virus, for which antibiotics are not an effective treatment.	1,439 patients with 2,171 outpatient and emergency department visits for the common cold (acute nasopharyngitis) from a random sample of 50,000 patients with at least one claim for care by a physician, dentist, or optometrist.	Kentucky Medicaid claims data, July 1, 1993, to June 30, 1994.	In 60% of encounters for the common cold, patients filled prescriptions for antibiotics.	Mainous et al., 1996
Same as above.	Patients ≥ 18 years old with a diagnosis of the common cold, exclusive of adults with underlying lung disease, from a nationally representative sample of 1,529 physicians representing 28,787 adult patient ambulatory care visits.	National Ambulatory Medical Care Survey (NAMCS), 1992.	51% of patients diagnosed with a cold were treated with antibiotics.	Gonzales et al., 1997

Same as above.	Children ≤ 18 years diagnosed with common colds from a total of 531 pediatric office visits with a primary diagnosis of cold, upper respiratory tract infection (URI), or bronchitis, exclusive of children with underlying lung disease, from a sample representative of the U.S. population.	Same as above.	Antibiotics were prescribed at 44% of visits of patients with common colds	Nyquist et al., 1998
Upper Respiratory Tract Infection Antimicrobial drugs do not shorten the course of viral URI, nor do they prevent secondary bacterial infections.	Physicians who participated from a nationally representative sample of 3,000 office-based physicians.	Same as above.	16% of all antimicrobial drug prescriptions (an estimated 17,922,000 prescriptions nationally) were written for upper respiratory tract infections in 1992.	McCaig and Hughes, 1995
Same as above.	Patients ≥ 18 years old with a diagnosis of URI, exclusive of adults with underlying lung disease, from a nationally representative sample of 1,529 physicians representing 28,787 adult patient ambulatory care visits.	Same as above.	52% of patients diagnosed with a URI were treated with antibiotics.	Gonzales et al., 1997

continues

TABLE A-2 Continued

Health Care Service[a]	Sample Description	Data Source	Quality of Care	Reference[b]
Same as above.	Children ≤ 18 years diagnosed with URIs from a total of 531 pediatric office visits with a primary diagnosis of cold, URI, or bronchitis, exclusive of children with underlying lung disease, from a sample representative of the U.S. population.	Same as above.	Antibiotics were prescribed at 46% of visits of patients with URIs.	Nyquist et al., 1998
Pharyngitis, Nasal Congestion, Common Cold, and Other Upper Respiratory Tract Infections				
Since most of these conditions are viral, antibiotics have no benefit.	Physicians who participated from a nationally representative sample of 3,000 office-based physicians.	Same as above.	Over 70% of patients received antibiotic prescriptions for pharyngitis (excluding streptococcal), over 50% received them for rhinitis, and over 30% received them for a nonspecific URI, cough, or cold.	Dowell and Schwartz, 1997

Bronchitis Most cases of bronchitis are caused by a virus, for which antibiotics are not an effective treatment.	Patients ≥ 18 years old with a diagnosis of bronchitis, exclusive of adults with underlying lung disease, from a nationally representative sample of 1,529 physicians representing 28,787 adult patient ambulatory care visits.	Same as above.	66% of patients diagnosed with bronchitis were treated with antibiotics.	Gonzales et al., 1997
Same as above.	Children ≤ 18 years diagnosed with bronchitis from a total of 531 pediatric office visits with a primary diagnosis of cold, URI, or bronchitis, exclusive of children with underlying lung disease, from a sample representative of the U.S. population.	Same as above.	Antibiotics were prescribed at 75% of visits of patients with bronchitis.	Nyquist et al., 1998
Respiratory Illness *Pneumonia* Hospital admissions for pneumonia are considered appropriate when, for example, a patient fails to improve with outpatient oral medication or has a pleural effusion or an empyema.	445 hospital admissions of children < 18 years old admitted with pneumonia.	Medical records for patients from 12 hospitals in five communities in Boston and nearby suburbs, July 1, 1985, to June 30, 1986.	9.4% of admissions were inappropriate.	Payne et al., 1995

continues

TABLE A-2 Continued

Health Care Service[a]	Sample Description	Data Source	Quality of Care	Reference[b]
Bronchitis/Asthma Hospital admissions for bronchitis/asthma are considered appropriate when, for example, a patient has failed to improve with outpatient therapy or has a pneumothorax.	1,038 hospital admissions of children < 18 years old admitted with bronchitis/asthma.	Same as above.	4.4% of admissions were inappropriate.	Payne et al., 1995
Otitis Media *Use of Tympanostomy Tubes* Indications for tympanostomy tube placement include refractory middle ear infection and chronic mastoiditis.	6,429 children < 16 years old with recurrent acute otitis media and/or persistent otitis media with effusion who were insured in health plans requiring precertification by a utilization review firm.	Interviews with physicians' office staff at otolaryngology practices from 49 states and the District of Columbia, January 1, 1990, to July 30, 1991; additional interviews were conducted with otolaryngologists to determine the existence of extenuating clinical circumstances.	41% of tube insertions were appropriate, 32% equivocal, and 27% inappropriate. If extenuating clinical circumstances were taken into account, 42% of tube insertions were appropriate, 35% equivocal, and 23% inappropriate.	Kleinman et al., 1994

Depression

Depression: Treatment

There is no evidence that minor tranquilizers are effective for depression, but there is evidence that antidepressant medications are effective for depression.	634 patients with current depressive disorder or depressive symptoms from a sample of 22,399 adult patients who visited one large HMO or several multispecialty, mixed-group practices in each city during the study period.	Medical Outcomes Study (MOS) in three cities (Boston, Chicago, Los Angeles); questionnaires completed February to October 1986; phone interviews completed May to December 1986.	19% of patients were treated with minor tranquilizers; 12% were treated with antidepressant medications; 11% were treated with a combination of minor tranquilizers and antidepressant medications; 59% received neither.	Wells et al., 1994a

Depression: Admission

Appropriate reasons for admission include depression, medical condition meriting acute care, comorbid major psychiatric disorder, or medical reasons precluding outpatient care for depression.	1,198 patients hospitalized with depression, representative of all Medicare elderly patients hospitalized in general medical hospitals with a discharge diagnosis of depression.	Medical records for Medicare patients from 297 hospitals in five states (California, Florida, Indiana, Pennsylvania, Texas), July 1, 1985, to June 30, 1986.	93% were admitted for clearly or possibly appropriate reasons, and 7% were admitted for inappropriate reasons.	Wells et al., 1993

Hysterectomy

Hysterectomy

Hysterectomy is the surgical removal of the uterus.	642 women ≥ 20 years old who underwent nonemergency, nononcologic hysterectomies.	Medical records for patients from seven managed care organizations, August 1, 1989, to July 31, 1990.	16% of hysterectomies were inappropriate, 25% were equivocal, and 58% were appropriate.	Bernstein et al., 1993b

continues

TABLE A-2 Continued

Health Care Service[a]	Sample Description	Data Source	Quality of Care	Reference[b]
Cardiovascular Disease				
Coronary Artery Disease: Coronary Angiography				
Coronary angiography is a method for evaluating coronary artery anatomy to determine whether a patient is a candidate for coronary artery bypass graft surgery or percutaneous transluminal coronary angioplasty.	Random sample of 1,335 patients who had coronary angiography.	Medical records from 15 nonfederal hospitals providing coronary angiography in New York State, selected through a stratified random sample (for location, volume of coronary angiography, and authorization to perform coronary artery bypass graft surgery), 1990.	4% of coronary angiographies were inappropriate, 20% were equivocal, and 76% were appropriate.	Bernstein et al., 1993a
Same as above.	Random sample of 1,677 cases of coronary angiography.	Medicare physician claims from three sites selected from 13 sites in eight states (Arizona, California, Colorado, Iowa, Massachusetts, Montana, Pennsylvania, South Carolina), 1981.	17% of coronary inappropriate, 9% were equivocal, and 74% were appropriate.	Chassin et al., 1987

Coronary Artery Disease: Coronary Artery Bypass Graft (CABG)
In CABG surgery, damaged blood vessels supplying the heart are replaced with vessels from elsewhere in the body.

Stratified random sample of 386 patients who underwent CABG surgery in the three hospitals.	Medical records from three hospitals (excluding Veterans Administration, other governmental, and specialty hospitals) selected through a stratified random sample (for size and teaching status) in a western state as part of the National Institutes of Health Consensus Development Program, 1979, 1980, and 1982	14% of CABG surgeries were inappropriate, 30% were equivocal, and 56% were appropriate.	Winslow et al., 1988
Random sample of 1,156 patients who had isolated CABG surgery.	Medical records for patients from 12 Academic Medical Center Consortium hospitals in 10 states (California, Iowa, Louisiana, Maryland, Massachusetts, Minnesota, New Hampshire, New York, North Carolina, Pennsylvania), 1990.	1.6% of CABG surgeries were inappropriate, 7% were equivocal, and 92% were appropriate.	Leape et al., 1996
Same as above.	Random sample of 1,338 patients who had isolated CABG surgery.	Medical records from 15 nonfederal hospitals providing CABG procedure in New York State, selected through a stratified random sample (for location and volume of CABG operations), 1990.	2.4% of CABG surgeries were inappropriate, 7% were equivocal, and 91% were appropriate.	Leape et al., 1993

continues

TABLE A-2 Continued

Health Care Service[a]	Sample Description	Data Source	Quality of Care	Reference[b]
Coronary Artery Disease: Percutaneous Transluminal Coronary Angioplasty (PTCA)				
PTCA uses a miniature balloon catheter to decrease stenosis (blockage) in blood vessels supplying the heart.	Random sample of 1,306 patients who had PTCA.	Medical records from 15 nonfederal hospitals providing PTCA in New York State, selected through a stratified random sample (for location and volume of PTCA), 1990.	4% of PTCAs were inappropriate, 38% were equivocal, and 58% were appropriate.	Hilborne et al., 1993
Myocardial Infarction (MI): Permanent Cardiac Pacemaker				
Pacemakers help regularize abnormal heart rates and rhythms.	Medicare patients who underwent a total of 382 pacemaker implantations.	Medical records from six university teaching hospitals, 11 university-affiliated hospitals, and 13 community hospitals in Philadelphia County, January 1, to June 30, 1983.	20% of pacemaker implantations were inappropriate, 36% were equivocal, and 44% were appropriate.	Greenspan et al., 1988
MI: Treatment with Lidocaine				
Lidocaine prophylaxis used to prevent ventricular fibrillation in patients treated for probable MI has been shown to increase mortality.	Subset of 2,938 patients with admitting diagnosis of MI.	Medical records from sixteen Minnesota hospitals for patients admitted August 1, 1995, to April 30, 1996.	The median percentage of patients ineligible for lidocaine who received it in the first 48 hours of hospitalization was 12%.	Soumerai et al., 1998

MI: Avoidance of Calcium Channel Blockers for Patients with a Contraindication

Calcium channel blockers should not be given to patients with certain conditions (e.g., low left ventricular ejection fraction, evidence of shock, or pulmonary edema during hospitalization).	785 patients with clear contraindication to calcium channel blockers from a sample of 16,124 Medicare patients hospitalized with a principal diagnosis of heart attack.	Medical records for Medicare beneficiaries who were hospitalized in four states (Alabama, Connecticut, Iowa, Wisconsin), as part of the Cooperative Cardiovascular Project Pilot, June 1, 1992, to February 28, 1993.	21% of those for whom calcium channel blockers were contraindicated received them.	Ellerbeck et al., 1995
Same as above.	220 patients with a contraindication for calcium channel blockers (i.e., a left ventricular ejection fraction < 40%) from a sample of 4,300 patients with MI.	Medical records from acute care hospitals in Maryland and the District of Columbia in Medicare's National Claims History File sampled during January 1994, to July 1995.	18% of those for whom calcium blockers were contraindicated received them.	Berger et al., 1998

Unstable Angina: Avoidance of Calcium Channel Blockers for Patients with a Contraindication

Same as above.	218 patients with contraindications for calcium channel blocking drugs, from a sample of 882 patients ≥ 65 years old with unstable angina.	Medical records of Medicare beneficiaries discharged from 16 hospitals in North Carolina between October 1, 1993, and September 30, 1994.	62% of those for whom calcium blockers were contraindicated received them.	Simpson et al., 1997

continues

TABLE A-2 Continued

Health Care Service[a]	Sample Description	Data Source	Quality of Care	Reference[b]
Carotid Arteries				
Carotid Endarterectomy				
Carotid endarterectomy is a procedure that opens up stenotic (blocked) carotid arteries (which supply blood to the brain).	Random sample of 1,302 cases of carotid endarterectomy.	Medicare physician claims data and medical records from three sites selected from thirteen sites in eight states (Arizona, California, Colorado, Iowa, Massachusetts, Montana, Pennsylvania, South Carolina), 1981.	32% of carotid endarterectomies were inappropriate, 32% were equivocal, and 35% were appropriate.	Chassin et al., 1987
Gastrointestinal Disease				
Upper Gastrointestinal Tract Endoscopy				
Endoscopy enables visualization of the gastrointestinal tract, and permits biopsy and brush cytologic examination.	Random sample of 1,585 cases of upper gastrointestinal tract endoscopy.	Same as above.	17% of upper gastrointestinal tract endoscopies were inappropriate, 11% were equivocal, and 72% were appropriate.	Chassin et al., 1987
Cataracts				
Cataract Surgery				
Cataract surgery is a commonly performed surgery in adults ≥ 65 years old. Cataract surgery should not be performed on people with certain conditions (e.g., macular degeneration or diabetic retinopathy).	1,020 patients who underwent a total of 1,139 cataract surgeries.	Medical records for patients from 10 academic medical centers, 1990.	2% of cataract surgeries were inappropriate, 7% were equivocal, and 91% were appropriate.	Tobacman et al. 1996

Low Back Pain

Chiropractic Spinal Manipulation

AHCPR has concluded that spinal manipulation hastens recovery from acute low back pain not caused by such conditions as fracture, tumor, infection, and cauda equina syndrome (AHCPR, 1994).	A random sample of 10 patients per office (920 patients) who sought chiropractic care for low back pain for the first time during the study period.	Medical records of patients from 92 chiropractic offices in or near Miami, Florida; Minneapolis-St. Paul, Minnesota; Portland, Oregon; and San Diego, California; who sought care for the first time between January 1, 1985, and December 31, 1991.	Initiation of spinal manipulation was inappropriate in 20%–40% of cases, uncertain in 20%–30% of cases, and appropriate in 40%–54% of cases (depending on city).	Shekelle et al., 1998

[a]If a description in the first column has no citation, it is covered by the citation in the reference column. [b]We contacted the authors of some of the articles to clarify details related to the sample and to the data analysis.

TABLE A-3 Examples of Quality of Health Care in the United States Misuse: Did Patients Receive Appropriate Care in a Manner That Could Have Caused Harm?

Health Care Service[a]	Sample Description	Data Source	Quality of Care	Reference[b]
Preventable Deaths				
Evaluation of preventable deaths				
A death is considered preventable when the patient received poor care, and the poor care probably resulted in the patient's death.	182 patients who died in hospitals from stroke, pneumonia, or heart attack.	Medical records for patients from 12 hospitals, 1985.	14% of deaths resulted from inadequate diagnosis or treatment and could have been prevented.	Dubois and Brook, 1988
Adverse Events				
Adverse Events				
An adverse event is an injury that is caused by medical management rather than the underlying disease and that prolongs hospitalization, produces a disability at discharge, or both.	30,121 medical records from a weighted sample of 31,429 records of hospitalized patients from a population of 2,671,863 nonpsychiatric discharged patients.	51 randomly selected acute care, nonpsychiatric hospitals in New York State, 1984.	There were 1,133 adverse events and 280 negligent events during 1984 admissions, representing a 3.7% statewide incidence rate of adverse events, and a 1.0% statewide incidence rate of adverse events due to negligence.	Brennan et al., 1991

Same as above.	30,121 medical records from a weighted sample of 31,429 records of hospitalized patients from a population of 2,671,863 nonpsychiatric discharged patients.	51 randomly selected acute care, nonpsychiatric hospitals in New York State, 1984.	17% of adverse events resulting from operations and 37% of other adverse events were due to negligence; 47% of physician errors leading to adverse events were due to negligence.	Leape et al., 1991

Adverse Drug Events

Same as above.	4,031 adult nonobstetric admissions to a stratified random sample of 11 medical and surgical units in two hospitals.	Medical records and reports of hospital staff for 2 tertiary care hospitals in Boston, February to July 1993.	There were 1.8 preventable adverse drugs events (ADEs) per 100 admissions (adjusted rate), of which 20% were life threatening, 43% were serious, and 37% were significant. There were an additional 5.5 potential ADEs per 100 admissions (adjusted rate).	Bates et al., 1995
Same as above.	4,031 patients admitted to 5 intensive care units (3 medical, 2 surgical) and 6 general care units (4 medical, 2 surgical) selected from a stratified random sample of units in 2 tertiary care hospitals in Boston.	Case-investigation reports (including staff interviews, medical record review, etc.) for patients admitted between February and July 1993.	There were 19 preventable or potential ADEs per 1000 patient days in the ICUs. There were 10 preventable or potential ADEs per 1000 patient days in general care units. Rates adjusted for number of medications per patient showed no significant differences for the two settings.	Cullen et al., 1997

continues

TABLE A-3 Continued

Health Care Service[a]	Sample Description	Data Source	Quality of Care	Reference[b]
Mental Health				
Depression: Treatment				
Includes treatment consistent with prevailing standards of care.	1,198 patients hospitalized with depression, representative of all Medicare elderly patients hospitalized in general medical hospitals with a discharge diagnosis of depression.	Medical records for Medicare patients from 297 hospitals in five states (California, Florida, Indiana, Pennsylvania, Texas), July 1, 1985, to June 30, 1986.	33% of patients discharged with antidepressants had doses below recommended level.	Wells et al., 1994b
Includes treatment consistent with prevailing standards of care.	64 patients with major depression from a sample of 2,592 consecutive primary care patients 18–65 years old who attended one of the study clinics.	Patient surveys and interviews, physician surveys, and computerized pharmacy records from 3 primary care clinics of Group Health Cooperative of Puget Sound in Washington.	Among patients with major depression who received antidepressant medications, 78% received dosages within the recommended ranges.	Simon and VonKorff, 1995

Tuberculosis

Tuberculosis: Treatment

People infected with tuberculosis (TB) in areas with ≥ 4% isoniazid resistance should be treated with a four-drug regimen.	1,230 culture-positive TB patients, 98% of whom were in counties for which a four-drug regimen is recommended.	Data from the Tuberculosis Control Program, New Jersey Department of Health and Senior Services, 1994 to 1995.	36% of patients were not initially treated with four or more drugs.	Liu et al., 1998

[a]If a description in the first column has no citation, it is covered by the citation in the reference column. [b]We contacted the authors of some of the articles to clarify details related to the sample and to the data analysis.

APPENDIX: Search Strategy for January 1997–July 1998 MEDLINE PLUS
Search

Search Type	Medical Subject Heading (MeSH) Search Term	Tree Number[a]	Boolean Operator
Subject	Quality of health care	N4.761	or
Subject	Guideline adherence	N4.761.337	or
Explode exact subject[b]	Outcome and process assessment, health care	N4.761.761.559	
Subject	Professional review organization	N4.761.673	or
Subject	Quality indicators, health care	N4.761.789	and
Language	English		and
Date	1997, 1998		

NOTE: As Boolean operators, "or" means that articles with one search term and/or another search term are included, and "and" means that articles must have both search terms (or strings of search terms) to be included. For this search, articles with any of the Medical Subject Headings (MeSH) were included, and only articles in English and from 1997 or 1998 were included.

[a]Tree Number is a National Library of Medicine alphanumerical code for indexing MeSH terms.

[b]The "Explode" search function includes the MeSH category as well as all the subcategorical branches connected to it. It is equivalent to typing out the MeSH term and each of its subcategorical branches separately. The subcategories included when exploding "Outcome and Process Assessment, Health Care" are: Outcome Assessment, Treatment Outcome, Medical Futility, Treatment Failure, and Process Assessment.

Appendix B

Redesigning Health Care with Insights from the Science of Complex Adaptive Systems

Paul Plsek

The task of building the 21st-century health care system is large and complex. In this appendix, we will lay a theoretical framework for approaching the design of complex systems and discuss the practical implications.

SYSTEMS THINKING

A "system" can be defined by the coming together of parts, interconnections, and purpose (see, for example, definitions proposed by von Bertalanffy [1968] and Capra [1996]). While systems can be broken down into parts which are interesting in and of themselves, the real power lies in the way the parts come together and are interconnected to fulfill some purpose.

The health care system of the United States consists of various parts (e.g., clinics, hospitals, pharmacies, laboratories) that are interconnected (via flows of patients and information) to fulfill a purpose (e.g., maintaining and improving health). Similarly, a thermostat and fan are a "system." Both parts can be understood independently, but when they are interconnected, they fulfill the purpose of maintaining a comfortable temperature in a given space.

The intuitive notion of various system "levels," such as the microsystem and macrosystem, has to do with the number and strength of interconnections between the elements of the systems. For example, a doctor's office or clinic can be described as a microsystem. It is small and self-contained, with relatively few interconnections. Patients, physicians, nurses, and office staff interact to produce

Consultant, Paul E. Plsek and Associates, Inc., Roswell, Georgia.

diagnoses, treatments, and information. In contrast, the health care system in a community is a macrosystem. It consists of numerous microsystems (doctor's offices, hospitals, long-term care facilities, pharmacies, Internet websites, and so on) that are linked to provide continuity and comprehensiveness of care. Similarly, a thermostat and fan comprise a relatively simple microsystem. Combine many of these, along with various boiler, refrigerant, and computer-control microsystems, and one has a macrosystem that can maintain an office building environment.

A distinction can also be made between systems that are largely mechanical in nature and those that are naturally adaptive (see Table B-1). The distinctions between mechanical and naturally adaptive systems are fundamental and key to the task of system design. In mechanical systems, we can know and predict in great detail what each of the parts will do in response to a given stimulus. Thus, it is possible to study and predict in great detail what the system will do in a variety of circumstances. Complex mechanical systems rarely exhibit surprising, emergent behavior. When they do—for example, an airplane explosion or computer network crash—experts study the phenomenon in detail to design surprise out of future systems.

In complex adaptive systems, on the other hand, the "parts" (in the case of the U.S. health care system, this includes human beings) have the freedom and ability to respond to stimuli in many different and fundamentally unpredictable ways. For this reason, emergent, surprising, creative behavior is a real possibility. Such behavior can be for better or for worse; that is, it can manifest itself as either innovation or error. Further, such emergent behavior can occur at both the microsystem and macrosystem levels. The evolving relationship of trust between a patient and clinician is an example of emergence at the microsystem level. The AIDS epidemic is an example of emergence that affects the macrosystem of care.

TABLE B-1   Mechanical Versus Naturally Adaptive Systems

Type of System	Mechanical	Naturally Adaptable
Simple	Thermostat and fan	Patient giving history information to a physician
Complex	Office building heating, ventilation and air conditioning	U.S. health care

The distinction between mechanical and naturally adaptive systems is obvious when given some thought. However, many system designers do not seem to take this distinction into account. Rather, they design complex human systems as if the parts and interconnections were predictable in their behavior, although fundamentally, they are not. When the human parts do not act as expected or hoped for, we say that people are being "unreasonable" or "resistant to change," their behavior is "wrong" or "inappropriate." The system designer's reaction typically is to specify behavior in even more detail via laws, regulations, structures, rules, guidelines, and so on. The unstated goal seems to be to make the human parts act more mechanical.

RECONCILING MECHANICAL AND ADAPTIVE SYSTEMS THINKING

This apparently misguided thinking arises from traditional science. In the Renaissance, Galileo, Newton, and others gave us the image of the clockwork universe (Capra, 1996). The paradigm of science for the last several hundred years has been one of reductionism; that is, further study of the parts of systems will lead to deeper understanding and predictability. Indeed, this tradition has led to great advances in knowledge.

Reductionist thinking has also been applied to organizations. Taylor (1911) introduced "scientific management" a century ago and changed our view of systems of work. Taylorism resulted in huge gains in productivity through the introduction of scientific study of time and motion in work. Taylor believed that if workers would do their work in the "one best way," everyone would benefit (Kanigel, 1997). These ideas form a continuing and deeply held paradigm today (Morgan, 1997; Zimmerman et al., 1998; Brown and Eisenhardt, 1998).

Mechanical systems thinking does work in many situations when applied to human systems, and it has led to great progress in the past century. It is precisely because mechanical systems thinking works in many situations that it has become such a strongly held paradigm.

Organizational theorist Ralph Stacey (1996) provides a way to think about this seeming paradox (Figure B-1). Zimmerman et al. (1998) further describe this concept and provides several examples of its application in health care. In the lower left portion of the diagram are issues in which there is a high degree of certainty (as to outcomes from actions) and a high degree of agreement (among the people involved in taking the actions). Here, mechanical systems thinking with detailed plans and controls is appropriate. An example in health care is a surgical team doing routine gall bladder surgery. Through experience and the accumulation of knowledge, there is a high degree of certainty about the surgical procedures that lead to successful outcomes. The members of the surgical team agree on the way they will operate. In a good surgical team, everyone's actions need to be relatively predictable and somewhat mechanical. Someone who behaved unpredictably would be expelled from the team. In this area it is important to fully specify behavior and reduce variation, and there are many such issues at both the micro- and macrosystem level in health care.

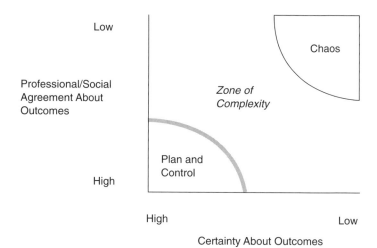

FIGURE B-1 Stacey Diagram: Zone of complexity. SOURCE: Stacey, 1996.

For other issues in human systems for which there is very little certainty and very little agreement (the area in the upper right of Figure B-1), chaos reigns and is to be avoided. A riot in the streets is an example.

Mechanical systems thinking (as intuitively applied by people designing and managing organizational systems) seems to allow only these two possibilities; it is necessary to plan and control, or there will be chaos. This seems so obvious to our mechanical-thinking mental model that it may not always be consciously acknowledged. Complex adaptive systems thinking allows for a third possibility.

There are many issues in human systems that lie in a "zone of complexity" (Langton, 1989; Zimmerman et al., 1998). These are issues for which there are only modest levels of certainty and agreement. Examples of such issues in health care might include: How should health care be financed? What is the best way to deliver primary care? For such issues there are many different models that have been successful in some situations and less successful in others; that is, only a modest level of "certainty" exists regarding what actions lead to what outcomes. Further, well-meaning, rational, intelligent people might not always agree as to the approach or outcome, meaning that there are only modest levels of agreement. For the most part the issues associated with designing the 21st-century health care system are in the zone of complexity where it would be more appropriate to use the paradigm of a complex adaptive system.

THE SCIENCE OF COMPLEX ADAPTIVE SYSTEMS

A complex adaptive system (CAS) is a collection of individual agents that have the freedom to act in ways that are not always predictable and whose actions are interconnected such that one agent's actions changes the context for other agents. Such systems have been the focus of intense study across a variety of scientific fields over the past 40 years (see Waldrop, 1992; Lewin, 1992; Wheatley, 1992; Kelly, 1994; Gell-Mann, 1995; Zimmerman et al., 1998; Brown and Eisenhardt, 1998). A major center of such research is the Santa Fe Institute, which includes several Nobel Prize winners among its faculty and associates (see Gell-Mann, 1995, p. xiv). Examples of systems that have been studied as a CAS include the human body's immune system (Varela and Coutinho, 1991); the mind (Morowitz and Singer, 1995); a colony of social insects such as termites or ants (Wilson, 1971); the stock market (Mandelbrot, 1999); and almost any collection of human beings (Brown and Eisenhardt 1998; Stacey, 1996; Zimmerman, et al. 1998).

The study of such systems reveals a number of properties. Although the list below is not a comprehensive description of the field, it illustrates some key elements of a way of thinking about complex organizational systems such as health care.

- *Adaptable elements.* The elements of the system can change themselves. Examples include antibiotic-resistant organisms and anyone who learns. In machines, change must be imposed, whereas under the right conditions in CAS, change can happen from within.
- *Simple rules.* Complex outcomes can emerge from a few simple rules that are locally applied.
- *Nonlinearity.* Small changes can have large effects; for example, a large program in an organization might have little actual impact, yet a rumor could touch off a union organizing effort.
- *Emergent behavior, novelty.* Continual creativity is a natural state of the system. Examples are ideas that spring up in the mind and the behavior of the stock market. In machines, new behavior is relatively rare, but in CAS it is an inherent property of the system.
- *Not predictable in detail.* Forecasting is inherently an inexact, yet bounded, art. For example, in weather forecasting, the fundamental laws governing pressure and temperature in gases are nonlinear. For this reason, despite reams of data and very powerful supercomputers, detailed, accurate long-range weather forecasting is fundamentally not possible. However, weather forecasting (and forecasting in general in any CAS) is bounded in the sense that we can make generally true statements about things like the average temperatures in a given season and place. The behavior of a machine is predictable in detail; it is just a matter of more study (reductionism). In a CAS, because the elements are changeable, the relations nonlinear, and the behavior creative and emergent, the only way to know what a CAS will do is to observe it.
- *Inherent order.* Systems can be orderly even without central control. Self-organization is the key idea in complexity science (Kaufmann, 1995; Holland,

1998; Prigogine, 1967, 1980). For example, termites build the largest structures on earth when compared with the height of the builders, yet there is no CEO termite. Similarly, there is no central controller for the stock market, the Internet, or the food supply of New York City.

• *Context and embeddedness.* Systems exist within systems, and this matters. For example, global stock markets are linked such that if the currency of Thailand falls, the U.S. stock market reacts. In a machine, one can extract the parts and characterize the response of a part to a stimulus. Although one can study the parts of a CAS independently, its context matters in fundamental ways.

• *Co-evolution.* A CAS moves forward through constant tension and balance. Fires, though destructive, are essential to a healthy, mature forest. Competition is good for industries. Tension, paradox, uncertainty, and anxiety are healthy things in a CAS. In machine thinking, they are to be avoided.

COMPLEXITY THINKING APPLIED TO THE DESIGN
OF THE 21ST-CENTURY HEALTH CARE SYSTEM

With challenges that naturally fall in the zone of complexity, such as the design of the 21st-century health care system, it is not surprising if the system does not act like a machine. CAS science and the Stacey diagram suggest additional metaphors to assist our thinking. Box-B-1 highlights some key ideas that emerge from the application of CAS science to the challenges of designing the 21st-century health care system.

Biological Approach and Evolutionary Design

It is more helpful to think like a farmer than an engineer or architect in designing a health care system. Engineers and architects need to design every detail of a system. This approach is possible because the responses of the component parts are mechanical and, therefore, predictable. In contrast, the farmer knows that he or she can do only so much. The farmer uses knowledge and

---

**BOX B-1   Key Elements in an Approach to
Complex Adaptive System Design**

• Use biological metaphors to guide thinking.
• Create conditions in which the system can evolve naturally over time.
• Provide simple rules and minimum specifications.
• Set forth a good enough vision and create a wide space for natural creativity to emerge from local actions within the system.

evidence from past experience, and desires an optimum crop. However, in the end, the farmer simply creates the conditions under which a good crop is possible. The outcome is an emergent property of the natural system and cannot be predicted in detail.

CAS science suggests that we cannot hope to understand a priori what a CAS will do or how to optimize it. A design cannot be completed on paper. Past attempts to do this in health care have not succeeded in part because they may not have been satisfactory designs, but mainly because a new understanding of "design" is needed.

Complex biological species (for example, human beings) get to be the way they are through evolutionary processes such as genetic mutation, and random variation. Changes that are useful to survival tend to persist. In a parallel manner, Holland (1995) points out that CAS need two processes in order to evolve: (1) processes that generate variation and (2) processes that "prune" the resulting evolutionary tree. Translating this insight to the task of designing the 21st-century health care system means combining the many ways to generate and test ideas with ways to enhance the spread of "good" ideas and impede the spread of "not so good" ideas. (Just as in biological evolution, seemingly harmful genetic variations do not die out completely in a generation; a not-so-fit characteristic might prove highly fit when combined with some other characteristic that evolves in a later generation.) These notions of evolutionary design are intuitively behind rapid-cycle plan-do-study-act (PDSA) improvement methods, which have been widely used in health care (Berwick, 1998).

Simple Rules, Good Enough Vision, and Wide Space for Innovation

A somewhat surprising finding from research on CAS is that relatively simple rules can lead to complex, emergent, innovative system behavior. For example, astrophysicists point out that all of the beauty and complexity we see in the universe emerges from two simple rules: (1) gravitational attraction and (2) the nonhomogeneity of matter in the early universe. In mathematics, the complexity and beauty of the Mandelbrot set (fractal mathematics) come from a very simple equation that is executed recursively. Reynolds (1987) showed that complex flocking, herding, and schooling behavior in animals could emerge from having each animal, such as a single fish in a school, apply three simple rules: (1) avoid collisions, (2) match speeds with your neighbors, and (3) move toward the center of mass of your neighbors. No central controller or director is needed; each animal can simply apply the rules locally. The behavior of the system emerges from the interactions, and this behavior is successful in avoiding predators. Holland (1998) shows how simple rules lead to emergent complexity in game theory, which models many situations in human interactions.

This idea of simple rules is counterintuitive to mechanical-systems thinking, in which if one needs a complex outcome, one needs a complex machine. There have been several past attempts to set out a complex set of rules to govern health care. When these have not yielded desired results, our instincts have been to create even more rules. CAS science asserts that these instincts take us in exactly the wrong direction.

The concept of complex system design using simple rules has also been demonstrated in organizations. The credit card company VISA built a trillion dollar business with very little central control. The banks that issue credit cards agree to only a few simple rules regarding card numbering, card appearance, electronic interface standards, and so forth. They are free to innovate and compete in all other aspects. There is no central control on new service development, and banks can go after each other's customers (Waldrop, 1996). In their study of high-tech firms, Brown and Eisenhardt (1998) found that the most successful firms had fewer rules, structures, and policies than their less successful competitors. Finally, the Internet is another example of a CAS. The few simple rules have to do with Hyper Text Markup Language (HTML), site naming conventions, and so on. Innovation is occurring daily in this arena. Zimmerman et al. (1998) provide several examples from early work applying these principles in the VHA, Inc. health care systems.

Again, the concept of simple rules clearly links to notions based on evolutionary genetics, game theory, innovation theory, and other sciences that are embracing new ideas about complexity. The concept provides wide boundaries for beginning the work of self-organization.

It is liberating to realize that the task of complex system design does not itself need to be complex. Although it has been suspected intuitively that it may not be possible to design in detail something as complex as the U.S. health care system, there is no need to fall victim to chaos. The answer is to create the conditions for self-organization through simple rules under which massive and diverse experimentation can happen.

Simple rules for human CAS tend to be of three types: (1) general direction pointing, (2) prohibitions, and (3) resource or permission providing. A good set of simple rules might include all three types. These three types of rules tend to match the predispositions of many systems designers. Those who would focus on leadership and aim setting are drawn to the simple rules of the first type.

Those who are drawn to regulation and boundary setting are comfortable with the second type. Those who would focus on incentives and resources are drawn to the third type. The theory honors all three points of view and suggests that it is best to have only a few such rules, so that no one point of view dominates.

Self-organizing innovation occurring in the health care system suggests that there is an implicit set of simple rules already in place. Experience in the fields of creativity and innovation suggests that changing these underlying rules might result in great innovation (Plsek, 1999).

Because the parts of a CAS are adaptable and embedded within a unique context, every change within a CAS can stimulate other changes that we could not expect. This approach to system design can never provide the assurance that is possible in a mechanical system. This is the nature of CAS. Therefore, rather than agonizing over plans, the goal is to generate a "good enough plan" and begin to observe what happens. Then, modifications can occur in an evolutionary fashion.

CONCLUSION

Complexity science provides a new paradigm to guide system design. Some key questions raised by a CAS-inspired approach to redesigning health care for the 21st century include:

• How can conditions in the health care system be established to allow many new ideas to emerge and mix into the existing system, while maintaining discipline to do just a little bit of nurturing, see what happens, then decide what to do next?

• How can diverse people be brought together, information shared, and forums convened among those to stimulate creative connections who do not normally come together to do so (similar to genetic cross-over and mutation)?

• How can desirable variation (innovation) be separated from the variation that ought to be reduced (error and waste)?

• What are the few simple rules that might guide the local development of the 21st-century health care system?

• What is the implicit, existing set of simple rules from which current innovations in health care emerge?

• How can these existing, implicit rules and underlying assumptions be modified?

• How can communication infrastructures be set up to disseminate the new simple rules?

• How can infrastructures be established in public policy to encourage experimentation and innovation under the new simple rules?

• How can experimentation be made highly visible so that the "fitness" of each evolution can be judged to quickly spread the best ideas?

• What is a "good enough plan" to begin the change?

• Who should take on the role of continuing to evolve the plan as the CAS plays itself out?

BIBLIOGRAPHY AND REFERENCES

Complex Systems Science

Arthur B.W. Increasing returns and the new world of business. *Harvard Business Review.* 74(4): 100–109, 1996.

Axelrod R.M. *The Complexity of Cooperation: Agent-Based Models of Competition and Collaboration.* Princeton, NJ: Princeton University Press, 1997.

Axelrod R.M. *The Evolution of Cooperation.* New York: Basic Books, 1984.

Briggs J. *Fractals: The Patterns of Chaos.* New York, NY: Simon & Schuster, 1992.

Brockman J. *The Third Culture: Beyond the Scientific Revolution.* New York: Simon and Schuster, 1995.

Capra F. *The Web of Life: The New Scientific Understanding of Living Systems.* New York: Anchor Books, 1996.

Cohen J. and Stewart I. *The Collapse of Chaos: Discovering Simplicity in a Complex World.* New York: Viking Penguin, 1994.

Dickinson M.H, Farley C.T, Full R.J, et al. How animals move: An integrative view. *Science.* 288(5463): 100–106, 2000.

Gabaix X. Zipf's law and the growth of cities. *AEA Papers and Proceedings: New Ideas on Economic Growth.* 89(2): 129–132, 1999.

Gell-Mann M. *The Quark and the Jaguar: Adventures in the Simple and Complex.* New York: W. H. Freeman, 1995.

Gladwell M. *The Tipping Point: How Little Things Can Make a Big Difference.* Boston: Little, Brown and Company, 2000.

Goodwin B. *How the Leopard Changed Its Spots: The Evolution of Complexity.* New York: Touchstone, 1994.

Holland J.H. *Emergence: From Chaos to Order.* Reading, MA: Addison-Wesley, 1998.

Holland J.H. *Hidden Order: How Adaptation Builds Complexity.* Reading, MA: Addison-Wesley, 1995.

Holldobler B. and Wilson E.O. *Journey of the Ants: A Story of Scientific Exploration.* Cambridge, MA: Harvard University Press, 1994.

Horgan J. From complexity to perplexity. *Scientific American.* 272(6):104–109, 1995.

Johnson G. Of mice and elephants: A matter of scale. *The New York Times.* January 12, 1999. F1.

Johnson G. Mindless creatures, acting mindfully: A few simple rules give rise to complex behavior. *The New York Times.* March 23, 1999. D1.

Kauffman S.A. Antichaos and adaptation. *Scientific American.* 265(2):78-84, 1991.

Kauffman S.A. *At Home in the Universe.* Oxford, England: Oxford University Press, 1995.

Langton C.G. Artificial Life. *Santa Fe Institute Studies in the Sciences of Complexity, Proceedings,* Vol. 6. Redwood City, CA: Addison-Wesley, 1989.

Lewin R. *Complexity: Life at the Edge of Chaos.* New York: Macmillan, 1992.

Lorenz E. *The Essence of Chaos.* Seattle: University of Washington Press, 1993.

Lovelock J. Gaia as seen through the atmosphere. *Atmospheric Environment.* 6:579. 1972.

Mandelbrot B. A fractal walk on Wall Street. *Scientific American.* 280(2), 70–73, 1999.

Mitchell M. *An Introduction to Genetic Algorithms.* Cambridge, MA: MIT Press, 1996.

Morowitz H.J. Metaphysics, meta-metaphor, and magic. *Complexity.* 3(4), 1998, 19–20.

Morowitz H.J. and Singer J.L. *The Mind, the Brain, and Complex Adaptive Systems.* Reading, MA: Addison-Wesley Publishing, 1995.

Prigogine I. Dissipative structures in chemical systems. In Claesson S. (ed.). *Fast Reactions and Primary Processes in Chemical Kinetics.* New York: Interscience, 1967.

Prigogine I. *From Being to Becoming.* San Francisco: W. H. Freeman, 1980.

Prigogine I. and Stengers I. *Order Out of Chaos: Man's New Dialogue with Nature.* New York: Bantam, 1984.

Resnick M. *Turtles, Termites, and Traffic Jams: Explorations in Massively Parallel Microworlds.* Cambridge, MA: MIT Press, 1997.

Reynolds C.W. Flocks, herds, and schools: A distributed behavioral model. *Computer Graphics.* 21(4):25–34, 1987.

Stewart I. and Cohen J. *Figments of Reality: The Evolution of the Curious Mind.* Cambridge, England: Cambridge University Press, 1997.

Valente T.W. *Network Models of the Diffusion of Innovations.* Cresskill, NJ: Hampton Press, 1995.

von Bertalanffy L. *General Systems Theory: Foundations, Development, and Applications, Revised Edition.* New York: George Braziller Publishers, 1968.

Waldrop MM. *Complexity: The Emerging Science at the Edge of Order and Chaos.* New York: Simon and Schuster, 1992.

Wilson E.O. *The Insect Societies.* Cambridge, MA: Harvard University Press, 1971.

Wyles J.S., Kimbel G. and Wilson A.C. Birds, behavior, and anatomical evolution. *Proceedings of the National Academy of Sciences.* 80(14):4394-4397, 1983.

Clinical Applications of Complexity Science

Armoni A. Use of neural networks in medical diagnosis. *MD Computing.* 15(2):100–4, 1998.

Bassingthwaighte J.B., Liebovitch L.S., and West B.J. *Fractal Physiology.* Oxford, England: Oxford University Press, 1994.

Coffey D.S. Self-organization, complexity, and chaos: The new biology of medicine. *Nature Medicine.* 4(8):882–885, 1998.

Cole C.R., Blackstone E.H., Pashkow F.J., et al. Heart-rate recovery immediately following exercise as a predictor of mortality. *The New England Journal of Medicine.* 341:1351–1357, 1999.

Dardik I.I. The origin of disease and health, heart waves: The single solution to heart rate variability and ischemic preconditioning. *Frontier Perspectives.* 6(2):18–32, 1997.

Fogel D.B., Wasson E.C., Boughton E.M., and Porto V.W. A step toward computer-assisted mammography using evolutionary programming and neural networks. *Cancer Letters.* 119:93-97, 1997.

Goertzel B. The complex mind/brain: The Psynet model of mental structure and dynamics. *Complexity.* 3(4): 51–58, 1998.

Goldberger A.L. Nonlinear dynamics for clinicians: Chaos theory, fractals, and complexity at the bedside. *Lancet.* 347:1312–14, 1996.

Goldberger A.L. Fractal variability versus pathologic periodicity: Complexity loss and stereotypy in disease. *Perspectives in Biology and Medicine.* 40(4):543–561, 1997.

Goldberger A.L., Rigney D.R., and West B.J. Chaos and fractals in human physiology. *Scientific American.* 262:42–49, 1990.

Goodwin J.S. Chaos, and the limits of modern medicine. *JAMA.* 278:1399–40, 1997.

Ivanov P.C., Amaral L.A.N., Goldberger A.L., et al. Multifractality in human heartbeat dynamics. *Nature.* 399:461–465, 1999.

Lipsitz L.A. and Goldberger A.L. Loss of complexity and aging: Potential applications of fractals and chaos theory to senescene. *JAMA.* 267:1806–1809, 1999.

Nelson T.R., West B.J., and Goldberger A.L. The fractal lung: Universal and species-related fractal patterns. *Experientia.* 46:251–254, 1990.

Pikkujamsa S.M., Makikallio T.H., Sourander L.F., et al. Cardiac interbeat interval dynamics from childhood to senescence: Comparison of conventional and new measures based on fractals and chaos theory. *Circulation.* 100:393–399, 1999.

Regaldo A. A gentle scheme for unleashing chaos. *Science.* 268:1848, 1995.

Schmidt G., Malick M., Barthel P., et al. Heart-rate turbulence after ventricular premature beats as a predictor of mortality after acute myocardial infarction. *Lancet.* 353:1390–1396, 1999.

Streufert S. and Satish U. Complexity theory: Predictions based on the confluence of science-wide and behavioral theories. *Journal of Applied Social Psychology.* 27(23):2096–2116, 1997.

Varela F. and Coutinho A. Second generation immune networks. *Immunology Today.* 12(5):159–166, 1991.

Varela F., Thompson E., and Rosch E. *The Embodied Mind.* Cambridge, MA: MIT Press, 1991.

Wagner C.D., Nafz B., Persson P.B. Chaos and blood pressure control. *Cardiovascular Research.* 31:380–7, 1996.

Weibel ER. Fractal geometry: A design principle for living organisms. *American Journal of Physiology.* 261:361–369, 1991.

Organizational Applications of Complexity Science

Anderson RA and McDaniel RR. RN participation in organizational decision making and improvements in resident outcomes. *Health Care Management Review.* 24(1):7–16, 1999.

Baskin K. *Corporate DNA: Learning from Life.* Boston: Butterworth Heinemann, 1998.

Baskin K., Goldstein J, and Lindberg C. Merging, de-merging, and emerging at Deaconess Billings Clinic. *The Physician Executive.* 20–5, 2000

Begun J.W. Chaos and complexity: Frontiers of organizational science. *Journal of Management Inquiry.* 3(3):29–335, 1994.

Beinhocker E.D. Robust adaptive strategies. *Sloan Management Review.* 40(3):95–106, 1999.

Beckman J.D. Change has changed: What the organism can teach the organization. *Health Care Forum Journal.* 60–62, 1998.

Beckman J.D. Embracing paradox: What the organism can teach the organization. *Health Care Forum Journal.* 66–68, 1998.

Berwick D.M. Developing and testing changes in delivery of care. *Annals of Internal Medicine.* 128:651–656, 1998.

Brown S.L. and Eisenhardt K.M. *Competing on the Edge: Strategy as Structured Chaos.* Cambridge, MA: Harvard Business School Press, 1998.

Clippinger J.H. *The Biology of Business: Decoding the Natural Laws of Enterprise.* San Francisco: Jossey-Bass, 1999.

Davidson S.N. Healthy chaos. *Health Care Forum Journal.* March–April:64–7, 1998.

Dooley K.J., Johnson T.L., and Bush D.H. TQM, chaos, and complexity. *Human Systems Management.* 14: 287–302, 1995.

Dooley K.J. A complex adaptive systems model of organizational change. *Nonlinear Dynamics, Psychology, and Life Science.* 1(1):69–97, 1997.

Eisenhardt K.M. and Brown S.L. Time pacing: Competing in markets that won't stand still. *Harvard Business Review.* March–April:59–69, 1998.

Eisenhardt K.M. and Brown S.L. Patching: Restitching business portfolios in dynamic markets. *Harvard Business Review.* May–June:72–82, 1999.

Eisenhardt K.M. and Galunic D.C. Coevolving: At last, a way to make synergies work. *Harvard Business Review.* 78(1):91–101, 2000.

Eoyang G.H. *Coping With Chaos: Seven Simple Tools.* Cheyenne, WY: Lagumo, 1997.

Goldstein J. *The Unshackled Organization: Facing the Challenge of Unpredictability Through Spontaneous Reorganization.* Portland, OR: Productivity Press, 1994.

Hamel G. Strategy as revolution. *Harvard Business Review.* 74(4):69–82, 1996.

Hamel G. Strategy innovation and the quest for value. *Sloan Management Review.* 39(2):7–14, 1998.

Hock D. *The Birth of the Chaordic Age.* San Francisco: Berrett-Koehler, 1999.

Hurst D. and Zimmerman BJ. From life cycle to ecocycle: A new perspective on the growth, maturity, destruction, and renewal of complex systems. *Journal of Management Inquiry.* 3(4):339–354, 1995.

Kanigel.R. *The One Best Way: Fredrick Winslow Taylor and the Enigma of Efficiency.* New York: Viking, 1997.

Kelly K. *Out of Control: The Rise of Neo-Biological Civilization.* Reading, MA: Addison-Wesley, 1994.

Kelly S. and Allison M.A. *The Complexity Advantage: How the Science of Complexity Can Help Your Business Achieve Peak Performance.* New York: McGraw-Hill, 1999.

Khurana A. Managing complex production processes. *Sloan Management Review.* 40(2):85–97, 1999.

Krackhardt D. and Hanson J.R. Informal networks: The company behind the chart. *Harvard Business Review.* July–August:104–111, 1993.

Kuo R.J. and Xue K.C. Fuzzy neural networks with application to sales forecasting. *Fuzzy Sets and Systems.* 108(2):123–143, 1999.

Lane D. and Maxfield R. Strategy under complexity: Fostering generative relationships. *Long Range Planning.* 29(2):215–231, 1996.

Lewin R. It's a jungle out there. *New Scientist.* November 29:30–34, 1997.

Lewin R., Parker T., and Regine B. Complexity theory and the organization: Beyond the metaphor. *Complexity.* 3(4):36–38.

Lewin R. and Regine B. *The Soul at Work: Embracing Complexity Science for Business Success.* New York: Simon and Schuster, 2000.

Lin G.Y.J. and Solberg J.J. Integrated shop floor control using autonomous agents. *IIE Transactions.* 24(3):57–71, 1992.

Lindberg C. and Taylor J. From the science of complexity to leading in uncertain times. *Journal of Innovative Management.* Summer:22–34, 1997.

Lindberg C., Herzog A., Merry M., Goldstein J. Life at the edge of chaos. *The Physician Executive.* January-February: 6–20, 1998.

Lissack M. and Roos J. *The Next Common Sense: Mastering Corporate Complexity through Coherence.* London: Nicholas Brealey, 1999.

Lorange P. and Probst G.J.B. Joint ventures as self-organizing ventures: A key to successful joint venture design and implementation. *Columbia Journal of World Business.* Summer:71–77, 1987.

McWinney W., Webber J.B., Smith D.M., and Novokowsky B.J. *Creating Paths of Change: Managing Issues and Resolving Problems in Organizations.* Venice, CA: Enthusion Press, 1996.

Morgan G. *Images of Organization, 2nd Edition.* Thousand Oaks, CA: Sage, 1997.

Parker D. and Stacey R.D. *Chaos, Management, and Economics: The Implications of Non-Linear Thinking.* Bournemouth, England: Bourne Press, 1994.

Pascale R.T. Surfing the edge of chaos. *Sloan Management Review.* 40(3):83–95, 1999.

Petrich C.H. Organizational science: Oxymoron or opportunity? *Complexity.* 3(4):23–26, 1998.

Petzinger T. Self-organization will free employees to act like bosses. *Wall Street Journal.* January 3, 1997. D1.

Petzinger T. A new model for the nature of business: It's alive! Forget the mechanical, today's leaders embrace the biological. *Wall Street Journal.* February 26, 1999. B1.

Petzinger T. *The New Pioneers: The Men and Women Who Are Transforming the Workplace and Marketplace.* New York: Simon and Schuster, 1999.

Plsek P.E. Innovative thinking for the improvement of medical systems. *Annals of Internal Medicine* 131(6),438–444, 1999.

Plsek P.E. and Kilo C.M. From resistance to attraction: A different approach to change. *Physician Executive.* 25(6):40-46,1999.

Resnick M. Unblocking the traffic jams in corporate thinking. *Complexity.* 3(4):27-30, 1998.

Roy B. Using agents to make and manage markets across a supply web. *Complexity.* 3(4):31–35, 1998.

Sanders T.I. *Strategic Thinking and the New Science: Planning in the Midst of Chaos, Complexity, and Change.* New York: Free Press, 1998.

Senge P.M. *The Fifth Discipline: The Art and Practice of the Learning Organization.* New York: Doubleday, 1990.

Sherman H. and Schultz R. *Open Boundaries: Creating Innovation Through Complexity.* Reading: MA: Perseus Books, 1998.

Spear S. and Bowen H.K. Decoding the DNA of the Toyota Production System. *Harvard Business Review.* 77(5):97–106, 1999.

Stacey R.D. *Complexity and Creativity in Organizations.* San Francisco, CA: Berrett-Koehler, 1996.

Stacey R.D. *Strategic Management and Organizational Dynamics.* London: Pitmann Publishing, 1996.

Taylor F.W. *The Principles of Scientific Management.* New York, NY: Harper & Brothers, 1911.

Waldrop M.M. The trillion dollar vision of Dee Hock. *Fast Company.* October–November:75–86, 1996.

Wells S.J. Forget the formal training: Try chatting at the water cooler. *The New York Times,* May 10, 1998.

Wheatley M.J. *Leadership and the New Science: Learning about Organization from an Orderly Universe.* San Francisco: Berrett-Koehler, 1992.

Wieck K.E. *Sense Making in Organizations.* Thousand Oaks, CA: Sage, 1995.

Zastocki D.K. A toolbox for managing in turbulent environments. *Journal of Innovative Management.* Summer:24–33, 1999.

Zimmerman B.J. Chaos and nonequilibrium: The flip side of strategic processes. *Organizational Development Journal.* 11(1):31–38, 1993.

Zimmerman B.J., Lindberg C, and Plsek PE. *Edgeware: Insights from Complexity Science for Health Care Leaders.* Dallas, TX: VHA Publishing, 1998.

Zimmerman B.J. Complexity science: A route through hard times and uncertainty. *The Health Forum Journal.* 42(2):42–46, 96, 1999.

Index